THE ARUBA PROJECT 2014

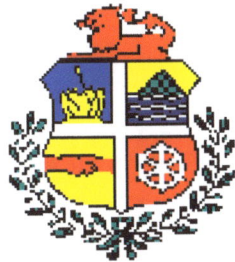

SPECIAL COMMITTEE ON OBESITY

R. W. M. Visser, DC, PhD., expert consultant NATIONAL PLAN ARUBA
2009–2018

The Aruba Project

Richard Visser, DC, PhD.

©Copyright 2018 Richard Visser

978-1-885-37703-6

DISLCAIMER

Care has been taken to confirm the accuracy of the information present and to describe generally accepted practices. However, the authors, editors, and publisher are not responsible for errors or omissions or for any consequences from application of the information in this publication and make no warranty, expressed or implied, with respect to the currency, completeness, or accuracy of the contents of the publication.

Application of this information in a particular situation remains the professional responsibility of the practitioner; the clinical treatments described and recommended may not be considered absolute and universal recommendations.

The authors, editors, and publisher have exerted every effort to ensure that drug selection and dosage set forth in this text are in accordance with the current recommendations and practice at the time of publication. However, in view of ongoing research, changes in government regulations, and the constant flow of information relating to drug therapy and drug reactions, the reader is urged to check the package insert for each drug for any change in indications and dosage and for added warnings and precautions. This is particularly important when the recommended agent is a new or infrequently employed drug. Some drugs and medical devices presented in this publication have Food and Drug Administration (FDA) clearance for limited use in restricted research settings. It is the responsibility of the health care provider to ascertain the FDA status of each drug or device planned for use in their clinical practice.

ACKNOWLEDGMENTS

Jan Visser, my father for the dream;

Celfa Lampe Visser for her relentless work ethic and believing in me (my biggest fan and supporter); Mother

My sister Monique for teaching me to live life all out;

My brothers Ed and John, for being my ying and yang;

Roger Jurriens for dreaming with me and being a true friend for life;

Donna and Robert Roos for teaching me lifestyle and believing in me;

Roger Putzel for being my coach and caretaker in Vermont;

Jason Araghi, the best Chiropractor I know and my friend for life;

Dave Munson/Chiropractic/NLP/Life Spring for showing me and pushing me to be the best;

Robin Anderson for nurturing the most important thing in life, my daughter;

Deepak Chopra for teaching me transcendental meditation and quantum healing;

Brian Weiss for teaching me past life regression;

Lin Young, for pushing me further, being my #1 fan, and giving me a son;

Akhter Ahsen for teaching me Eidetic Imaging and Psychotherapy;

Lin Yung, my Black Sekt Buddhist Feng Shui teacher from Tibet;

My Cuban top team: Troadto Gonzales and Angel Caballero "Hasta la Victoria Siempre" — from green room to incubating the ideas that would drive the change;

Monica Kock for playing a crucial role in charting this new path for change and being a true friend;

Cabinet Mike Eman1, AVP and my team 2009-13, for letting me do my thing and giving me a political platform;

Dick Souge for being a friend/advisor, and holding down the fort while we change a country;

WHO-PAHO 2009–2013 for believing in my leadership in bringing the fight against Obesity "The Aruba call to action" to the Americas and the World;

The people of Aruba for believing in me and for the change we created together;

My kids Savannah and Kai, whom I love to the moon and back; they push me to be and do better every day

The family business and all the hard working members at Visser Holding NV and it's subsidiaries in Aruba, Curacao and St Martin

My life partner Aysel Erbudak for embarking with me on creating the future of health care in VERA Health and Education

— Thank you.

CONTENT

iv

INTRODUCTION

In this paper a compilation of documents is presented that reflect various efforts related to the fields of Health and Sports in Aruba, from November 1, 2009, to October 31, 2013.

This introduction is a brief review of these documents for the purposes of consolidating the most important information in a single publication, so it can be consulted by those interested in working in or with the field of public health in general and particularly in the prevention of obesity and noncommunicable diseases.

In August 2013 a review of these efforts was carried out by experts of the PAHO / WHO. The experts published a report reflecting the specific achievements identified in the nation.

These achievements have an even greater significance considering that until 2009 there was no proper prioritization of disease prevention and health promotion. This further underlines the considerable improvement realized during the four years discussed here.

For Aruba this is evidence of the current recognition of the importance of this priority, as a result of the underlying policy and its correspondence to contemporary international public health strategies.

The most important direct legal precedent of this ministerial policy is the National Plan for Aruba 2009–2018, which was approved by parliament and by the government as the essential guide to address obesity and chronic noncommunicable diseases in a time when they were not yet recognized as health and developmental problems.

Among other things, the creation of the Institute for Healthy and Active Living (IBiSA), 'educational bikeways', the Health Bus, the 'health-promoting schools' program and the use of the guide to healthy living, are all activities that contributed to positive change in the health environment in Aruba.

These efforts were endorsed and further supported by the Pan American Conference on Obesity (PACO), with special attention to Childhood Obesity, also helping to address this problem in other countries.

The first of these conferences, PACO I, resulted in a document that was part of the preparations for the UN Summit on non-communicable diseases in 2011. This paper is published in this compilation along with other documents produced during this event, as well as the ones produced in PACO II and PACO III. All these documents were sent to all the Ministers of Health of the Americas.

To strengthen disease prevention and health promotion in Aruba, a Health Monitor and Healthy and Active Lifestyle were developed, which are both also presented in this compilation to provide an overview of the primary results of various efforts and changes in health indicators in the Aruban population. Some of the most important of these are a significant reduction of sedentary lifestyles and a clear change in the development of the obesity epidemic, which no longer showed the upward trend it had experienced in previous decades.

Dr. Visser contributed the scientific basis for prioritizing the prevention of childhood obesity in a publication that explains why a dedicated platform should be developed to prevent this disease. The publication also lays down a guide for promoting healthy eating habits and an active lifestyle, in addition to the philosophical principles that should accompany these actions. Given the importance of these contributions, it was deemed necessary to include them in this compilation.

In 2014 Dr. Richard Visser's proposal was nominated for the Award of Excellence in Public Health, seeking endorsement for the results of his efforts and dedication to improve the state of health in Aruba and in the Pan-American region as a whole.

2014 MEMORANDUM ON THE PAHO/WHO EVALUATION

A team of eight officials of the PAHO/WHO visited Aruba in August of 2013, producing a report outlining their findings regarding the following achievements:

- Recognition of and attention to the problem of noncommunicable diseases (NCDs) and the importance of health promotion and the prevention of these diseases and their risk factors (RF).

- Implementation of the Aruba National Plan for 2009 to 2018. The plan was approved by parliament and enjoys widespread acceptance of the society as a whole.

- Establishment of legislation and public infrastructure to develop health promotion and prevention of NCDs and their risk factors, with a comprehensive population vision.

- The experiences and progress on issues related to physical activity, diet, nutrition and prevention of overweight and obesity, especially in children, are political and technical contributions of Aruba to other countries in the Americas.

- The organization of three Pan American Conferences on Obesity with special emphasis on childhood obesity, (PACO I, II and III) particularly stands out.

- Creation of the Institute for Healthy and Active Living (IBiSA) under the Ministry of Health and Sports, which has implemented innovative strategies and practices of health promotion and prevention of NCDs and their risk factors. Highlights include the Health Bus, and the initiation of partnerships and networks involving NGOs, community leaders and schools. A notable increase in registered institutions and individuals involved in sports and physical activity was reported.

- Leadership of the Ministry of Health and Sports in intersectoral efforts towards health promotion and disease prevention, changing lifestyles and addressing the determinants of health. Some examples are the creation of parks and bike paths; eliminating taxes on the import of fruits and vegetables; availability of healthy foods in supermarkets and hotels; and a new law giving working mothers two hours a day off for breastfeeding during nine months after childbirth.

- The White-Yellow Cross Foundation and the Health Bus have developed measures for health education and prevention of NCDs in homes, schools, communities and public and private work centers. For this initiative, they established partnerships with various stakeholders, in which the incentives to private companies to achieve better health in their workforce particularly stand out.

- Recognition of drug addiction as a public health problem and not merely as a legal issue; attention shifted from the Ministry of Justice to the Ministry of

Health and Sports, which implements strategies and programs for prevention and comprehensive care. In the prevention component, the incorporation of the 'No Apologies' Program into the curriculum of schools stands out.

- Data collection and analysis and the production of the 'Health Monitor,' with the commitment to generate this report every four years to guide and evaluate policies, plans and programs.

- The implemented strategy of 'Healthy Schools', under the supervision of the Ministry of Health and Sports in cooperation with the Ministry of Education.

- The prevalence of obesity in the population of preschool and fifth grade children did not increase in the period of 2011 and 2012, compared to 2008 and 2009. In the same period the regular 'overweight' percentage increased only slightly.

- The existence of managers, professionals and technicians committed to the priorities of the Ministry of Health and Sports, motivated to develop complex projects of high importance.

- Expansion, modernization and reorientation of San Nicolás Medical Institute (ImSan) as a comprehensive national center for the prevention and treatment of NCDs, with a focus on promotion, prevention, diagnosis, control, treatment and rehabilitation. The center is outfitted with high tech equipment for the detection and diagnosis of certain types of cancer, kidney failure and diabetes, providing services to local and foreign patients, in close cooperation with Baptist Health International.

- Leadership of the Ministry of Health and Sports in recognizing both sectoral and extra-sectoral institutions for their contributions to a holistic concept of health, wellness and quality of life of the population.

- Existence of an financial health coverage, safeguarding the population's right to good health.

- Second- and third-level services apply innovative ideas, complementing and reinforcing the system of primary health care, in an effort to achieve greater efficiency and quality of care.

- Implementation of an academic training program for family physicians, expanding their performance skills. In the past year, seven health care professionals have successfully graduated from the program, producing specialized physicians for primary and geriatric care. In addition, dedicated nurse practitioners were assigned to these primary care physicians, to support in the prevention and control of NCDs.

- A notable increase in the number of people engaging in physical activities and exercise. However, it is necessary to continue working on changing eating habits combined with exercise, in order to further fight overweight and obesity.

Chapter 1

FIGHTING AGAINST OBESITY AND RELATED HEALTH ISSUES: THE NATIONAL PLAN FOR ARUBA 2009-2018

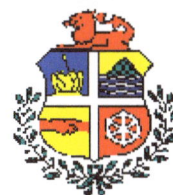

Dr. Timothy Armstrong, Coordinator Surveillance and Population-based Prevention Chronic Diseases and Health Promotion, WHO and Dr. Caroline Bollars, World Health Organization, Regional Office for Europe, WHO – EU endorsed this document in basis of the following:

"This National Plan and its objectives are in line with the implementation of the Global Strategy on Diet, Physical Activity and Health and the implementation of the World Health Organization Action Plan for the Global Strategy for the Prevention and Control of Non-Communicable Diseases."

CONTENTS

1. INTRODUCTION

In the past thirty years, the prevalence of overweight and obesity has risen drastically in Aruban society, especially among children, with an estimated prevalence of overweight from 15% (2001) to 37% (2004) among our children, and from 52% (1993) to 73% (2001) to 77% (2006) among our adult population.

These figures are even higher than those of the United States and indicate a deteriorating trend of poor eating habits and little physical exercise, in consequence whereof some chronic diseases are expected to increase in the future, such as cardiovascular diseases and hypertension, diabetes mellitus type 2, strokes, certain types of cancer, musculoskeletal system disorders, and even some mental health disorders. In the long term, this trend will have a negative impact on life expectancy in Aruba and reduce the quality of life for many. It is disturbing that life expectancy has already decreased by 1 year, viz.: among men from 71.1 years (1991) to 70.1 years (2000), and among women from 77.12 years (1991) to 76.02 years (2000).

As a result of the health data, the Special Committee on Obesity of Aruban Parliament was established on May 9, 2008. The task of this Committee will be to prepare a national plan for the fight against overweight and obesity.

Several studies in Aruba showed alarming results, i.a. STEPS Aruba 2006 of the Department of Public Health, according to which the prevalence of overweight among adults was 77%, and the Childhood Obesity Study 2004 of Dr. Richard Visser, according to which the prevalence of overweight among children ages 6–11 was 37%. This made Aruba one of the highest risk groups in the world and indicated that urgent attention had to be paid to the prevention and intervention of overweight and obesity and, thus, related health issues.

These alarming data led the problem of overweight and obesity to be placed on the agenda of the Bipartite Parliamentary Consultations Kingdom Relations Netherlands Antilles and Aruba in Curacao from May 14 through 18, 2007. During the Tripartite Parliamentary Consultations Kingdom Relations the Netherlands, Netherlands Antilles and Aruba, from June 25 through 29, 2007, it also was requested to pay attention to the problem of overweight. During the Bipartite Parliamentary Consultations Kingdom Relations Netherlands Antilles and Aruba in Oranjestad, from November 12 through 14, 2007, it was decided to establish a (special) committee that would be charged with preparing a national plan, as approved on page 2, footnote a, of the Final Declaration. On the part of Aruban Parliament, the Special Committee on Obesity was established on May 9, 2008, consisting of the following members: Mr. M.H.J. Kock, member of Parliament, Mr. J.E. Thijsen, member of Parliament, and Dr. R.W.M. Visser, expert.

The purpose of the National Plan Aruba 2009–2018 is to set out an integrated Aruban approach to contribute to the reduction of health problems caused by poor nutrition, overweight, and obesity. Internationally, it has been confirmed that education, intervention, and very specific prevention are the best methods to tackle this pandemy. The most important aspect of these methods is to promote health.

It is extremely important to develop information and activities related to the accomplishment of a balanced nutrition by stimulating healthy eating habits to promote a healthy body. At the same time, a lifestyle consisting of a healthy exercise pattern should be promoted.

Healthy physical activity and balanced nutrition contribute to a good development of young children and, when they are older, will be an important source for an active and independent life in our community. Furthermore, healthy physical activity and balanced nutrition enhance resistance to infections, limit sickness-related absenteeism, and are related to an increase in productivity and intellectual capacity. It has been proven that the rate of overweight and obesity as well as chronic diseases, such as cancer, cardiovascular diseases, obesity, diabetes type 2, hypertension, (alcoholic) fatty liver disease, and osteoporosis, declines (Alberti et al., 2007, U.S. Department of Health and Human Services, 2000). In addition to a biological function, eating and exercising also have a strong social and cultural function. The impact thereof on the development of people and society cannot be neglected (Meydani, 2001; Health Canada, 2002; Walters et al., 1999; Van der Bij et al., 2002; Shephard, 1997). Furthermore, an enormous increase of obesity is observed worldwide, caused by a disturbance in the energy balance. Further to the recommendations of the WHO and the European institutions, the National Plan Aruba 2009–2018 also pays special attention to the surveillance of a healthy weight (WHO, 2007; Commission of the European Communities, 2007).

The epidemiological data indicate that our current nutrition and physical activity pattern contains bottlenecks. The National Plan Aruba 2009–2018 and the strategies it contains should enable our country and the community to achieve the objective, i.e., the reduction of overweight and obesity among the Aruban population. The strategies and the concrete interventions within the strategies, proposed by the Special Committee on Obesity, should lead to the achievement of the health objective.

With the National Plan Aruba 2009–2018 Aruba follows the recommendations of the World Health Organization and recent European policy initiatives against obesity and promoting a lifestyle encompassing balanced nutrition and sufficient physical activity.

2. BACKGROUND

The purpose of the National Plan Aruba 2009–2018 is to set out an integrated Aruban approach to contribute to the reduction of health problems caused by poor nutrition, little exercise, overweight, and obesity. The National Plan Aruba 2009–2018 also builds on recent initiatives arising from the various studies, international guidelines, government information, and information from society's stakeholders.

2.1. Documentation examined by the Special Committee on Obesity

A. Studies

1) STEPS Aruba 2006, Chronic Disease Risk Factor Surveillance Data Book, carried out in the period of October through December 2006, the main objective of which was to monitor behavioral risk factors for chronic non-transmittable diseases in Aruba among persons between the ages of 25–64. For the study, use was made of the 'WHO STEPwise approach to chronic disease risk factor surveillance'. Result: 77% of the citizens between the ages of 25-64 are overweight, of whom 40.8% obese.

2) Summary study number of diabetics in 'AZV' [General Health Insurance] file 2005, (March 14, 2007, Executive Body AZV). The percentage of diabetics in Aruba amounts to 6.4%, i.e., 6,000 persons. They cause 20% of all AZV medical expenses. This amount has not been adjusted for possible exceptional medical expenses not related to diabetes; this requires a more thorough study.

   It is suspected that there is a large group of "undisclosed diabetics," amounting to 5 to 6% of the population.

3) Childhood Obesity Study 2004 of Dr. Richard Visser, is a study among 3,952 children ages 6–11 as to the prevalence of overweight and obesity among the study population, the identification of health disorders, and the determination of factors related to this problem. Result: 37% of the children between the ages of 6 and 11 are overweight.

4) Health Study Aruba 2001 of the Department of Public Health. Prevalence of overweight among the population 20 years and up amounted to 73%. The prevalence of overweight among elementary schoolchildren amounted to 15%.

5) Aruba, One Heavy Island 1993 of the Department of Public Health. Prevalence of overweight among the population 20 years and up amounted to 52%, of which 28% obese.

B. Government budgets

1) Budget of the Minister of Public Health for the financial year 2009 and 2008.

2) Budget of the Minister of Sports for the financial year 2009 and 2008.

3) Budget of the Minister of Education for the financial year 2009 and 2008.

C. Special documents

1) Central Bureau of Statistics. Statistical Yearbook 2007, May 2008.

2) "Obesidad ta hiba nos na Mortalidad" [Obesity will lead us to Mortality], White Yellow Cross 2008.

3) "Verslag van de Resultaten van het Onderzoek naar BMI en Glucosegehalte bij Leerlingen van de EPI" [Report on the Results of the Study on BMI and Glucose Content among Students of the 'EPI'], Diabetic Center Aruba, March 2008.

4) Department of Public Health, Obesity Programs, November 2007.

5) Policy document: Diabetic Center Aruba, November 7, 2007.

6) Annual report of the AZV Executive Body 2007.

7) "Trabou y Salud 2007, Jaarverslag ziekteverzuim en arbeidsomstandigheden 2004-2007" [Work and Health 2007, Annual report on sickness absenteeism and working conditions], 'BGD' [Industrial Medical Service] Aruba.

8) Impact of Obesity on Mortality and Morbidity, Netherlands Interdisciplinary Demographic Institute, April 19, 2005

9) "From One Heavy Island to One Healthy Island," 'Commission Plataforma Alimentacion Nacional' [National Committee Platform on Nutrition].

10) "KABP-onderzoek Borstvoeding Aruba 2003" [KABP Study Breastfeeding Aruba 2003] of the Department of Public Health.

11) "Borstvoedingsonderzoek 2002" [Breastfeeding Study 2002] of the Department of Public Health.

12) "Aruba ban cana" [Aruba, let's walk], IDEFRE December 2001.

D. International documentation

1) Dietary habits in the Caribbean and Central and South America, Richard Visser Institute, IASO Genève, May 14, 2008.

2) White Paper, A Strategy for Europe on nutrition, overweight and obesity related health issues, Commission of the European Communities, May 30, 2007.

3) Commission Staff Working Document of the White Paper, Commission of the European Communities, May 30, 2007

4) Draft Report on the White Paper on nutrition, overweight and obesity related health issues, European Parliament, December 19, 2007.

5) Workers' health: Global Action Plan 2008–2017 (WHO, 2007).

6) Second Action Plan 2007–2012 (WHO, 2007).

7) Obesity in children and young people: a crisis in public health. IASO International Obesity Taskforce.

8) "Preventie Overgewicht" [Overweight Prevention], 'RIVM' [National Institute of Public Health and Environmental Protection] V/260301/01/OG.

9) "Signaleringsprotocol overgewicht jeugdgezondheidszorg" [Identification Protocol Overweight Youth Healthcare], 'VUmc' [Free University Medical Center] Amsterdam.

10) "Het aanbod van levensmiddelen op middelbare scholen" [The offer of food in secondary schools], 'Voedsel en Waren Autoriteit' [Dutch Food and Non-Food Authority], January 2007.

11) "De kosteneffectiviteit en gezondheidswinst van behalen beleidsdoelen bewegen en overgewicht, Onderbouwing Nationaal Actieplan Sport en Bewegen" [Cost effectiveness and health benefits of achieving policy objectives physical activity and overweight, Substantiation National Action Plan Sports and Physical Activity], 'Rijksinstituut voor Volksgezondheid en Milieu' [National Institute of Public Health and Environmental Protection].

12) Nutrition Enhancement Program (NEP), Choices, Unilever.

13) "Werkdocument De Gezonde School Methode in Nederland" [Working Document The Healthy School Method in the Netherlands], October 2005.

14) "Op weg naar een gezonde schoolkantine" [Towards a healthy school cafeteria], 'Stichting Voedingscentrum Nederland' [Netherlands Nutrition Center Foundation].

2.2. Involvement European Parliament

On June 23 and 24, 2008, the Special Committee on Obesity had meetings with several agencies, experts, and members of European Parliament on the problem of obesity in Brussels.

- A briefing with the Netherlands Permanent Representative to the European Union, Mr. Jos Draijer. Topics were i.a. the insurance system, advertising ban, medical impact studies, legislation, and health policy at school.

- Meeting with Euro MP Ms. Dorette Corbey, representing the 'PVDA' and spokesperson labeling and obesity. Topics were guidelines on labeling, labeling system of England, and research into the effects of labeling on purchasing behavior.

- Meeting with Ms. Stephanie Bodenbach, European Commission DG SANCO. Topics consisted of explanation of the White Paper, impact assessment, labeling, sports, and transportation.

- Meeting with Ms. Carolina Bollaers, EU policy manager at European Health Alliance (EPHA). Various projects supported and created by the agency were discussed in detail. The agency cooperates with the Bill Gates Foundation and provides support in the area of health.

- Documentation regarding the results of Aruban studies was also submitted. Since then, the Special Committee on Obesity and the EPHA have had a working relationship in support of the National Plan Aruba 2009–2018.

- Meeting with assistant of Euro MP, Katalijne Buitenweg, 'Groen Links' and shadow report White Paper Obesity. Topics consisted of healthy products at a lower price, children and physical activity, stop light labeling system of England.

- Meeting with Euro MP Lambert van Nistelrooy, 'CDA' and spokesperson obesity. Topics of discussion were free school fruit, ban on the sponsoring of candy during sports, the healthy school.

- Furthermore, 10 amendments were submitted to the Commission.

2.3. Cooperation with the Ad Hoc Committee on Overweight and Obesity Netherlands Antilles

During the meetings of the Bipartite Parliamentary Consultations Kingdom Relations Netherlands Antilles and Aruba in Oranjestad, on November 12–14,

2007, it was decided to establish a (special) committee that will be charged with the preparation of a national plan, as approved on page 2, footnote a, of the Final Declaration.

In implementation of this decision, Aruban Parliament established the Special Committee on Obesity on May 9, 2008, and the Netherlands Antilles established the Ad Hoc Committee on Overweight and Obesity Netherlands Antilles.

The meeting between the Ad Hoc Committee on Overweight and Obesity Netherlands Antilles and the Special Committee on Obesity Aruba took place in Curacao, on September 4, 2008. Although, originally, both committees had to arrive at a joint prevention plan, the Special Committee on Obesity, established by Aruban Parliament, proposed to draw up a prevention plan for each island separately, as the healthcare structure and problems of each island differ. Taking into account the request of the President of Parliament of the Netherlands Antilles to submit to both Parliaments a joint document containing "guidelines" during the Bipartite Parliamentary Consultations Kingdom Relations, the committees decided to offer Parliament a document containing "guidelines" during the Bipartite Parliamentary Consultations Kingdom Relations in October 2008. The guidelines can be found in Chapter 4.

2.4. Involvement of society

The Special Committee on Obesity counts on society's involvement. Several stakeholders have been selected, with which the problem has been discussed in order to arrive at a combined approach regarding the preparation of the National Plan 2009–2018.

The following topics and activities were discussed with the stakeholders:

- Consumer education, advertising and marketing with special attention for children.
- Offer of foodstuffs, physical activity, and health information at work.
- Integration of the prevention and treatment of overweight and obesity into healthcare.
- Fighting the "obese" society (lifestyle).
- Socio-economic inequality.
- An integrated and broad approach to promote healthy nutrition and physical activity.
- Recommendations for the nutrition intake and for the preparation of nutrition guidelines.

During the consultations with the stakeholders regarding the National Plan to be prepared, there was very wide consensus on the opinion that the community should contribute by working with different types of stakeholders at a national level. The stakeholders underlined the necessity of consistency and coherence in the community policy and the importance of a multisectoral approach. They emphasized the usefulness of the Committee's task to prepare a national plan for the fight against overweight and obesity and the coordination of the actions, such as the collection of, and familiarization with good practices, and the necessity of an action plan and a strong unambiguous message to the persons concerned. It was considered important that the information is the same across the board.

Furthermore, the stakeholders concerned are of the opinion that one series of coordinated actions is preferable to a large number of individual actions. In Aruba, there are many separate projects, which mostly are nonrecurring and, therefore, have less effective results in the long term. It is important to create a central unit that coordinates all preventative actions. This central unit should also dispose of all information regarding the actions and overweight problem. Thus, certain projects can be expanded to obtain betters results for larger groups.

At present, most sports programs are fully, at any rate partially sponsored financially by means of donations from the private sector. The sports sector and the stakeholders have expressed their concern about the fact that, since the amendment to the law on taxes in respect of donations, the support by the private sector to the sports clubs has been influenced negatively. As a result of the amendment, the tax deduction for donations has been set at a maximum of Afl. 10,000 = per year. Furthermore, the donation can only be deducted, if it has been made to an agency designated by the Minister of Economic Affairs. This has led to a decrease in the financial support by the private sector to the sports clubs. The sports clubs argue that, at present, it is even more difficult to offer sports activities at a low rate. Due to this amendment, sports or physical activity are curbed instead of being stimulated.

In Aruba, there is a clear correlation between stopping breastfeeding and returning to work. A 2002 study shows that more than 54.2% of the new mothers do not begin breastfeeding. Many mothers worry that their child is receiving sufficient milk, so that the mothers start to give supplements of formula prematurely. Risk groups are mothers with low incomes, born in Aruba, who have given birth via cesarean, or who are not supported by their partners. In order to promote continued breastfeeding during the first six months, despite returning to work, the right to breastfeed has become effective in Aruba, meanwhile, since May 2007. The Foundation indicated that too little information is available to the employers and employees about the new law in actual practice. The Foundation also indicated that only 17.1% of the new mothers breastfed within 48 hours after the delivery. According to the Foundation, the bottleneck is that the hospital does not sufficiently stimulate breastfeeding and rather promotes bottle-feeding. The policy in the hospital on the promotion of breastfeeding as of birth should be changed.

The summary study number of diabetics in AZV file 2005 shows that identified MED-DIAB insured persons amount to 6.4% of the insured persons, i.e., 6,000 persons. They are responsible for approximately 20% of all AZV medical expenses. The age group 50–80 incurs most expenses (medication, hospitalization, and amputations). Diabetes is a disease with enormous financial consequences for the AZV Fund. The demand for care will continue to increase in the years to come, given the prevalence of overweight in Aruba and the expected aging of the population. The demand for care will also increase because of necessarily catching up, as, apparently, a large number of insured persons with diabetes do not receive proper diabetes care at present. There also is reason to believe that there is a large group of "undisclosed diabetics." The document is focused on primary prevention, mainly encompassing the fight against overweight and the promotion of physical activity. Specific information and prevention for the youth, 'the healthy school' project. Consultation with the business community and schools. Government plays a decisive role. Intensifying physical activity at schools, increasing the excise tax on sugar and alcohol in order to obtain funds for the purpose of prevention. Cooperation between the Government, AZV, schools, business community, and physicians is required and is a critical success factor in the fight against overweight.

It was understood that the possibility to undergo a gastric bypass exists in Aruba for persons with a BMI between 50–55. According to the specialist in charge of these treatments, it has turned out that, in certain cases, the costs of the treatment will be recovered within a period of approximately 3 years. At present, the AZV only reimburses 20 treatments per year, despite the fact that 100 persons are waiting. An integral treatment procedure should be developed, so that more of these extreme cases will receive the medically necessary intervention.

The topics most frequently brought forward by the stakeholders are the following:

- Prevention as part of health.
- Prevention through information about proper physical activity and balanced nutrition by means of television shows, brochures, newsletters, cooking shows, etc.
- An integral national plan with an unambiguous message is necessary.
- A central unit where all information and treatments against overweight are available.
- Amendment to the State Ordinance General Health Insurance, so that prevention is reimbursed.
- More sports at school and after school.
- More small recreational facilities in the districts. Reactivating the district centers.

- Reducing the price of vegetables and fruits and promoting the consumption of vegetables and fruits.

- Food labeling of the products.

- Banning the sale of soft drinks and "pastechis" [pastries] at school.

- Offering healthy food at school.

- More dieticians, notably for children.

- Closing roads for family bicycle and hiking activities during the weekend.

- Repeal of the state ordinance on donations.

- Great interest in the blood sample taking actions of the White Yellow Cross.

- Cooperation between education and sports.

- Increasing excise tax on candy.

3. VISION

When tackling the problem of overweight and obesity, three factors should be taken into account.

First, the individual is ultimately responsible for his way of living and that of his children, although the importance of the environment and the effect hereof on his behavior are recognized.

Secondly, only a well-informed consumer/individual is able to make well thought-out decisions.

Finally, an optimal response in this area will be accomplished by promoting complementarity and integration of the Government in the different relevant policy areas (horizontal approach) and the different action levels (vertical approach).

4. GUIDELINES ON OVERWEIGHT AND OBESITY

4.1. Promoting healthy physical activity and balanced nutrition

To tackle the problem of overweight and obesity it is extremely important to promote healthy physical activity and balanced nutrition. These issues are decisive for a change in lifestyle and the promotion of a healthy body, which should lead to a decrease in the overweight and obesity figures in Aruba. The approach should be focused on several target groups or environments, viz.:

A) the community;

B) the living environment of infants and young children;

C) school, and

D) the workplace.

A: The community

Interventions should take place in the community or the "bario" [district] to promote a balanced nutrition and physical exercise among all residents. Targeted attention to interventions in the immediate living and residential environment does not exist in Aruba. Still, an important part of the eating and exercising habits takes place there: at home, during leisure time, in the district. To approach the community the stakeholders are of importance to have an effect on the behavior of people or on their environment. Health promotion in the local community will be effective only in the long term, if the various actors cooperate and/or spread the same message. It is necessary to create a central information center for the coordination of the projects and information. Special attention should be paid to social risk groups and the elderly.

One of the complaints of the sports clubs is that, since the entry into effect of the act on taxes in respect of donations, these clubs have seen a decrease in donations, which, of course, curbs the promotion of sports. It is necessary to initiate a study as regards the statutory amendment concerning donations, in order to assess whether it should be tackled or modified.

B: The living environment of infants and young children

Priority should be given to children ages 0–6 and their mothers. The first year of life is of crucial importance to a healthy life. Furthermore, the circumstances for the mother in these first years are heavy and expensive. Providing support to mother and child is important. One possibility is the program "Hallo Wereld" [Hello World], which is willing to broadcast this show in Aruba.

Stimulating mothers to breastfeed. Breastfeeding is the most natural way to feed a newborn. In the long term, breastfeeding offers protection against i.a. obesity. It turns out that most parents make their choice for the type of feeding before the pregnancy already. Therefore, it is important that women and their partners will already be informed before becoming pregnant about the importance of exclusively breastfeeding the child as of birth.

In addition, attention is paid to young children in childcare. The first years of life are important to familiarize oneself with a healthy lifestyle, consisting of balanced and varied eating habits and sufficient exercise. In Aruba, obesity already increases as of childhood. Therefore, it is important to watch over good eating habits and sufficient physical activity in this age group. As regards infants and toddlers, childcare is the main factor of influence in their immediate social environment, apart from the parents and grandparents. Therefore, additional attention is paid to the role these organizations can play in the promotion of balanced nutrition in young children.

C: School

The eating pattern of children, young people, and young adults, notably as regards breakfast, beverages, snacks, consumption of vegetables and fruits, simply is problematical. The Childhood Obesity Study 2004 shows that 71.9% of the children between the ages of 6 and 11 do not eat breakfast on a regular basis.

This also applies to the extent to which schoolchildren and students exercise. The Childhood Obesity Study 2004 shows that 77.4% of the children between the ages of 6 and 11 do not arrive at the minimum quota of physical activity.

Changing eating and exercising habits is of crucial importance to prevent overweight and obesity at a later age.

Of course, school is an important living environment for this target group. The impact thereof on the behavior of its pupils or students should not be underestimated. The prevention, promotion, and stimulation with regard to the children and youth should take place through education.

Furthermore, the SER report of January 2005 has also shown that afterschool care is not adequate in Aruba, and that children are often alone, without supervision, after school. An integral approach entails that there should be a structural change, such as keeping the children at school longer to create the possibility that the children are looked after and are not lonely. In addition, these additional hours should be used to offer i.a. health classes, to promote sports up to three times per week, while also offering healthy food. There should also be possibilities to build up one's ability to do things independently and self-esteem. It is important that each school has a room for physical activity/gymnastics and promotes interscholastic games. In this way, a healthy school will be created. For this purpose, Aruba can enlist the help of the Netherlands Healthy School Institute. The project "healthy school cafeterias" of the Netherlands Nutrition Center is a concrete example of how healthy food can become a focus at school. An integral approach is used as a starting point, and not only the offer in the school cafeteria is looked at, but substantive support in the classes is also provided. The snack tents surrounding these schools play an important role.

D: The workplace

Promoting balanced nutrition and sufficient physical activity at the workplace refers to every effort of employers, employees, and of society to strengthen the patterns of living of working people.

A person working fulltime eats 1/2 to 1/3 of his daily meals at work. However, the workplace often does not offer the possibility to apply healthy living habits. Programs should be prepared to educate and promote exercising at the companies.

4.2. Promoting breastfeeding

The promotion of breastfeeding requires a structural approach. The study "KABP-onderzoek Borstvoeding Aruba 2003" [KABP Study Breastfeeding Aruba 2003] of the Department of Public Health has shown that only 17% of the mothers exclusively breastfeed during the first 48 hours (KAPB-Study 2003). The approach should be focused on stimulating and facilitating breastfeeding. This can be done by having the hospital promote exclusive breastfeeding for 6 months after the birth of the child. The implementation of the National Breastfeeding Policy Plan Aruba ("NBBA") is desirable.

Research has shown that there is a correlation between stopping breastfeeding and returning to work. The 2002 breastfeeding study of the Department of Public Health has shown that 66% of the new mothers stop breastfeeding when they return to work again. Recently, an act has also been adopted, which makes it legally possible to breastfeed and/or to pump in the workplace. It has turned out, however, that there is not sufficient information for the employer and employee as to how this should take place. Targeted information should be given to the employer and employee. An employee who breastfeeds is more productive. Besides, breastfeeding promotes the health of the mother/employee.

4.3. Promoting unambiguous information by the healthcare providers

General practitioners, dieticians, exercise experts, (homecare) registered nurses, general dentists, pharmacists, gynecologists, pediatricians, and other care providers are inevitably confronted in their practices with all sorts of questions about nutrition and physical activity. They have the important task to make the patient aware of the importance of a balanced eating pattern and healthy exercising. In Aruba, care providers are one of the most important sources of information for people as regards balanced nutrition, as well as the most reliable one. It has turned out that the healthcare providers do not give unambiguous information as regards the approach of overweight and obesity. To properly inform and refer people, care providers should dispose of the appropriate knowledge and be able to make use of practical tools when giving advice. Therefore, it is necessary to draw up unambiguous information and to adopt guidelines for this group. As most of the prevention will depend on the first line, support to the general practitioners is necessary. This support has to consist of highly educated nurses, who can provide the information. Dieticians and exercise experts should be hired in the near future.

4.4. Good nutritional information

It has turned out that many groups are not aware of what balanced nutrition means, nor are they familiar with nutritional information. It is necessary that the consumer receives clear and non-contradictory information in a positive and attractive manner. Within this framework, it is important to introduce a food-labeling system, as well as to exchange good practices with the European Union and the Netherlands. A good example is a clear food-labeling policy, such as the system of a 4-color label on the front of the product, e.g. the "Sailboat Design for the Region".

The information will automatically influence the purchasing behavior and promote the purchase of healthy food. This policy should be implemented in cooperation with the various supermarkets. Thus, a healthier purchasing pattern and eating habits can be created. The service clubs are working on a pilot project in this area. A labeling policy should be combined with a general information campaign.

4.5. Media and communication

There are *other actors* that are of importance to communicating about balanced nutrition and healthy physical activity. First, it is endeavored to involve the media sector, the food outlets/supermarkets, restaurants, snack bars. Within this framework, it is important to avoid advertising for candy and soft drinks during the children's shows on television. The media can contribute to this. Information programs and messages regarding the promotion of balanced nutrition and healthy physical activity should become part of the media. A complete large-scale awareness and prevention program in cooperation with the healthcare sector, education, sports, nongovernmental organizations, and the private sector, coordinated by a central unit, such as a central prevention institute/foundation, is of vital importance to the success of the National Plan Aruba 2009–2018. Information can be provided via text-messaging and advertising on Cable TV.

Aforementioned guidelines have been drawn up based on WHO, IOTF, and the European White Paper, taking into account the *information* of the stakeholders, our culture and traditions. and the strong influence of other countries.

In 2007, the European Commission proposes its *'White Paper'* (Commission of the European Communities, 2007) on a 'Strategy for Europe on Nutrition, Overweight, and Obesity related Health Issues.' It contains the following areas of interest for private actors, as well as the recommendation for a shared approach and the strengthening of local action networks:

- making the healthy option available and affordable;

- keeping consumers informed;

- encouraging physical activity

- priority groups and settings:

  - schools bear a great responsibility in ensuring that children not only understand the importance of good nutrition and exercise but can actually benefit from both;

  - businesses can also support the development of healthy lifestyles in the workplace;

- developing a picture of good and best practice.

In 2007, the WHO adopted the following objectives:

Workers' health: global plan of action 2008–2017 (WHO, 2007):

1. to devise and implement policy instruments on workers' health;

2. to promote health at the workplace, i.e., by promoting healthy food and physical activity;

3. to improve the performance of and access to occupational health services;

4. to provide and communicate evidence for action and practice;

5. to incorporate workers' health into other policies.

At the end of 2007, the WHO proposes the *Second Plan of Action 2007–2012*, consisting of six actions areas (WHO, 2007), which each country integrates into its policy at several levels and adjusts to its own situation:

1. supporting a healthy start: the care for mothers and children;

2. ensuring a safe, healthy, and sustainable food supply: sufficient good and safe food for everyone;

3. providing comprehensive information and education to consumers: know what you eat and how to avoid risks;

4. taking integrated action to address related determinants: taking into account other risk factors;

5. strengthening nutrition and food safety in the health sector: involving health professionals in the improvement of the health services;

6. monitoring, evaluation, and research: actions based on facts and gathering new knowledge.

The IOTF, or International Obesity Task Force, drew up a schedule called:

"The opportunities for influencing a child's environment."

From	Social policies and national legislation
to	organizational and commercial practices
to	planning controls and regional strategies
to	community and cultural traditions
to	school practices and peer influence
to	family customs and choices
to	individual self-control
'til	THE CHILD

"It is clear from these suggestions that policies and actions will be needed at a variety of levels, some local and individually based, some national or internationally based. All of them will require the support and involvement of departments across the broad range of government and may include education, social and welfare services, environment and planning, transport, food preparation and marketing, advertising and media, and international trading and standard-setting bodies.

Government and inter-governmental activities in all departments, including education, agriculture, transport, trade, the environment and social welfare policies are assessed for their health impact, and Government food purchases, e.g. for departmental staff, for the military, police, prisons, hospitals and schools and other agencies involved in public sector supply contracts are consistent with health and nutrition policies."

5. PHYSICAL ACTIVITY AND EATING HABITS IN ARUBAN SOCIETY

5.1. Demographic data

- The Aruban population amounts to 104,494, of which 49,844 female and 54,650 men (*CBS, Statistical Yearbook 2007*). Graph 1F shows the composition of the population and how this composition will be in the year 2023.

- The composition of the population according to age is as follows (*CBS, Statistical Yearbook 2007*):

  - < 14 years   20.3%
  - 15–65 years   70.6%
  - > 65 years   9.1%

Graph 1F. Population Pyramid, 1960, 2007, 2023

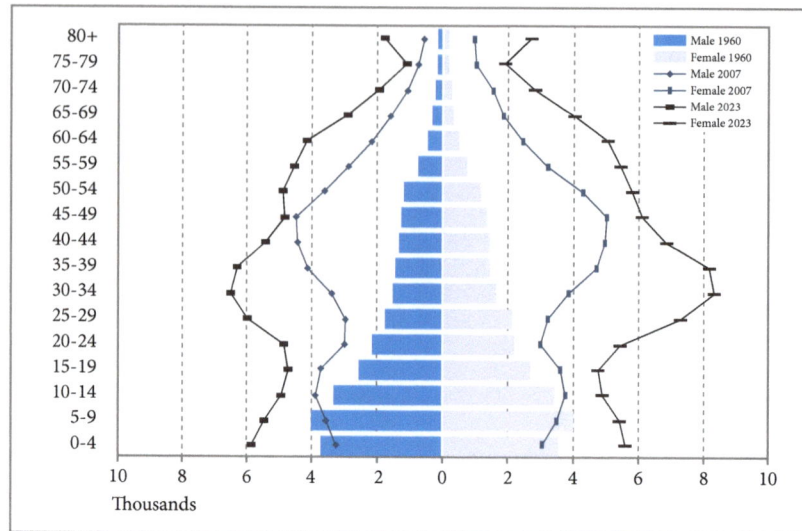

- The population density per km² land is 581 (*CBS, Statistical Yearbook 2007*).

- Aruban society is multicultural, as 40% of the population were not born in Aruba.

- The educational level of the Aruban community is composed as follows. Only 8% of the population enjoyed education at a 'HBO' [*university of professional education*] or a university (*CBS, Statistical Yearbook 2007*).

- The GDP rate has decreased. The standard is 6% (*CBS, Statistical Yearbook 2007*).

- Living zone of children according to age (*CBS, Statistical Yearbook 2007*).

- The gross income of the population (*CBS, Statistical Yearbook 2007*).

- Life expectancy for men is 70.1 years (2000), compared to 71.1 years previously (1991). Life expectancy for women is 76.2 years (2000), compared to 77.12 years previously (1991). Life expectancy has decreased by one year in a period of less than 10 years.

- Passenger transportation is equal to half the population. There are 50,211 passenger vehicles with a population of 75,817 aged 20 years and up (*CBS, Statistical Yearbook 2007*).

Population[1] by level of education obtained by age category in percentage

Level of education	Age category					Total
	15–24	25–34	35–44	45–54	55–64	
Primary education or less	37%	29%	33%	45%	62%	39%
Secondary education	53%	50%	48%	39%	25%	44%
Vocational middle level	8%	12%	10%	6%	5%	9%
Higher level and University level	2%	8%	9%	9%	7%	8%
Not reported	1%	–	1%	–	1%	1%
Total	100%	100%	100%	100%	100%	100%

Source: *"Onderwijs op Aruba, Context on Output."*

[1]*Population 15–65 years, not visiting school.*

Graph 5D. Government expenditures on education as % of GDP and expenditures per student

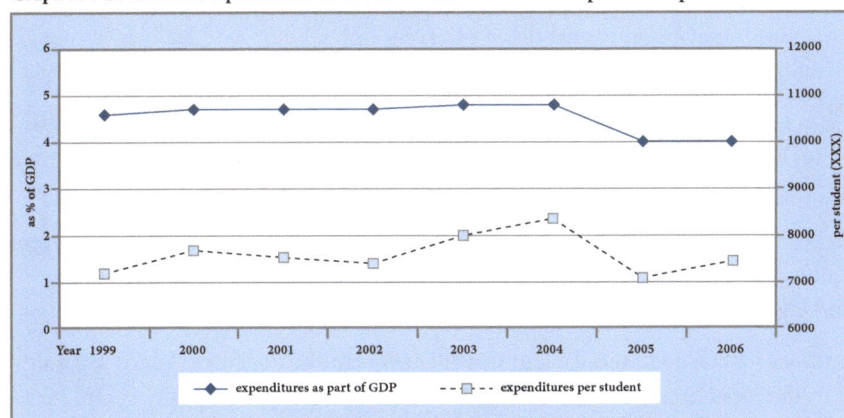

5. Average gross wages and salaries by income categories and gender, ave. 1999-2004

Income class	1999 - 2004			
	Tot. % of Employees	Cumulative	Male	Female
Afls.				
< 20,000	17.1%	17.1%	7.0%	10.1%
20,001 ≤ 25,000	14.2%	31.3%	7.0%	7.2%
25,001 ≤ 30,000	12.5%	43.9%	6.6%	6.0%
30,001 ≤ 35,000	10.6%	54.5%	5.9%	4.7%
35,001 ≤ 40,000	7.4%	61.8%	4.3%	3.1%
40,001 ≤ 50,000	11.7%	73.0%	6.0%	4.9%
50,001 ≤ 75,000	16.2%	89.8%	9.9%	6.3%
75,001 ≥	10.2%	100.0%	7.5%	2.6%

Source: C.B.S.

5.2. Eating habits in Aruba

A. Breastfeeding

The *Childhood Obesity Study 2004* shows that 90.8% of the overweight children and 93.3% of the obese children were not exclusively breastfed during a period of six months.

This is also confirmed by the "KABP-onderzoek 2003" [KAPB *Study 2003*], showing that only 17% of the children are exclusively breastfed within the first 48 hours after birth.

Of the group that does begin breastfeeding (45.8%) 66% stops when returning to work again, usually within six weeks after the delivery. Not giving exclusive breastfeeding for six months is one of the risk factors related to overweight, *Childhood Obesity Study 2004*.

Special attention to breastfeeding in the hospital, by the health care providers, and at work is really necessary.

B. Breakfast habits among schoolchildren

The *Childhood Obesity Study 2004* shows that 71.9% of the elementary school-going children do not eat breakfast regularly. The parents of this group hardly set an example. This means that 2/3 of our children skip breakfast. It has also turned out that the children who do eat breakfast often eat unhealthy foods, such as 'pastechi' or 'empana'.

The first meal of the children who do not have breakfast does not take place until 10:30 or 11:30, usually consisting of a 'pastechi' or another deep-fried snack with a soft drink.

Breakfast is the most important meal of the day, because it is the first meal the body gets after a long night's rest. The IOTF concluded that 25% of one's daily energy should come from breakfast.

A healthy breakfast will reduce and possibly prevent the consumption of unhealthy food in the morning. A healthy breakfast will also stimulate the physical and mental capacities of the child. Skipping breakfast is one of the largest risk factors related to overweight.

C. Consumption of fruits and vegetables

STEPS *Aruba 2006* shows that the consumption *of fruit* amounts to 0.8 fruits per day per *adult*. The usual recommendation of fruit consumption according to the WHO and IOTF amounts to 250 gr. or two servings of fruit each day. The fruit consumption of *children* is even less, whereas the recommendation of fruit consumption amounts to at least 350 grams or three servings daily.

Age Group	Number of servings of fruit per day[1]			Number of servings of vegetables per day[1]			Number of servings of fruit and/or vegetables per day[1]		
	Men No. 664 Max. 95% CI	Women No. 895 Max. 95% CI	Both Sexes No. 1559 Max. 95% CI	Men No. 661 Max. 95% CI	Women No. 895 Max. 95% CI	Both Sexes No. 1556 Max. 95% CI	Men No. 665 Max. 95% CI	Women No. 896 Max. 95% CI	Both Sexes No. 1561 Max. 95% CI
25-34 years	0.6 (0.5 0.7)	0.5 (0.1 0.9)	0.7 (0.6 0.8)	0.9 (0.8 1.1)	1.0 (0.9 1.1)	1.0 (0.9 1.1)	1.6 (1.4 1.8)	1.8 (1.6 2.0)	1.7 (1.6 1.8)
35-44 years	0.7 (0.6 0.8)	0.5 (0.7 0.9)	0.7 (0.6 0.8)	1.0 (0.9 1.1)	1.0 (0.9 1.1)	1.4 (1.0 1.1)	1.7 (1.6 1.8)	1.8 (1.6 1.9)	1.8 (1.7 1.9)
45-54 years	0.7 (0.6 0.8)	0.8 (0.8 0.9)	0.8 (0.7 0.9)	0.9 (0.8 1.0)	1.0 (1.0 1.1)	1.4 (0.9 1.1)	1.6 (1.4 1.8)	1.9 (1.7 2.0)	1.8 (1.7 1.9)
55-64 years	0.9 (0.7 7.0)	1.0 (0.9 1.1)	0.9 (0.8 1.0)	1.0 (0.9 1.1)	1.0 (1.0 1.1)	1.0 (1.0 1.1)	1.9 (1.7 2.1)	2.0 (1.9 2.2)	2.0 (1.8 2.1)
25-64 years	0.7 (0.6 0.8)	0.8 (0.8 0.9)	0.8 (0.7 0.8)	1.0 (0.9 1.1)	1.0 (1.0 1.1)	1.0 (1.0 1.0)	1.7 (1.6 1.8)	1.9 (1.8 1.9)	1.8 (1.7 1.8)

[1]Corr. Numbers of Servings per Day as Days Concerned

The *vegetable consumption* by adults in Aruba amounts to 1.0 serving daily (*STEPS Aruba 2006*). This is far below the quantity recommended by the WHO and IOTF, viz.: 300 grams per day.

Vegetables and fruits contain most of the vitamins, minerals, and fibers the body needs to stay healthy. They have a preventative effect with regard to oxidative stress and, therefore, improve the immune system. Not eating sufficient fruits and vegetables is a risk factor for overweight and being healthy.

D. Excessive consumption of soft drinks and sugar-sweetened drinks

Several local studies have shown that the consumption of soft drinks and other sugar-sweetened drinks by children and youngsters is so high that problems related to i.a. sugar level, dentistry, and overweight have grown excessively. At the same time, the consumption of water has decreased considerably, especially among the most vulnerable group of the population, viz.: the children. Attention should also be paid to the sale of soft drinks and other sugar-sweetened drinks in and around our schools. The consumption of water should be promoted, and the 'WEB' [*Water and Electricity Company*], in cooperation with the Richard Visser Institute, is working on the preparation of a national campaign to promote the consumption of water.

E. Local and international fast foods

The Aruban meals and snacks are high in fat content, because the meals and snacks, such as 'pastechi', 'crocket', cheese balls, etc., are deep-fried. In addition, there is an abundance of international fast food chains, which also focus on our children by means of their influence through the media.

School cafeterias mostly only sell local junk food, candy, chocolate, chips, etc. The school cafeterias that do not do this have to deal with competition from snack bars in the surroundings of the school.

Social life and culture largely revolve around food, given the birthday culture. Nowadays, the celebration of a birthday entails complete meals at work. Eating is used as a reward for children and parents. Except for local snack bars and fast food chains, it turns out that the takeaway meals of the Chinese restaurants have become a weekly habit for the population. Most takeaway meals are high in caloric value, salt and fat content, and low in nutritional value.

Summarized:

- We do not breastfeed enough.
- We eat too little breakfast.
- We eat too little vegetables, too little fruits.
- We drink too little water and too many sugar-sweetened drinks.
- We eat too much junk food or unhealthy food.

5.3. Physical activity in Aruba

Healthy exercise is understood to be a level of physical activity leading to positive health effects. This corresponds to a PAL value of more than 1.60 (Bouchard et al., 2007). Adults are recommended to get at least 30 minutes of moderate to intensive exercise per day, children and youngsters at least 60 minutes. To reduce the chance of obesity, this should be increased to 60 and 90 minutes, respectively, per day. This corresponds to a PAL value of 1.75 (Ross, 2007, Institute of Medicine, 2002). Given the dose-response relationship between physical activity and health, more will be gained when exceeding this minimum standard (Strong et al., 2005; Nelson et al., 2007; Haskell WL et al., 2007). To get a complete picture of the amount of physical activity per day, the PAL value, the physical activity level, is a good parameter or indicator. The PAL value is the factor by which the basal metabolism (= energy expended at rest) should be multiplied to calculate the total energy use per day. In theory, this index can range between 1.0 for extremely sedentary individuals and approx. 2.5 for very physically active persons.

This value encompasses both professional activities, quiet activities, sports activities, and sedentary activities. Internationally, it is assumed that a daily amount of physical activity corresponding to a PAL value exceeding 1.75 (combined with a low-fat diet) is required for acting preventively against obesity and diabetes type 2. Individuals with a PAL value of 1.40 or less show a sedentary lifestyle.

The *Childhood Obesity Study 2004* showed that 77.4% of the schoolchildren do not regularly exercise and/or participate in sports. They walked less than 10 minutes per day, spent three to four hours before the television and computer. This group is classified as sedentary. *STEPS Aruba 2006* shows that only 9.5% of the group ages 25–64 gets a high level of physical activity.

Age Group	Men (No. 653)			Women (No. 886)			Both Sexes (No. 1,539)		
	Low level of activity % 95% CI	Moderate level of activity % 95% CI	High level of activity % 95% CI	Low level of activity % 95% CI	Moderate level of activity % 95% CI	High level of activity % 95% CI	Low level of activity % 95% CI	Moderate level of activity % 95% CI	High level of activity % 95% CI
25-34 years	27.9 (18.5 – 37.4)	52.8 (42.4 – 63.3)	29.2 (11.8 – 26.7)	41.1 (32.4 – 49.8)	53.8 (42.9 – 60.6)	7.1 (2.6 – 11.6)	35.5 (29.0 – 42.0)	52.2 (45.5 – 59.0)	22.3 (1.2 – 26.4)
35-44 years	44.5 (36.8 – 52.2)	37.9 (30.5 – 45.3)	27.6 (11.8 – 23.4)	46.8 (43.2 – 55.3)	47.3 (40.7 – 53.8)	5.9 (2.9 – 9.0)	46.8 (40.8 – 50.7)	43.2 (38.3 – 48.1)	11.0 (7.9 – 24.1)
45-54 years	49.5 (41.1 – 57.9)	42.5 (33.5 – 49.6)	8.9 (4.7 – 13.1)	56.7 (50.1 – 63.2)	37.3 (31.0 – 43.6)	6.0 (2.6 – 9.5)	53.3 (48.1 – 58.5)	39.3 (34.3 – 44.4)	7.1 (4.7 – 20.1)
55-64 years	43.2 (35.2 – 52.2)	51.0 (42.9 – 58.1)	6.5 (2.9 – 10.7)	57.2 (50.2 – 64.2)	39.7 (32.8 – 46.6)	3.1 (0.7 – 5.5)	53.2 (45.3 – 56.6)	44.3 (33.8 – 49.4)	4.7 (2.5 – 6.9)
25-64 years	41.6 (37.0 – 46.1)	44.4 (39.8 – 49.0)	14.0 (11.0 – 17.0)	49.2 (45.4 – 53.2)	44.8 (41.0 – 48.6)	5.9 (4.1 – 7.8)	45.8 (42.9 – 48.8)	44.6 (41.7 – 47.6)	9.5 (7.8 – 11.2)

The elementary schools in Aruba do not teach special gym classes. In cooperation with IDEFRE, 1½ hours of sports classes are taught to the 4th-, 5th-, and 6th-graders per week. Swimming lessons are given to the 3rd-graders once per week. There are no gym or sports classes for the 1st-and 2nd-graders. The elementary schools also have a problem with the facilities. Some do not have a gym, others have an indoor gym. Hardly any physical activity takes place during school hours. Given the duration of the school hours, there also is too little time to expand further sports possibilities, as school ends at 01:03 p.m.

It is difficult for children to participate in afterschool sports activities, because of transportation difficulties and the parents' working hours. Furthermore, the costs involved cannot be afforded by the part of the population earning a minimum income. The sports sector still has not been structured properly. Both education and sports work independently of each other, and each pursues its own policy.

It can be observed, however, that there are various projects to promote physical activity among children, such as Extreme H Games of the Richard Visser Institute, Fit Kids of IDEFRE, etc. Reference is made to the budget of the Minister of Sports.

Summarized:

- 77.4% of the schoolchildren do not regularly exercise.
- These children have a sedentary lifestyle (3 to 4 hours television/computer games).
- Only 9.5% of the population gets at least 60 minutes of intensive physical exercise per day.
- Not all schools dispose of sports facilities.
- The 1st- and 2nd-graders are not taught any sports.
- The 3rd-, 4th-, 5th- and 6th-graders are taught sports 1x per week.
- Access to afterschool activities is difficult.

5.4. BMI results

CHILDREN:

The *Childhood Obesity Study 2004* shows that:

WHO tables according to gender and age	OverweightBMI	Obesity BMI	Overweight + Obesity
Boys 6–11 years	11.4%	28.4%	37.8%
Girls 6–11 years	9.7%	24.5%	34.2%

YOUTH:

	Overweight BMI	Obesity BMI	Overweight + Obesity
17–24 years	22.11%	20%	42%

ADULTS:

	Overweight + Obesity	Of whom obese BMI > 29.9
Health survey 1993	52%	28 %
Health survey 2001	73.5%	38%
STEPS Aruba 2006	77%	40.8%

The 1993, 2001, 2004, and 2006 health surveys show an increasing trend among all age groups. The increase of overweight among children is notably disturbing, viz.: from 15.0% to 37% in 2004. These figures are higher than those of the Netherlands and the United States.

The surveys show that people are not aware that they are overweight. They have a completely wrong self-image. 61% of the persons with overweight in 2001 thought that they had a normal weight.

Summarized:

- 77% of the adults age 25 and up have an unhealthy weight.
- 42% of […?] (17–24 years) are overweight and obese.
- 37% of the children ages 6–11 are overweight and obese.
- There is question of an increasing trend among all age groups.

5.5. Conclusion

In general, it can be concluded that the average Aruban exercises insufficiently and has an unbalanced eating pattern. The information about what we eat and how much we exercise clearly indicates that the recommendations are not met in several respects. This notably applies to children, youngsters, the elderly, and underprivileged groups. It has also been established that the overweight and obesity figures are excessively high in Aruba compared to the United States and the Netherlands. What is even more disturbing is that most people do not realize that they are overweight or obese.

It is the ambition of the National Plan Aruba 2009–2018 to rectify these shortcomings and to harmonize the physical activity and eating pattern of the Aruban and the recommendations.

This was the starting point for deciding on the concrete details of the healthy food and physical activity objective for the period 2008–2015.

6. THE NATIONAL PLAN ARUBA 2009-2018

6.1. Objective

The main objective is to achieve health gain for the entire population by creating an increase in the number of people that are sufficiently active, have a balanced diet, and strive for a healthy weight.

6.2. Achievement of the objective

It is clear that health gain can be achieved by promoting a balanced diet and healthy exercise. This requires a change demanding enormous social effort. The question arises 'which effort will lead to the best result?'

An unbalanced diet, too little physical activity, and the consequences thereof are enabled by various factors. It has been demonstrated that the causes are related both to people's lifestyle and to their environment (National Heart, Lung and Blood Institute, 2004; Law, 2007). What people do or do not do is influenced by their opinions, preferences, or skills, as well as by their intentions, knowledge, risk assessment, and experienced social influence, or their expectations as regards the new behavior.

Behavior can never be seen separately: it occurs in a specific environment, with physical, social, cultural, political, and economic characteristics. The more this environment invites people to make healthy choices, the bigger the chance that they will also actually opt for the healthy alternative.

The starting point is to make the healthy choice the most obvious choice: easily available, at an acceptable price, in accordance with rules, and supported by the opinions and standards of the environment.

The objects pursued for 2018:

1. Children. Promoting sufficient physical activity from 22.6% to 45% to achieve health gain.

2. Adults. Promoting the number of people that are physically active to achieve health gain by increasing moderate activity from 44.6% to 55% and intensive activity from 9.5% to 15%.

3. The population's inactivity should decrease from 45.8% to 30%.

4. Promoting exclusive breastfeeding for six months from 15% (2003) to 30% and for four months from 37% to 60%.

5. School cafeterias should comply with the Healthy School System in the majority of our schools, and there should be a policy on the prevention of the sale of unhealthy food outside and around the schools.

6. Identification and examination policy, pursuant to which all school-going children are examined and advised on BMI and weight each year.

7. Gym classes for all schools and grades for at least 1 hour and three times per week.

8. Weekly health class.

9. Daily breakfast before school from 28.1% to 56%.

10. The number of people having a healthy weight should increase by at least 5%.

A multifactoral cause pleads for a multifactoral solution. High consensus exists that the best results are obtained by taking an integral series of mutually supporting measures at the same time. The World Health Organization (WHO) and several European institutions argue that each country should elaborate a balanced nutrition and physical activity policy, adjusted to its own culture, region, and standards. This entails a mixture of interventions and measures, in which all policy levels find and support each other. The various international initiatives to promote a balanced diet and health physical activity are based on this same integral approach. They plead for wide consumer information and for working with priority groups, for education and for adjustments in the environment, for involvement of various social actors, and for an engagement from the private sector, for interventions responding to the needs of the population, and for a sustainable policy.

6.3. Preconditions

A basic condition to be able to put in place the National Plan Aruba 2009–2018 and, thus, to achieve the new health objectives is the involvement of the Government in playing its condition-creating role. This role consists of creating an environment, together with all parties concerned, which encourages individuals, families, and communities in a positive way to opt continuously for balanced nutrition and an active lifestyle.

Preconditions

- Implementation of the National Plan Aruba 2009–2018 requires a clear division of tasks and sufficient structural financing.

- Allocation of funds for prevention in the government budgets.

- Preparation of a prevention policy document and a prevention policy by the Government, so that all actors are familiar with the prevention policy and the objectives thereof, as indicated in this National Plan Aruba 2009–2018.

- An integral approach entails that the various policy areas, such as education, public health, sports, culture, youth, traffic, are involved and take responsibility, in order to influence the entire community.

- An integral approach requires the designation or creation of an institute/organization as a central unit and a coordinating body that exclusively provides all information and coordinates activities.

- Implementation of the healthy school policy, in order to arrive at a healthy basis for children and teachers at school.

- Better coordination with regard to the various initiatives, and messages regarding sufficient physical activity and balanced nutrition should be integrated into them.

- Cooperation between actors in the social sector should be initiated, and primary and secondary prevention should be in line with each other.

- Reimbursement by the AZV of the treatment by dieticians and expansion of the number of dieticians, notably for children.

- The themes 'healthy physical activity and balanced nutrition' should be integrated into the curricula, and there should be adjusted education for all actors.

- There should be a sufficiently powerful investment in projects in support of the achievement of these health objectives, which meet the criteria of sustainability, intersectoral coordination, and a structural basis.

- Amendment to the act on donations, in order to increase the financial support from the private sector to the sports sector again.

- Additional funds should be obtained by increasing the excise duty on candy and soft drinks.

- The Socio-Economic Council should be requested to prepare an economic impact study with regard to the consequences of overweight and obesity on our economy, labor market, and labor productivity. The Free University of Amsterdam can be of assistance.

7. STRATEGIES

7.1. Promoting healthy physical activity and balanced nutrition

To tackle the problem of overweight and obesity it is extremely important to promote healthy physical activity and balanced nutrition. These issues are decisive the promotion of a healthy body and a change in lifestyle, which should lead to a decrease in the figures in Aruba. The approach should be focused on several target groups or environments, viz.: A) the community, B) the living environment of infants and young children, C) school, and D) the workplace.

A. The community

Interventions to take place will encompass all efforts made in district, 'bario', or the city to preserve or improve a healthy lifestyle in a healthy environment for all residents. The Government will provide for a (integral) policy. The numerous organizations in the city or the district can help with the implementation of the actions.

A nutrition and physical activity action plan focused on the entire population, and interventions focused on specific target groups (youth, the elderly, young mothers, underprivileged groups) should be prepared.

Health promotion in our small island will mainly be effective in the long term, if the various actors cooperate and spread the same message. The Government is the designated partner to draw up an action plan for sufficient physical activity and balanced nutrition, in cooperation with the actors (to be sensibilized first) and, if possible, with the participation of the residents. Such an action plan falls within the framework of the policy to protect and promote the citizens' health.

In concrete terms, this means that this theme will be embodied in the government policy, in which the other social rights, with many of the same actors, are also safeguarded to guarantee each citizen maximum chances of health. To decide on the concrete details hereof, methods are required and support should be provided in the preparation of a nutrition and physical activity action plan. The degree of physical activity and eating habits in our community depend on the district one lives in, the cultural community one belongs to, and the social status, all entailing a different lifestyle. Depending on the age category, we see important behavioral differences leading to other health risks.

Strategies for specific target groups and in specific settings within the local community should be developed in detail with the involvement of the relevant organizations.

Possible actors: Government, Public Health, AZV, 'SVB' [Social Insurance Bank], other policy areas, such as sports (IDEFRE), education, infrastructure, first-line care providers, health centers, White Yellow Cross, and various non-governmental organizations, sports clubs and their federations, sports organizations, such as COA and ASU, the hospital, medical and paramedical groups, trade unions, private sector, tourist sector, distribution sector, hospitality industry, service clubs, etc.

IMPLEMENTATION:

1. A political commitment on the part of the Government is essential to the successful implementation of the National Plan Aruba 20092018. Cooperation between and partnerships of groups or organizations should also exist. A central unit, e.g. an institute/foundation, should be created as a prevention center.

2. A national campaign to promote healthy physical activity and balanced nutrition among the population. This campaign should be initiated by the Government, in cooperation with the various actors. The campaign should consist of education and activities. The campaign should raise awareness in the following areas:

- exercising more, at least 60 minutes per day;
- curbing a sedentary lifestyle, such as television and computer programs;
- increasing the consumption of fruits and vegetables;
- reducing the consumption of soft drinks and sugar-sweetened drinks;
- promoting the consumption of water;
- promoting breakfast;
- it is better to eat smaller servings several times per day (6);
- providing clear information about food. It is extremely important that all actors spread the same message in a national campaign.

3. In addition to education and activities, certain preconditions and the policy should be adjusted, such as maintenance of our parks, sports facilities. More areas should be created to promote physical activity, such as playgrounds for children and clubs for youngsters, so that they can be used frequently.

4. Stimulating the district centers to become more active, so that possibilities to exercise will be created in the living and residential environment, which are easily accessible to avoid transportation difficulties.

5. Closing certain roads during the weekend, so that the population can walk and exercise safely, e.g. Irausquin Boulevard (Eagle), San Nicolaas, and Oranjestad. This can take place in cooperation with IDEFRE, which already organizes many walking and running tours. This stimulates the entire family to exercise, so that exercising becomes a family affair.

6. Cooperation between the Government and the private sector to promote the sale of healthy food.

7. Increasing the financial support to the White Yellow Cross for projects, such blood sample taking actions, as education, and prevention.

8. Amendment to the act on donations to promote the financial support from the private sector to sports clubs and organizations.

B. The living environment of infants and young children

Priority should be given to children ages 0-6 and their mothers. The first year of life is of crucial importance to a healthy life. Furthermore, the circumstances for the mother in these first years are heavy and expensive. Providing support to mother and child is important.

Stimulating mothers to *breastfeed*. Breastfeeding is the most natural way to feed a newborn. In the long term, breastfeeding offers protection against i.a. obesity. It turns out that most parents make their choice for the type of feeding before the pregnancy already. Therefore, it is important that women and their partners will already be informed before becoming pregnant about the importance of exclusively breastfeeding the child as of birth. Babies who are breastfed have health benefits in the short term, such as a reduced risk of acute otitis media, atopic dermatitis,

IMPLEMENTATION:

1. It is extremely important to support the 'Stiching Pro Lechi Mama' for the implementation of the National Breastfeeding Policy Plan Aruba ('NBBA').

2. Interventions relating to the prenatal and postnatal period, including the crucial days around the delivery, such as the program 'Hallo Wereld', seem to be more effective than interventions focusing on only one period.

3. Multifaceted interventions are notably effective, when they are focused on both the beginning, the duration, and the exclusiveness of breastfeeding.

4. Optimizing the essential social support to underprivileged groups.

gastrointestinal infections, lower respiratory tract infections, asthma, and necrotizing enterocolitis (this last only in premature children).

In the long term, breastfeeding protects against chronic disorders, such as obesity, diabetes mellitus, celiac disease, leukemia (ESPHGAN Committee on Nutrition, 2007; Canadian Institute for Health Promotion, 2006; Arenz et al., 2004). To increase the number of mothers that begins breastfeeding, information should notably be provided about the benefits of breastfeeding. This raises knowledge and awareness, leading to a stronger motivation to begin and see through.

In addition, attention is paid to young children in childcare/daycare centers. The first years of life are important to acquire a healthy lifestyle with balanced and varied eating habits and sufficient physical activity. In Aruba, obesity already increases as of childhood. Therefore, it is important to watch over good eating habits and sufficient physical exercise in this age group. As regards infants and toddlers, childcare is the main factor of influence, in addition to the parents and grandparents, in their immediate social environment. Therefore, additional attention is paid to the role these organizations can play in the promotion of balanced nutrition for young children. Toddlers really enjoy running, jumping, and climbing and should have the freedom to do so. Exercising forms part of the child's development. Young children should have sufficient possibilities to exercise and develop. In Aruba, there is no supervision over the daycare centers, so that there is no integral policy on the quality and contents of childcare.

IMPLEMENTATION:

1. Laying down by law the requirements for and supervision over the child daycare centers to protect the children as soon as possible. Supervision over the quality and contents of daycare should be guaranteed.

2. Working out supporting measures for childcare to draw up balanced menus (meals and beverages) and, thus, to promote a balanced and healthy offer. This can take place by means of e.g. brochures, work instruments, a website, education with attention for good practical examples.

3. Promoting parent participation in as far as healthy food in childcare is concerned by informing daycare facilities about how they can educate parents and involve them in the food offered and the composition of the menu. This can take place by making available brochures, a website, work instruments.

4. Informing daycare facilities about how they can stimulate children to exercise and enjoy exercising. This can take place by means of brochures, a website, work instruments.

5. Working out the active sailboat model for toddlers and preschoolers. The knowledge hereof should be transferred to the communities and care providers in cooperation with the services for integration.

6. Working on healthy nutrition together with the toddlers in a playful manner.

C. School

The eating pattern of children, young people, and young adults, notably as regards breakfast, beverages, snacks, consumption of vegetables and fruits, simply is problematical. This also applies to the extent to which pupils and students exercise. Even more so, now that physical exercise classes are not taught in each grade. Changing eating and exercising habits is of crucial importance to prevent overweight and obesity at a later age.

Of course, school is an important living environment for this target group. The impact thereof on the behavior of its pupils or students should not be underestimated. The prevention, promotion, and stimulation with regard to the children and youth should take place through education. The implementation of a food and physical activity policy at school, embodied in a broader health policy, is an effective way to promote balanced nutrition and healthy physical activity (www.gezondeschool.ned). International studies clearly show that the promotion of health at school yields a return (Stewart-Brown, 2006). Gain is actually achieved on both public health, healthy behavior, and the educational performances (Allensworth, 1997).

Studies show the following:

- Interventions through the school for children and young people are effective to reduce weight (Bessems et al., 2006).

- Daily physical education (increasing frequency, duration and intensity of gym classes), improving motor skills, physical education classes should be based on theoretic models, physical education teachers should be requested to inform and stimulate students, daily classes should be integrated into the school curriculum, and encouraging leisure time exercising is effective. Even a small increase in physical education classes is useful to reduce overweight (CIHI, 2006; Sharma, 2006).

- Interventions through school for children and young people are effective to increase leisure time physical activity (Bessems et al., 2006).

- Education to reduce screen-watching (television, games, DVD) is effective (Doak, C.M. et al., 2006; Sharma, 2006).

- Nutritional education (i.a. discouraging the consumption of soft drinks (including diet soft drinks), encouraging the intake of fruits and promoting the consumption of water) is effective (Doak, 2006).

Furthermore, the SER report of January 2005 has also shown that afterschool care is not sufficient in Aruba, and that children are often alone, without supervision, after school. The participation and active involvement of parents in a behavioral change of the child is an important success factor for school interventions. Parents can be involved in several ways by making the parents more skilled in actively stimulating and encouraging physical activity among their children, offer of vegetables and fruits, creating a positive framework, and encouraging physical activity among their children. The best way to involve the parents is through parent-teacher contact, e.g. via newsletters, homework assignments, and sending material to the parents' home (Van Sluijs, 2007; Blanchette & Brug, 2005).

It is important that the same messages are spread and the same actions are taken at different levels: both in the classroom and at school and towards the parents. Only an ongoing, long-term effect leads to sustainable results. The school should explicitly opt for and work on health. The involvement of the students and especially the parents leads to broad support.

An integral approach entails that there should be a structural change, such as keeping the children at school longer to make it possible that the children are looked after and are not lonely. In addition, these additional hours should be used to offer i.a. health classes, to promote sports up to three times per week, while also offering healthy food. There should also be possibilities to build up one's ability to do things independently and self-esteem. It is important that each school has a room for exercise/gymnastics and promotes interscholastic games. In this way, a healthy school will be created. For this purpose, Aruba can enlist the help of the Netherlands Institute Healthy School. The project "healthy school cafeterias" of the Netherlands Nutrition Center is a concrete example of how healthy food can become an area of interest at school. An integral approach is used as a starting point, and not only the offer in the school cafeteria is looked at, but substantive support in the classes is also provided. The snack tents surrounding these schools play an important role.

The offer of meals, beverages, and snacks at the schools is a weak point. The policy should be focused on a more limited offer with less options and mainly 'healthy' choices, including i.a. a ban on soft drinks.

IMPLEMENTATION:

1. Implementing the healthy school.

2. Making sure that the 1st and 2nd grades attend physical education classes.

3. Increasing the number of physical education classes per week.

4. Implementing an integrated nutrition and physical activity policy.

5. Structural annual health education on all points.

6. Further developing and supporting school policy on nutrition and physical activity. Introducing the sailboat model.

7. Stimulating a balanced offer of school meals by increasing fruits and vegetables in the meals and as a snack.

8. Promoting expertise among the kitchen staff.

9. Stimulating a balanced offer of beverages, consisting of water and beverages of low sugar content.

10. Offering each grade free drinking water.

11. Banning soft drinks and beverages of high sugar content.

12. Prolonging the school hours, so that there is afterschool care, during which physical activity is stimulated by sports organizations (broad school system).

13. Implementing 'exercise snacks' throughout the school day.

14. Promoting active playgrounds, gyms to increase physical activity among elementary schoolchildren.

15. Implementing, screening, and steering educational material in the area of physical activity and nutrition.

16. Stimulating the teacher-training course 'Movecion y Salud' [*Exercise and Health*] ('IPA').

17. Promoting the expertise of school teams, management, teachers, school staff members (kitchen staff and educators) in the area of nutrition and physical activity.

18. Identification protocol with the schools for an annual measurement of weight, height, BMI, and waist circumference of all school-going children.

D. The workplace

Promoting balanced nutrition and sufficient physical activity at the *workplace* refers to every effort of employers, employees, and of society to strengthen the patterns of living of working people. Apart from the work or the working conditions, unhealthy living patterns have their own share in the occurrence of sicknesses and absenteeism. An unbalanced nutrition and insufficient physical activity lead to a considerable personal and social loss due to a decrease in the quality of life, loss of productivity, or premature incapacity for work.

Together with the Government, the employers are responsible for the indirect costs related to unhealthy eating and exercising habits, through medical expenses for hospitalization, medication, laboratory tests, and social benefits. On the other hand, a healthy weight and an improved physical condition lead to better concentration and an increased daily productivity. A balanced eating and exercising pattern also benefits the company. At present, physical inactivity is internationally recognized as a new labor risk (European Agency for Safety and Health at Work, 2005).

A person working fulltime eats ½ to ⅓ of his daily meals at work. However, the workplace often does not offer the possibility to bring healthy living habits into practice. Moreover, it turns out that working people tend to skip breakfast more often due to a lack of time in the morning.

The involvement of the employer in the employee's health is essential. Thus, the blood sample taking actions of the White Yellow Cross should be promoted by the employers. Programs should be prepared to educate and promote physical activity at the companies.

IMPLEMENTATION:

1. Stimulating employers to have the company participate in the preventative blood sample taking actions of the White Yellow Cross. Additional financial support to the White Yellow Cross is necessary.

2. Programs linked to the blood sample taking actions of the White Yellow Cross, including an incentive package for the participants, so that continuity in physical activity and nutrition programs is created.

3. Stimulating and having available fruits as a snack at work.

4. Avoiding the presence of soft drinks and beverages of high sugar content in the office.

5. Rooms for pumping and other changes to meet mother and child (environment).

6. Promoting the possible cooperation between companies, so that the smaller companies can participate in larger projects.

7. Exchanging intracompany and intercompany information (newsletter) as regards the activities in the area of physical activity and nutrition education.

8. Promoting company sports and tournaments between companies.

9. Family days, during which the entire family exercises and learns how to eat healthy– also stimulating healthy food/nutrition classes in the workplace.

7.2. Promoting breastfeeding

The promotion of breastfeeding requires a structural approach. The study "KABP-onderzoek Borstvoeding Aruba 2003" [*KABP Study Breastfeeding Aruba 2003*] of the Department of Public Health has shown that only 17% of the mothers exclusively breastfed during the first 48 hours (*KAPB-Study 2003*). The approach should be focused on stimulating and facilitating breastfeeding. This can be done by having the hospital promote exclusive breastfeeding for 6 months after the birth of the child. The implementation of the National Breastfeeding Policy Plan Aruba ("NBBA") is desirable.

Research has shown that there is a correlation between stopping breastfeeding and returning to work. The new mothers stop breastfeeding when they return to work again. Recently, an act has been adopted, which makes it legally possible to breastfeed and/or to pump in the workplace. It has turned out, however, that there is not sufficient information for the employer and employee as to how this should take place. Targeted information should be given to the employer and employee.

An employee who breastfeeds is more productive. Besides, breastfeeding promotes the health of the mother/employee. The health benefits are: a reduced risk of diabetes mellitus type 2, breast and ovarian cancer, quicker recuperation of the womb, less bleeding. Women who do not breastfeed or prematurely stop breastfeeding, run an increased risk of postnatal depression. ("Voedingscel Vlaamse Vereniging Kindergeneeskunde", 2006; Agency for Healthcare Research and Quality, 2007).

In addition to health benefits, breastfeeding also entails *economic benefits*. Breastfeeding reduces the costs of healthcare and decreases absenteeism. According to a study in the Netherlands, each increase of 10% in breastfeeding results in a direct savings of approx. 1 million. Furthermore, the employee is more productive.

Many mothers worry that their child is receiving sufficient milk, so that the mothers start to give supplements of formula prematurely. Risk groups are mothers with low incomes, born in Aruba, who have given birth via cesarean, or who are not supported by their partners.

The duration of the period of rest after the delivery is an important predictor of the duration of breastfeeding. If the mother stays home longer than the assumed duration of maternity leave, the chance of longterm breastfeeding increases considerably. Therefore, it is important to provide supporting information. Offering breastfeeding information to parents-to-be or young mothers without personal contact or with very brief contact (folders or telephone advice) is less effective than offering information combined with in-depth one-on-one communication. Using to increase the number of women that begins breastfeeding and to support and stimulate mothers when breastfeeding in the first days and weeks.

The actors of importance are: "Fundacion Pro Lechi Mama", White Yellow Cross, hospital, Department of Public Health, midwifes, gynecologists, and pediatricians.

IMPLEMENTATION:

1. Implementing the National Breastfeeding Policy Plan Aruba ("NBBA").

2. Protocol with the hospital that exclusive breastfeeding for six months is promoted in the maternity ward. Also prohibition on offering new mothers free formula products. This can take place by means of a protocol with the formula agents.

3. Inserting the right to breastfeed and/or pump in the State Ordinance Substantive Civil Servants' Law.

4. Informing employer and employee as to how the newly implemented act on breastfeeding and/or pumping works in actual practice by means of brochures.

5. Continuing the distribution of information (brochures), advice, and education with regard to breastfeeding to parents and among the actors.

6. Setting up mothers' groups to share experiences with breastfeeding. Offering information with personal contact is more effective.

7. Interventions in healthcare in the form of a combined approach, consisting of refresher courses for the staff, appointing a breastfeeding consultant, or a lactation expert, making available written information to staff and clients.

8. Recognizing the lactation expert diploma.

7.3. Promoting unambiguous information by the healthcare providers

General practitioners, dieticians, exercise experts, (homecare) registered nurses, general dentists, pharmacists, gynecologists, pediatricians, and other care providers are inevitably confronted in their practices with all sorts of questions about nutrition and physical activity. They have the eating pattern and healthy exercising. In Aruba, care providers are one of the most important sources of information for people as regards balanced nutrition, as well as the most reliable one. It has turned out that the healthcare providers are aware of the usefulness hereof but do not have time to discuss this during the consult. The knowledge of nutritional aspects can be improved. It has turned out that the general practitioners do not give unambiguous information as regards the approach of overweight and obesity. To properly inform and refer people, care providers should dispose of the appropriate knowledge and be able to make use of practical tools when giving advice. Therefore, it is necessary to draw up unambiguous information and to adopt guidelines for this group. As most of the prevention will depend on the first line, support to general practitioners is necessary. It is not the intention to turn the general practitioners into nutrition and physical activity experts. It is important that they recognize the problem and are able to provide relatively simple information. The support has to consist of highly educated nurses, who can provide the information. Dieticians and physical activity experts should be hired in the near future.

As regards morbid obesity, there should be a treatment protocol with competent central unit for the treatment of these cases. At present, the AZV only reimburses 20 gastric bypass interventions per year for patients with an average BMI between 50–55. This causes a waiting list of approximately 100 patients per year, who are eligible for this treatment, but who do not receive treatment due to the current policy. An integral treatment procedure should be developed, so that more of these extreme cases will receive the medically necessary intervention.

The *summary study number of diabetics in AZV file 2005* shows that identified MED-DIAB insured persons amount to 6.4% of the insured persons, i.e. 6,000 persons. They are responsible for approximately 20% of all AZV medical expenses. The age group 50-80 incurs most expenses (medication, hospitalization, and amputations). Diabetes is a disease with enormous financial consequences for the AZV Fund. The demand for care will continue increasing in the years to come, given the prevalence of overweight in Aruba and the expected aging of the population. The demand for care will also increase because of necessarily catching up, as, apparently, a large number of insured persons with diabetes do not receive proper diabetes care at present. There also is reason to believe that there is a large group of "undisclosed diabetics." The document is focused on primary prevention, mainly encompassing the fight against overweight and the promotion of physical activity. Specific information and prevention for the youth, 'the healthy school' project. Consultation with the business community and schools. Government plays a decisive role. Intensifying physical activity at schools, increasing the excise tax on sugar and alcohol in order to obtain funds for the purpose of prevention. Cooperation between the Government, AZV, schools, business community, and physicians is required and is a critical success factor in the fight against overweight.

IMPLEMENTATION:

1. Preparing a scenario with agreements between the care providers, the AZV, and the Department of Public Health as regards preventative and curative care.

2. Providing for courses and information for general practitioners and/or HAVA.

3. Elaborating preventative guidelines for care providers to promote balanced nutrition and physical activity.

4. Preparing a prevention package for the care providers, based on the sailboat model, with direct tools to measure waist circumference and BMI.

5. Stimulating the general practitioner to systematically measure weight, height, and waist circumference.

6. Encouraging the engagement of multidisciplinary teams, such as a nurse, dietician providing information to the patient.

7. Providing unambiguous information both horizontally and vertically in the care sector.

8. Expanding surgical and other treatments of morbid obese patients.

9. Expanding and strengthening youth healthcare and several other divisions within the Department of Public Health.

10. Ensuring that financial funds are available for the Department of Public Health to implement projects for the promotion of balanced nutrition and healthy physical activity.

7.4. Good nutritional information

It has turned out that many groups are not aware of what balanced nutrition means, nor are they familiar with nutritional information. It is necessary that the consumer receives clear and non-contradictory information in a positive and attractive manner.

Within this framework, it is important to introduce a food-labeling system, as well as to exchange good practices with the European Union and the Netherlands.

A good example is a clear food-labeling policy, such as the system of a 4-color label on the front of the product, e.g. the "Sailboat Design for the Region".

The information will automatically influence the purchasing behavior and promote the purchase of healthy food. This policy should be implemented in cooperation with the various supermarkets. Thus, a healthier purchasing pattern and eating habits can be created.

The service clubs, in cooperation with the Richard Visser Institute, are working on a pilot project in this area. This project will be examined by the Free University Medical Center of Amsterdam. A labeling policy should be combined with a general information campaign.

A new Aruban information model "Sailing towards a healthy society."

The Balanced Diet Ship

The "Balanced Diet Ship," with its five sails, reflects this concept as it moves through a sea of plenty filled with sunshine, clean air, healthy food and physical activity on its journey toward a longer and healthier life.

Each of the sails propelling the Balanced Diet Ship forward represents a distinct food group. The three large sails represent the consumption of water, fruits and vegetables, and carbohydrates; the medium sail represents proteins; and the small sail represents fats. The size of each sail is correlated with the amount of food that should be consumed from the food group it represents.

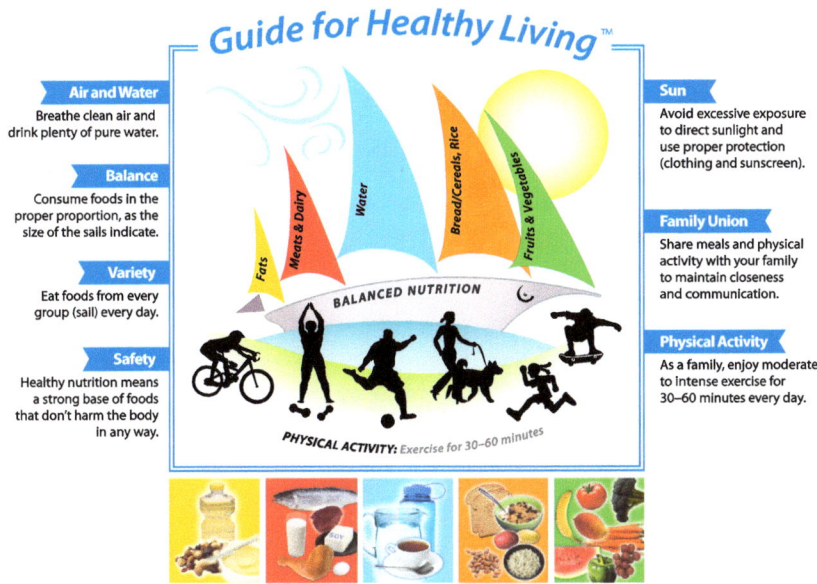

Guide for Healthy Living™

Air and Water
Breathe clean air and drink plenty of pure water.

Balance
Consume foods in the proper proportion, as the size of the sails indicate.

Variety
Eat foods from every group (sail) every day.

Safety
Healthy nutrition means a strong base of foods that don't harm the body in any way.

Sun
Avoid excessive exposure to direct sunlight and use proper protection (clothing and sunscreen).

Family Union
Share meals and physical activity with your family to maintain closeness and communication.

Physical Activity
As a family, enjoy moderate to intense exercise for 30–60 minutes every day.

Fats · Meats & Dairy · Water · Bread/Cereals, Rice · Fruits & Vegetables

BALANCED NUTRITION

PHYSICAL ACTIVITY: Exercise for 30–60 minutes

Water

*(Represented by a large **blue sail** on the Balanced Diet Ship)*

Water is the principal component and most important element of every living organism, representing 50% or more of our total body weight. The importance of water as a nutrient is only exceeded by the importance of oxygen. Water is therefore represented by a large sail, reflecting the need to drink as much water as possible.

The physical and chemical characteristics of water make it an ideal medium for the distribution of chemical substances found in the body substances which are important to the metabolic process. Given its role as a general transport medium, water plays a direct part in enabling various biological functions to operate effectively. transport medium, water plays a direct part in enabling various biological functions to operate effectively.

The total amount of water found in the body changes with age. In the newborn, it comprises up to 75% of total body weight. The percentage of water decreases as one grows older, down to 55–65% of body content in adult men and 50–55% in adult women. This difference between men and women is due to the fact that women have less muscle and more fat tissue. In a physiologically ideal situation, a male individual 20 years old and 1.83 m tall, with a body weight of 70 kg and in good health should have a body water content of about 40 liters.

Total body water content remains relatively constant due to the action of two powerful reflex mechanisms: the sensation of thirst and a reduction in the volume of urine eliminated when total body water volume begins to diminish. Should the total body water content increase for any reason, the sensation of thirst tends to wane and the volume of water eliminated through the kidneys increases as well, producing the desired balance of body water content.

There are three principal sources of body water: water ingested as such; water found in food; and water generated by one's cells as a by-product of the metabolism of carbohydrates, fats and proteins. The total amount of water ingested by an individual, either as water or as water contained in his diet, can vary widely, depending upon factors such as climate and type of food consumed. For example, oranges, watermelons, cantaloupe and similar fruits have a high water content per unit of weight, while the water content per unit mass of other foods, such as grains, legumes and tubers, is much lower. The need for water also increases in hot, dry climates and in situations involving increased respiration or what is known as "alveolar ventilation".

Urine is the principal channel through which water is lost from the body. The amount of water lost through the skin is extremely variable and may occur as sweat, which is noticeable, or "insensible perspiration", which is

unnoticeable. It can also occur through fecal matter, the lungs and exhaled air.

It has been suggested that at least 1.5 liters of water should be consumed each day, but it is practically impossible to determine one's true water needs in a given situation with any degree of precision because of the large number of factors that can increase or decrease water loss. Water nourishment requirements have been established with this in mind. Of these water requirements, over half are obtained from the water content of food with the remainder coming from the water we drink.

Water must be clean and drinkable and must not contain any physical, chemical or biological agents in significant quantities or any harmful characteristics that could adversely affect one's health. Mineral content, or hardness, is also of particular importance and must be kept within certain limits. Consumption of so-called "hard water", or mineral-rich water, places an excessive functional load on the kidneys which can cause severe balance disorders in the body if certain limits are exceeded. It can even lead to death which would occur if an individual were to drink sea water, for example.

At the other extreme, we find distilled or completely de-mineralized water which, in addition to causing other disorders, can have a negative impact on the dynamic equilibrium that exists between various mineral components of the cells that make up body tissues. It too can lead to death if allowed to persist for a sufficient period of time.

Fruits and Vegetables

(*Represented by a large **green sail** on the balanced diet ship*)

Fresh fruits and vegetables must be part of a varied, nutritious diet. These foods provide significant amounts of the vitamins, minerals, trace elements, dietary fiber and antioxidant nutrients that protect an individual's health and are active in the prevention of disease. A diet consisting of large quantities of fruits and vegetables is one that is high in both taste and nutrition. Fruits and vegetables are therefore represented by a large sail, indicating the need to consume large portions of these types of foods in your diet.

Consumption of fruits and vegetables increases the antioxidant content of one's diet which is currently thought to be a basic dietary requirement. Nutrition experts now recognize the contribution of fresh fruits and vegetables in helping to destroy or neutralize the oxygen-based free radicals generated as part of the human metabolic process, supporting the defense systems that reduce the adverse effects of these free radicals. The damage caused by free radicals, if extensive enough can harm the body's cells and makes it difficult for them to adapt to change. It can even lead to cell death. The consequences of these changes can be severe, and have

been linked to the development of arteriosclerosis, cancer, inflammatory bowel disease, neuro-degenerative diseases, autoimmune problems such as rheumatoid arthritis, and the complications of diabetes.

Fruits should be eaten fresh in their natural state, and salads should be eaten raw due to the loss of vitamins and minerals that occurs during the cooking process.

Preference should be given to dark-green and yellow or orange vegetables, and to fresh, unstrained vegetable juices with no salt or sugar added.

Fruits and vegetables also play a significant role in providing the required amount of *dietary fiber*. Not long ago, dietary fiber was thought to be an inert substance consisting largely of cellulose and having an insignificant influence on human health. However, it is currently suggested that insufficient fiber in the diet may contribute to the development of many diseases including colon and rectal cancer; diverticulitis; appendicitis; constipation; hemorrhoids; diabetes; and obesity.

Much research has been done on the relative importance of dietary fiber, and some contro-versy exists as to which foods should, or should not, be defined as dietary fiber. However, there is general agreement on the value of a number of properties characteristic of this element.

One important property of dietary fiber is its ability to retain water. This property makes a major contribution toward a well-functioning digestive system. Dietary fiber also has the ability to form gels in the gastrointestinal tract, leading toward increased glucose tolerance and lessening the absorption of cholesterol and salt. Another important property attributed to dietary fiber is its ability to absorb calcium, magnesium, zinc and iron. The fermentation of dietary fiber in the colon also produces two elements, gas and energy, that are necessary for proper colon function.

The consumption of a sufficient amount of dietary fiber therefore has a positive effect on the digestive system through increased fecal mass; increased stool fluidity; shortened intestinal passage time; dilution of solids found in the large intestine; excretion of nitrogen, fatty acids, cholesterol and salt through the feces; and the stimulated growth of beneficial bacteria. It also helps to reduce the absorption of carbohydrates which increases glucose tolerance, reduces insulin requirements after meals, and increases the efficiency of glucose metabolism.

Currently, there is no definite agreement among researchers on the amount of dietary fiber that should be consumed daily, and there is even less agreement as to the type and variety of fiber that should be eaten. It has been suggested that consumption of 15–30 grams daily is sufficient for a healthy adult, and 3–4 grams a day is recommended for children two years of age or older. No recommendations have been made for younger children. Diets providing 6 grams of fiber or more are considered to be rich in this nutrient which should form a regular part of every person's diet.

Vegetables that should be eaten include chard, cabbage, lettuce, carrots, squash, beets, beans, peppers, onions, pumpkin, cucumbers, radishes, tomatoes, celery, eggplant, broccoli and okra, among others. Fruits that should be eaten include oranges, lemons, limes, grapefruit, mangos, papaya, bananas, guava, apples, pineapple, pears, grapes, apricots, peaches, coconut, cherries, mandarin, mango, anon, sour sop, pineapple pear, coco, prunes, red currants, mamoncillo, medlar, strawberries, cantaloupe and watermelon, among others.

The importance of consuming large amounts of fruits and vegetables is reflected in the large size of the green sail representing this food group.

Carbohydrates

(*Represented by a large **orange sail** on the Balanced Diet Ship*)

Foods containing carbohydrates are critical in that they provide the energy we need to function well and to lead an active life style. Of all of the dietary elements, carbohydrates, represented by a large orange sail, has to be consumed most frequently in order to meet the body's energy needs. Sixty percent or more of an individual's total energy needs must be satisfied through this food group.

There are two basic types of carbohydrates: *complex carbohydrates* such as starch, and *simple or refined carbohydrates* such as sucrose, maltose, or lactose. Carbohydrates should preferably be eaten in the form of starch which is absorbed into the bloodstream more slowly than simple carbohydrates. This slower absorption, as compared with the rapid absorption of simple carbohydrates, is beneficial because it does not produce the concentrated peaks of large glucose production that simple carbohydrates does and therefore does not require the production of large quantities of insulin by the pancreas. When combined with adequate amounts of soluble dietary fiber, carbohydrates will be digested more slowly, thereby improving glucose tolerance so critical to the prevention and control of diabetes.

No less than 85% of carbohydrates eaten must come from starch, with the remaining 15% consumed through simple or refined carbohydrates. Foods containing high levels of starch include rice, wheat, corn, barley and rye. It is important that these foods be designated as "whole grain," that is, grains that have not had their shell completely removed or depleted through industrial processing. Pasta is also an excellent source of carbohydrates, and pastas too should

be "whole grain." Other sources of carbohydrates include potatoes, yucca, and bananas, among others. Foods containing high concentrations of simple or refined carbohydrates, which should be consumed in limited quantities, include jam, candy, donuts, cakes, cookies, sugary beverages and other foods containing large quantities of sucrose, maltose or lactose. Priority should be given to low glycimic index carbohydrates.

Proteins

(*Represented by a medium **red sail** on the Balanced Diet ship*)

Foods containing large amounts of protein are represented by a medium red sail.

Foods containing protein should satisfy 10-15% of an individual's total energy needs. However, the fundamental nutritional purpose for consuming proteins is not their use as an energy source but rather their role in theprocess of cell multiplication and the repair of body tissues.

Proteins are made up of simpler structural units known as amino acids. There are currently 22 different types of amino acids.

Amino acids too are classified as essential and non-essential. Non-essential amino acids can be synthesized from carbohydrate and nitrogen residues, whereas essential amino acids cannot be produced this way and must be obtained through one's diet.

Proteins must be digested before their constituent amino acids can be released and subsequently absorbed. The digestion of protein begins in the stomach and is completed in the small intestine, with help from the pancreas. The nutritional quality of the proteins found in food depends, among other things, upon their digestibility and upon their biological use and importance once they have been digested and their constituent amino acids absorbed. A protein is considered complete from a nutritional perspective if it contains all essential amino acids in the correct proportions, as is true for milk and egg proteins.

Dietary proteins can also be of animal or plant origin. Animal proteins tend to have a higher amino acid score and a higher level of digestibility, adding to their nutritional value.

Many experts believe that 50% of the total amount of protein consumed should be of animal origin and the remaining 50% of plant origin, although this may vary depending on the individual's life style, functional capacity and health.

Excellent sources of animal protein include milk, meat and meat products, free-range poultry, fish, eggs and internal organs such as the heart, liver and spleen. Plant-based foods, such as grains and legumes or beans, make the greatest quantitative contribution in

meeting an individual's protein needs, especially in developing countries. When grains and legumes are combined in appropriate proportions, amino acid mixtures that significantly reduce the actual need for animal-based proteins can be achieved. Vegetables, tubers and other starchy foods provide very little protein, and any protein obtained from these foods is of poor nutritional quality.

Foods of animal origin are often related to food-borne illnesses caused by biological contaminants. It is therefore important to be sure that these types of foods are fully and evenly cooked by applying enough heat to allow the thermal center of these foods to reach 70 degrees. You should also avoid cross contamination from other uncooked foods or contaminated surfaces.

Fats

*(Represented by a small **yellow sail**)*

Fats are represented by a small yellow sail, indicating that 25–30% of an individual's total energy needs should be met through this type of food.

The most common fats in the human diet are *triglycerides* and *cholesterol esters*. Triglycerides may be *saturated* or *unsaturated*, depending on the presence or absence of what are called "double bonds." If a fatty acid contains only one double bond between two carbon atoms, the fat is considered to be mono-unsaturated. Fat containing two or more double bonds are considered to be poly-unsaturated.

Of the total energy received through the ingestion of fat, 5–10% should be in the form of saturated fats; another 10% in the form of mono-saturated fats; and the remaining 10% as poly-saturated fats.

Fats may have an *animal or plant origin*. Animal fats are generally saturated fats. Foods containing this type of fat are also generally rich in cholesterol. With the exception of coconut and palm oil, fats originating in plants, known as oils, contain a greater amount of unsaturated fat.

The fats we consume may be *visible* or *invisible*. Visible fats include fats used for cooking, such as oils, lard or bacon, or those served at the table, such as butter, cream cheese or margarine. Because this type of fat is visible, it can be easily avoided. Non-visible fat, on the other hand, cannot be seen, even though it is present in many of the foods we eat. These fats can be found in meat, fish, eggs, milk, and nuts, among others.

Fats are also classified as being *non-essential* or *essential*, depending upon the body's capacity to synthesize its own fatty acids. The non-essential group consists of fat produced by one's own body; essential fatty acids must be supplied through one's diet in quantities equivalent to 3–5% of an individual's total energy needs.

Excessive fat consumption is associated with many medium and long-term health implications. This is especially true of foods rich in saturated fat and fatty acids. Limited consumption of pork, beef, lamb, bacon, lard, butter, chicken skin, cream cheese, whole milk and fatty cheeses is therefore recommended. Coconut, palm and avocado oils also have a high saturated fat content. Fats that are liquid at room temperature, in contrast, are rich in polyunsaturated fats and can be found in vegetable oils such as olive, soy, corn, sunflower, sesame and peanut oils. chicken skin, cream cheese, whole milk and fatty cheeses is therefore recommended. Coconut, palm and avocado oils also have a high saturated fat content. Fats that are liquid at room temperature, in contrast, are rich in polyunsaturated fats and can be found in vegetable oils such as olive, soy, corn, sunflower, sesame and peanut oils.

When preparing food rich in fat, especially fried foods, it is important to avoid overheating the fat or reusing it to the point where its essential qualities are altered. This can produce toxic substances in the fat leading tovarious illnesses, including cancer.

This instructional guide is designed to go together with a colored "front of Label" food labeling system — to ensure change in the publics buying habits.

7.5. Media and communication

There are *other actors* that are of importance to communicating about balanced nutrition and healthy physical activity. First, it is endeavored to involve the media sector, the food outlets/supermarkets, restaurants, snack bars.

Information programs and messages regarding the promotion of balanced nutrition and healthy physical activity should become part of the media. A complete large-scale awareness and prevention program in cooperation with the healthcare sector, education, sports, nongovernmental organizations, and the private sector, coordinated by a central unit, such as a central prevention institute/foundation, is of vital importance to the success of the National Plan Aruba 2009–2018. Information can be provided via text-messaging and advertising on Cable TV. Furthermore, several stakeholders, such as ATIA, Chamber of Commerce, OPPA (1200), SNBA, FTA, SETAR, etc., have indicated to be willing to provide information to their members through their newsletters.

The central prevention institute should take care of the distribution of information to all actors, so that the same information and messages are spread in the entire island and at each level. If messages are contradictory, the consumer gets confused and threatens to lose interest in healthy physical activity and balanced nutrition.

IMPLEMENTATION:

1. Establishing a central prevention institute.

2. Organizing a large-scale campaign on balanced nutrition and healthy physical activity.

3. Entering into a protocol with the media in connection with the campaign.

4. Providing information to the actors that have a newsletter to pass on the message to their members.

5. Promoting recreational physical activity in addition to sports on television.

6. Supervision and legislation as regards commercials during children's shows.

7. Teaching to cook healthy and affordably by means of television shows.

8. Special rates of the media for information campaigns on balanced and healthy nutrition.

9. Creating special information segments in all media and stimulating interactivity among the population.

By repeatedly campaigning under the same "brand name" of the central institute, the public profile will be raised.

It is easier to change the exercising and eating habits of children and young people, because their behavioral patterns have not yet or not entirely set in. This also indicates that commercials for candy and soft drinks during children's shows on television should be avoided. The media can contribute to this.

October 2008

Drawn up by Dr. Richard W.M. Visser, DC., PhD.

Chapter 2

HEALTH MONITOR ARUBA 2013

Lifestyle

Life expectancy

MENTALHEALTH and deaths

Provision, demand and supply of to the Aruban People of particular FOCUS

CONTENTS

PREFACE

It is with great pleasure that as the Minister of Health and Sports I can present to you the very first edition of the Health Monitor 2013 Aruba.

We are living in an age where the overall wellbeing of our citizens and the economy of the nation are being challenged by the effects of chronic diseases, reemerging infectious diseases, and rising health care costs among other factors. In order to be able to address these issues responsibly and effectively and to develop "healthy" policies and programs it is, therefore, critical not only to have a mechanism in place that systematically monitors the health status and behavior of the population but also to present these in an overview.

The Health Monitor 2013 has been developed having the above in mind and following the strategic direction mentioned in the "Kaderbrief Publieke Gezondheid 2011–2013" which states the need for an overview of health data and information that will assist the decision-making process regarding healthcare in general and also the development of health policies. This document will be published every four years and will provide invaluable information regarding factors associated with the health of our inhabitants such as lifestyle, health care, health care providers, mental health and the social environment.

The health gains acquired by the various applied health policies and preventive programs will be visible by upcoming publications of this Health Monitor. However, the measurement of health gains and progress obviously varies by subject. It is of utmost importance to monitor the trend of the health of the Aruban population in time.

This publication has been coordinated by the Epidemiology and Research unit of the Department of Public Health in cooperation with the Ministry of Health and also with the valuable contribution of the different representatives of the various units and services within the Department of Public Health, Central Bureau of Statistics (CBS) and the National Health Insurance (AZV). I am grateful for everyone's participation in this magnificent publication.

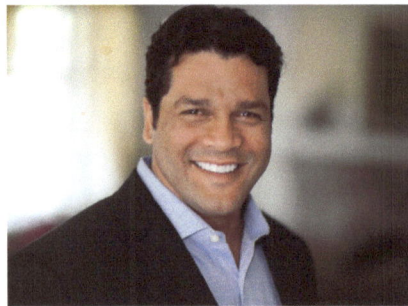

I would encourage all organizations whether they are governmental or private to use this document not only as a basis for prioritizing and making the right choices regarding health policies and programs, but also as a compass for rational planning, implementation, and intervention regarding the prevention and control of disease and injury.

Dr. Richard Visser
Minister of Public Health and Sports

INTRODUCTION

In front of you lies the first Health Monitor for Aruba. This Health Monitor will be published every 4 years and will give an overall impression of the health of the Aruban population.

This monitor not only provides vital information about the physical health and lifestyle of the total population, but it also gives you an overview of the health and/or risk behavior of specific population groups.

Aruba has known a rapid economic development which brought all types of influences from around the world, together with the phenomenon of globalization. The same as in many countries worldwide, these developments had their positive influence on health with its scientific and technical advances for earlier detection of diseases or improving care. But on the other hand it also had its negative influence on the health of the population. With the introduction of fast food chains, a considerable growth in tourism among other factors, Aruba has been exposed to all types of cultures, norms and values and consequently a drastic change in lifestyle. As a result Aruba faces an overweight epidemic that has been in development for the past 10 years and continues to maintain its course. Infectious diseases that were forgotten have been reemerging. Not to mention the pressure of this development on the mental health of the Aruban population.

This Health Monitor represents a valuable tool which will give the necessary information and guidance in order to prioritize processes for effective policy development at the Department of Public Health but also to provide guidance to other Governmental departments and services.

The Department of Public Health has developed a strategic policy for Health Promotion 2011–2015: From facts to actions. Hereby the Department of Public Health aims mainly at using population targeted prevention strategies to minimize the risk factors the Aruban population is exposed to which stimulates the development of e.g. non-communicable diseases. The information provided in the Health Monitor underscores the strategies

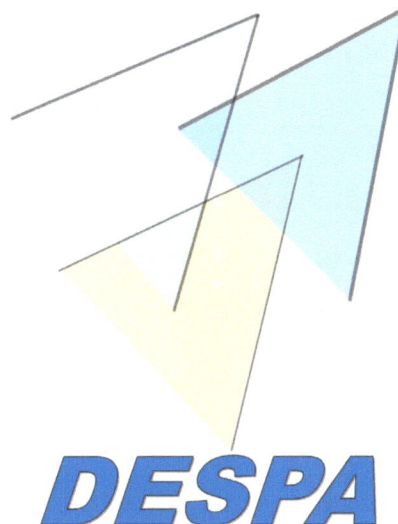

DESPA

Management Team
Department Of Public Health Aruba, 2013

developed in this document and the decision of the Department of Public Health to focus on targeted prevention.

Management Team
Department of Public Heath Aruba, 2013

ACKNOWLEDGMENTS

The Department of Public Health of Aruba would like to thank the steering committee, the work group and all who were involved in the development of this Health Monitor Aruba 2013. Without the support and motivation for realizing this publication, it would not have been achievable.

Also the Ministry of Health and Sports who believed in the capacities of both committees for the development of this document, which is the first one ever developed and published.

Members of Steering Committee

Management Team Department of Public Health:

- Mrs. Sharline Koolman
- Mrs. Nivia Doolabi
- Mr. Wilmer Salazar

Ministry of Health and Sports

- Mrs. Chanin Boekhoudt

Members of the Work Group

Department of Public Health:

- Mrs. Maribelle Tromp
- Mr. Eugène Maduro
- Mrs. Gisela de Veer
- Mrs. Latifa Mercera
- Mrs. Arnelda Els
- Mrs. Hella Wehberg
- Mrs. Janice Hoofd
- Mrs. Patricia Angela
- Mr. Guido Wever

Central Bureau of Statistics:

- Mrs. Desiree Helder

Algemene Ziektekosten Verzekering:

- Mrs. Merreldeth Curie

Technical Assistance, Public Health Services, The Hague - GGD Den Haag:

- Mrs. G. Ariëns
- Mrs. M. Bakker

LIST OF ABBREVIATIONS

AIDS: Acquired Immunodeficiency Syndrome

AMIS: Aruba Migration and Integration Survey

AZV: Algemene Ziektekosten Verzekering

BMI: Body Mass Index

CA: Cancer

CBDB: Coördinatie Bureau Drugsbestrijding

CDC: Centre of Disease Control

CVD: Cerebrovascular heart disease

DALY's: Disability-adjusted Years of Life

DEN: Dengue

DOW: Dienst Openbare Wegen

DP: Diphtheria and Polio Vaccine

DPH: Department of Public Health

DPT: Diphtheria, Polio, Tetanus

DPTP: Diphtheria, Polio, Tetanus and Pertusis vaccine

EU: European Union

FCSW: Female Commercial Sex Workers

g: grams

GDP: Gross Domestic Product

GP: General Physicians

HBV: Hepatitis B virus

Hep B: Hepatitis B

HIB: Hemophilus Influenza B type vaccine

HIV: Human Immunodeficiency Virus

IARC: International Agency for the Research on Cancer

ICD-10: International Statistical Classification for Diseases and Related Health Problems; 10th revision

IHD: Ischemic Heart Disease

IPV: Polio vaccine

LBW: Low Birth Weight

MAVO: Middelbaar Algemeen Voortgezet Onderwijs

MMR: Measles, Mumps and Rubella vaccine

PAAZ: Psychiatrische Afdeling Algemeen Ziekenhuis

PAHO: Pan American Health Organization

PCV: Pneumococcal conjugate vaccine

PEP: Post exposure Prophylaxis

PLHIV: People Living with HIV

PYLL: Potential Years of Life Lost

SPD: Sociaal Psychiatrische Dienst

STI's: Sexual Transmitted Infections

ULBW: Ultra Low Birth Rate

USA: United States of America

VLBW: Very Low Birth Weight

WHO: World Health Organization

WYC: White Yellow Cross

YDC: Youth Dental Care

LIST OF FIGURES

LIST OF TABLES

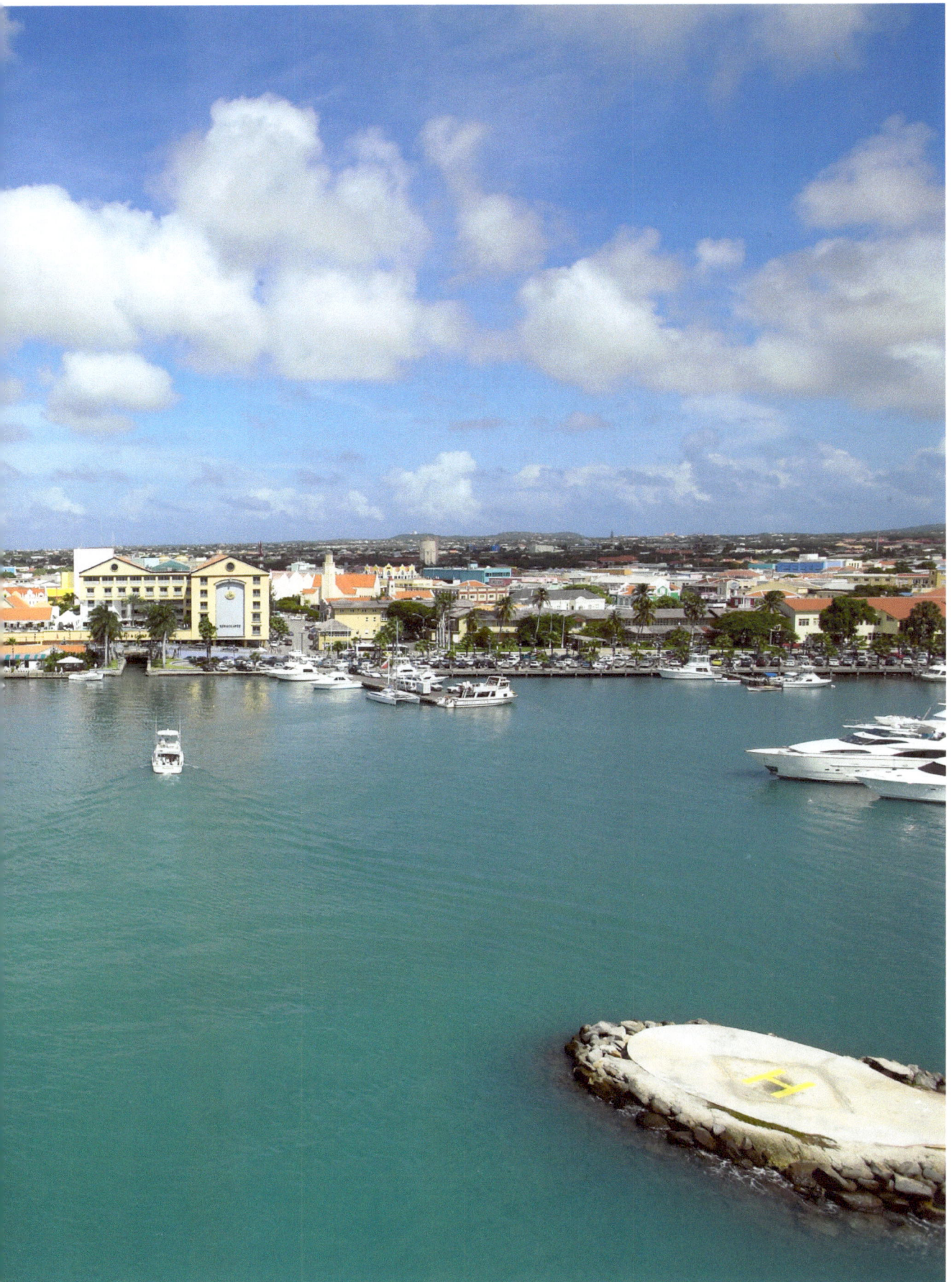

1. DEMOGRAPHICS

1.1 The Population of Aruba by Age and Sex

On December 31st 2011, the population of Aruba consisted of 103,504 inhabitants, of which 49,075 (47.4%) were male and 54,429 (52.6%) female. Aruba is a densely populated island with an average of 575 persons per km2, the majority living on the northern side of the island (see Figure 1).

The age composition of the population of Aruba shows a binominal distribution. The largest segment of the population consists of inhabitants between 5 and 19 years of age and inhabitants between 40 and 54 years of age. Between these two segments a significant gap is formed, in particular, by a lack of inhabitants between ages 20 and 34 years (see Figure 2). The marked lack of women in the childbearing ages will almost certainly impact the number of newborns in the years to come, following the national and global trend of a declining fertility rate.

On the other hand, the proportion of 65+ in the population of Aruba has been rising rapidly. According to the 2010 Census, 10.4 percent of the population is 65+, compared to 7.3 percent in the year 2000, an increase of 45.2 percent.

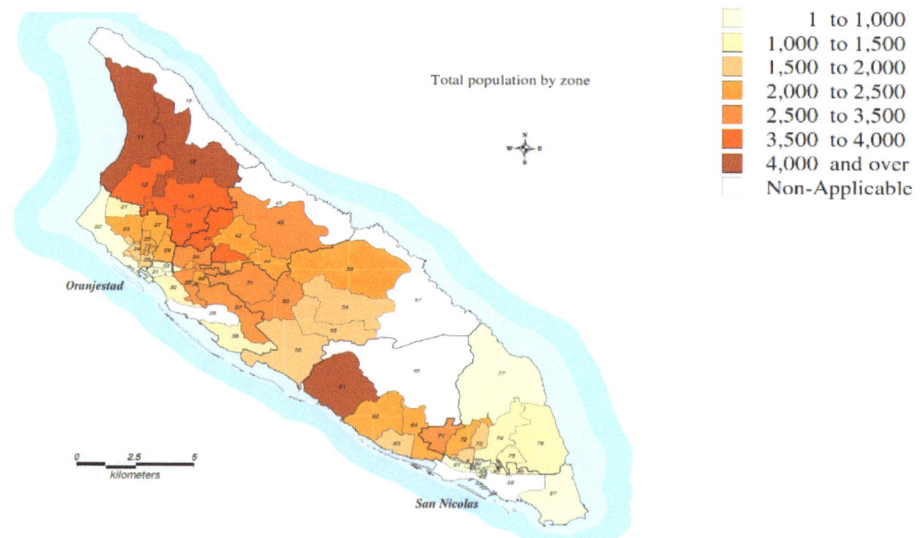

Figure 1. Population density Aruba, 2011.

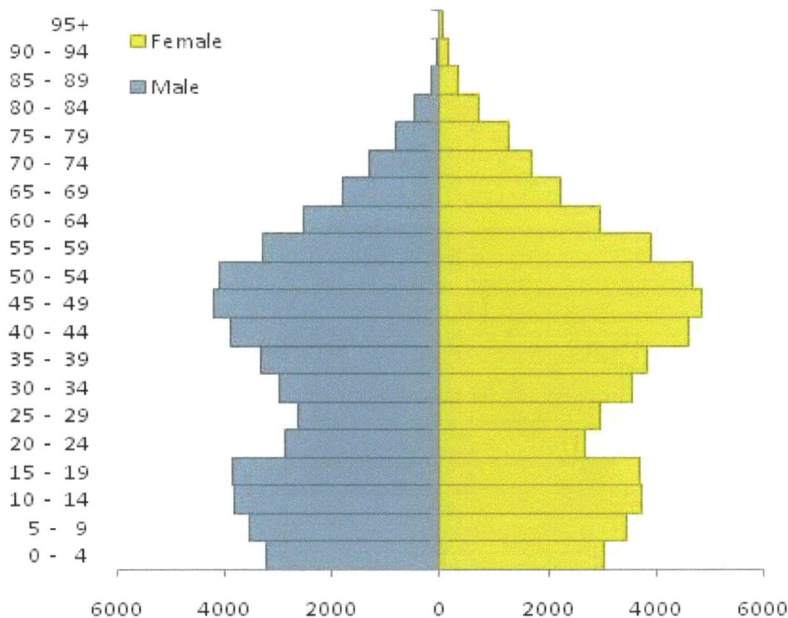

Figure 2. Population Pyramid of the Population of Aruba, 2011.

1.2 Population Projections

With fairly constant levels of fertility and mortality, population dynamics in Aruba are largely dependent on levels of immigration and emigration, which are linked to the performance of the local economy. Based on 2010 Census data, information about key economic parameters provided by the Department of Economic Affairs, Trade and Industry, and migration characteristics retrieved from the 2003 Aruba Migration and Integration Survey (AMIS), three scenarios were created by the Central Bureau of Statistics for a twenty-year period (2010-2030) with four five-year progressions: a low scenario, a medium scenario, and a high scenario (see Figure 3 A, B & C).

The three scenarios show two important trends. Firstly, the aging of the population will continue at a quick pace during the next twenty years, having serious consequences for the Aruban society in the next twenty years. More and more people will be using services that are geared towards the elderly, the number of persons with chronic diseases will grow rapidly, as the prevalence of many of these diseases is higher among the elderly, and pension schemes will have to deal with more and more persons who reach retirement age.

Secondly, because of the aging of the population of Aruba and the consistent low levels of fertility, an insufficient number of local laborers will be available to fill all the positions created by a growing economy. A moderate to rapid growth of real GDP will lead to a high demand of laborers and consequently to high levels of immigration.

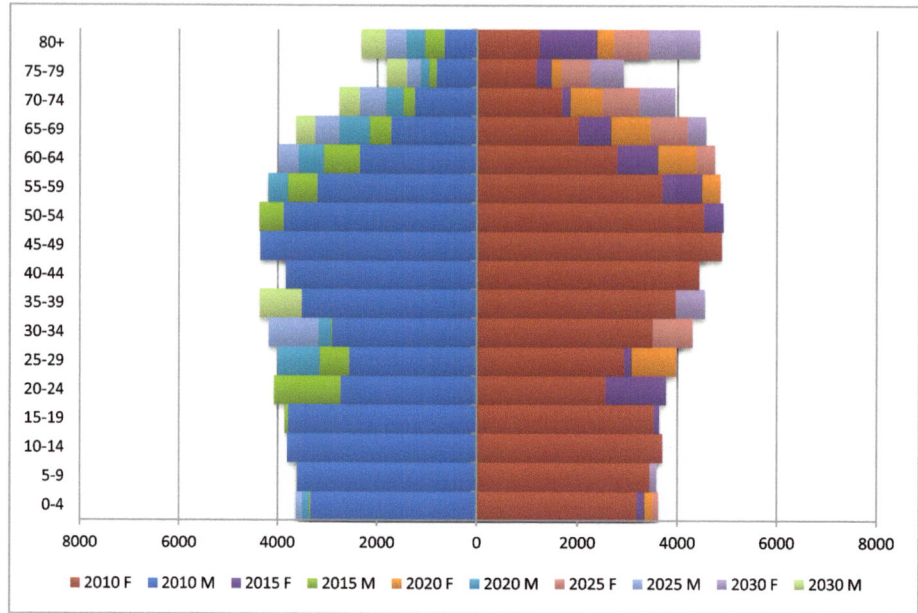

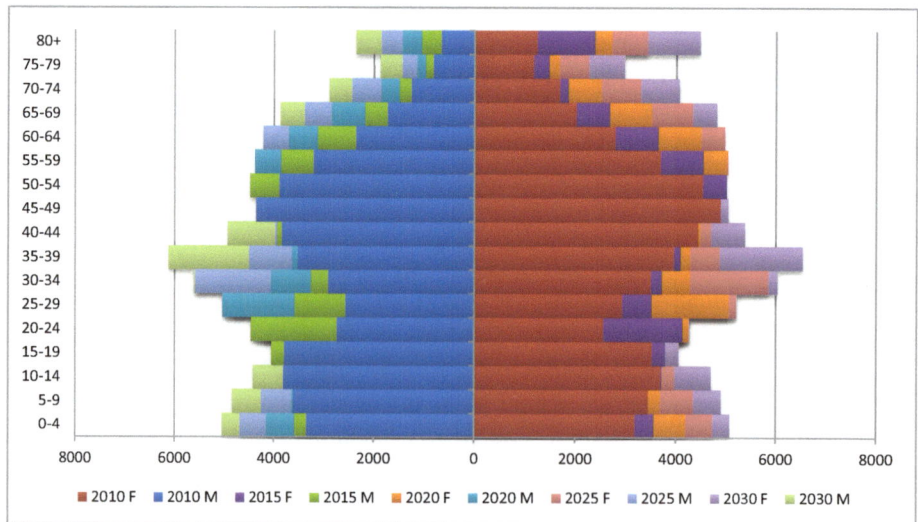

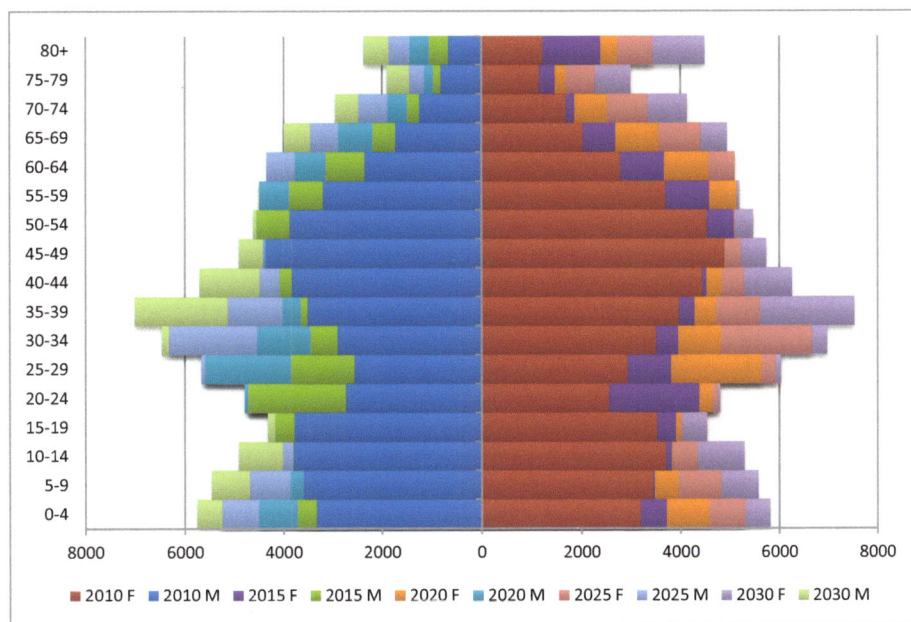

Figure 3. Population Projections, 2010–2030: A. Low scenario; B. Medium scenario; C. High scenario

1.3 Level of Education

The school participation rate in Aruba is high and has been that way for decades (see Table 1.). However, after completing secondary education, a significant number of young adults leave the island to continue their studies abroad. Only a few return to the island after obtaining their diploma. This may be the reason why, according to data gathered during the 2010 Census, 69.1 percent of the population of Aruba 14 years and older did not attend school and has a lower secondary education, MAVO level or lower (see Figure 4).

Females between 14 and 34 years of age are the most educated group of people in Aruba, with 27.2 percent having an education at an intermediate level and 14.3 percent having a higher education.

Table 1. School participation rate of the population of Aruba by age category and sex, Aruba 1991–2010.

Year	Age (years)	Male (%)	Females (%) 1991
1991	0–5	55	56.2
	6–11	99	99
	12–17	93.4	92.9
	18+	3.7	3.3
2000	0–5	57.9	56.3
	6–11	98.3	98.1
	12–17	94.5	94.4
	18+	4.2	4.6
2010	0–5	64.0	64.8
	6–11	98.7	98.9
	12–17	95.7	96.4
	18+	5.5	5.7

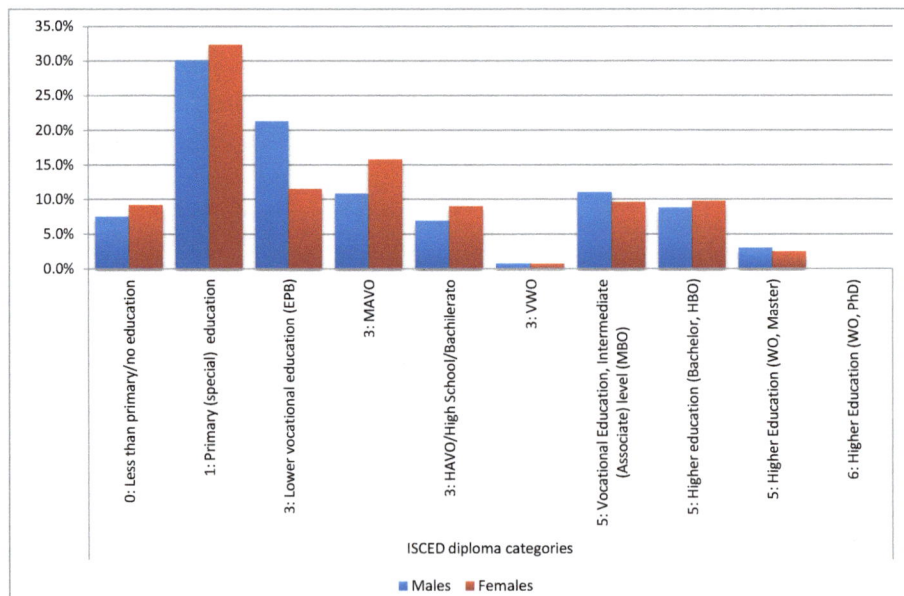

Figure 4 Level of education attainment of the population of Aruba not attending school by sex, 2010.

1.4 Household Composition

Households in Aruba consist, on average, of 2.9 persons. Large households consisting of 5 persons or more are in the minority, representing less than 15 percent (14.8 percent) of the total number of non-collective households. The majority of persons live in a nuclear household (46 percent), composed in most cases of a married couple with children (22 percent, see Figure 5). In total, 62.6 percent of children (up to 17 years of age) live with both parents.

As age increases, the type of household persons live in, is subject to important changes. The proportion of the population living in a one-person household increases dramatically as age increases, as well as the proportion of the population living in extended households.

Compared to a decade ago, the composition of households in Aruba has changed significantly:

- The size of households has decreased from an average of 3.1 persons to an average of 2.9 persons per household.

- The share of one person households has increased from 19 percent in 2000 to 21 percent in 2010.

- The share of married couples with children has decreased from 26 percent in 2000, to 22 percent in 2010.

- There are more mothers with children.

- There are more fathers with children.

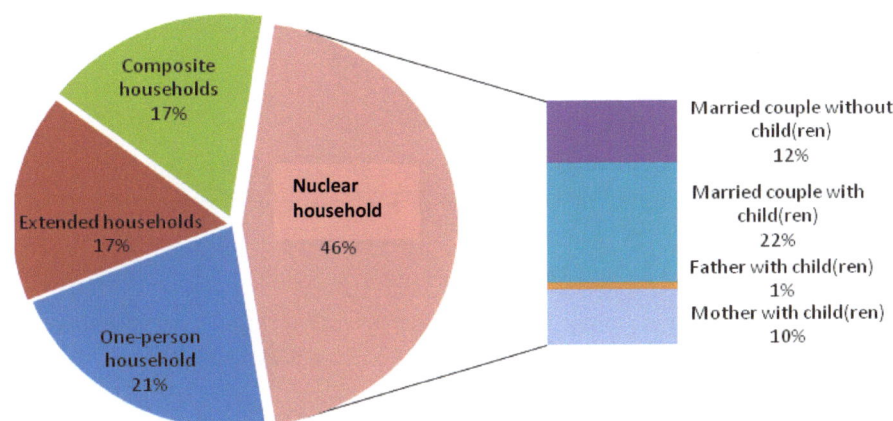

Figure 5. Percentage of the population by type of (non-collective) household.

1.5 Employed/not Employed Population

In total, in 2010, 58.2 percent of the population of Aruba (15 years and older) was employed, 6.9 percent was unemployed and 34.9 percent was inactive. It is important to mention that, in 2010, there were more females in the labor market than males (n = 22,761 and n = 22,676, respectively, see Figure 6).

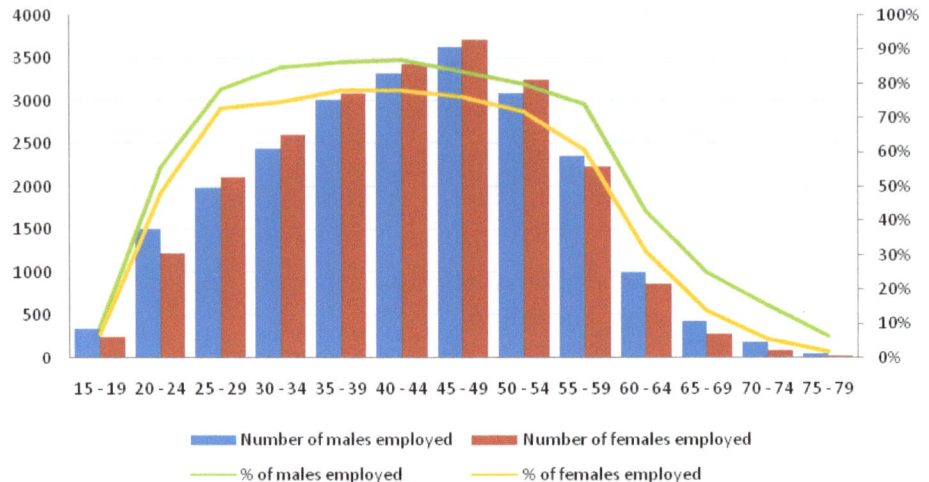

Figure 6. Employed population by age and sex, 2010.

The top five sectors employing persons in Aruba were, in order of importance: hotels and restaurants, trade, public administration, real estate, and construction, employing respectively 20.6 percent, 16.2 percent, 9.9 percent, 9.1 percent and 8.3 percent of the employed population.

1.6 Immigration/Emigration

In 2010, 34 percent of the population of Aruba was foreign-born. The percentage of foreign-born was highest in the population of working age 15 to 64 years, 41.6 percent. Between ages 35 and 44 years more than 50 percent (53.9 percent) of the population of Aruba was foreign-born (see Figure 7).

On the other hand, the percentage foreign born was relatively low in the young and in the elderly. In children up to 14 years of age, 11.4 percent was foreign-born. In the group of 65 years and older, 28.8 percent was foreign-born.

The foreign-born population consisted primarily of persons born in Colombia, who represented 26.9 percent of the foreign-born population, persons born in the Netherlands (12.7 percent), and persons born in the Dominican Republic (11.9 percent; see Figure 8).

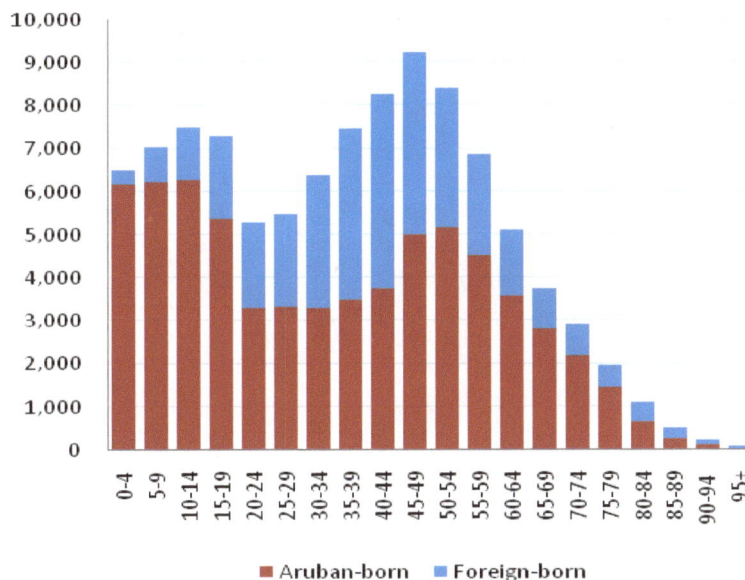

Figure 7. The Aruban- and foreign-born population by age, 2010.

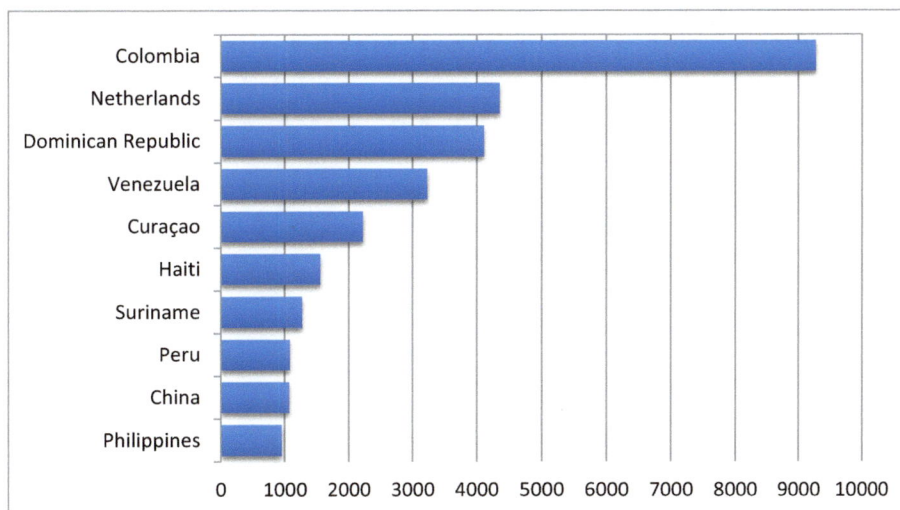

Figure 8. Foreign-born population (top 10 Countries), 2010.

In ten years (2000 to 2010), the percentage of persons born in China and in Haiti increased the most, with 68 percent ($n = 1,071$) and 52 percent ($n = 1,551$), respectively, whereas persons born in Colombia increased the most in numbers (with 2088 persons). In 2010, 52.2 percent of foreign-born persons had a Dutch nationality.

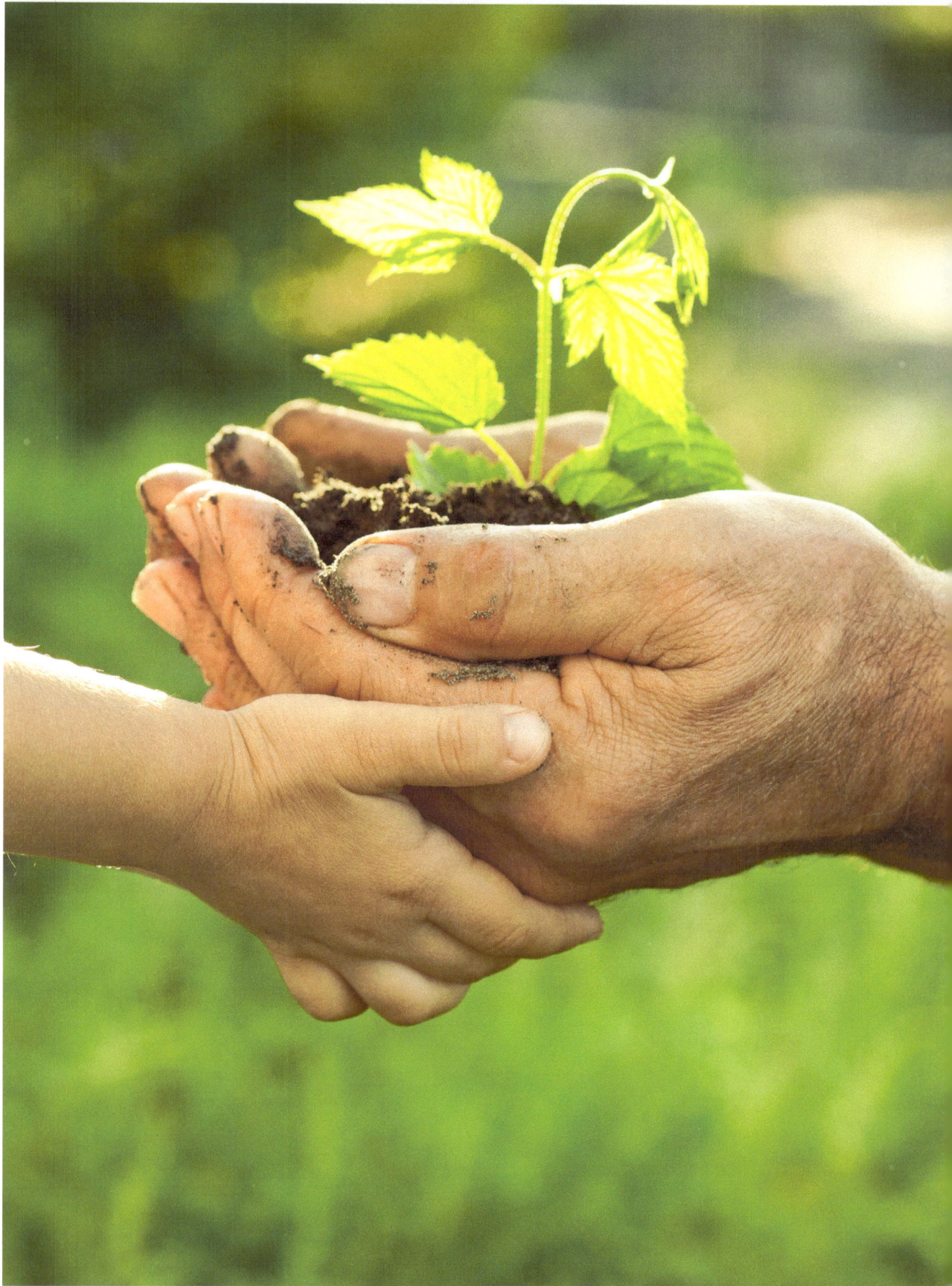

2. LIFE EXPECTANCY AND DEATHS

2.1 Life Expectancy

Life expectancy is the average number of years a person is expected to live. It is a good indicator of the standard of living in a country and of the overall health of the inhabitants. Important societal changes combined with significant advances in medicine, improved access to health care services, better access to clean water and better hygiene have contributed to a dramatic increase in life expectancy, worldwide.

2.1.1 Life Expectancy At birth

The life expectancy at birth reflects the overall mortality level of a population. In 2009, the global life expectancy at birth was 68 years, 57 years in low-income countries and 80 years in high income countries. In Aruba, in 2010, the life expectancy at birth was 76.9 years. Females were expected to live 6.1 years longer than males, living to become 79.8 years, compared to 73.9 years in males, Figure 9 illustrates that with increasing age, the difference in life expectancy between males and females showed a gradual decrease.

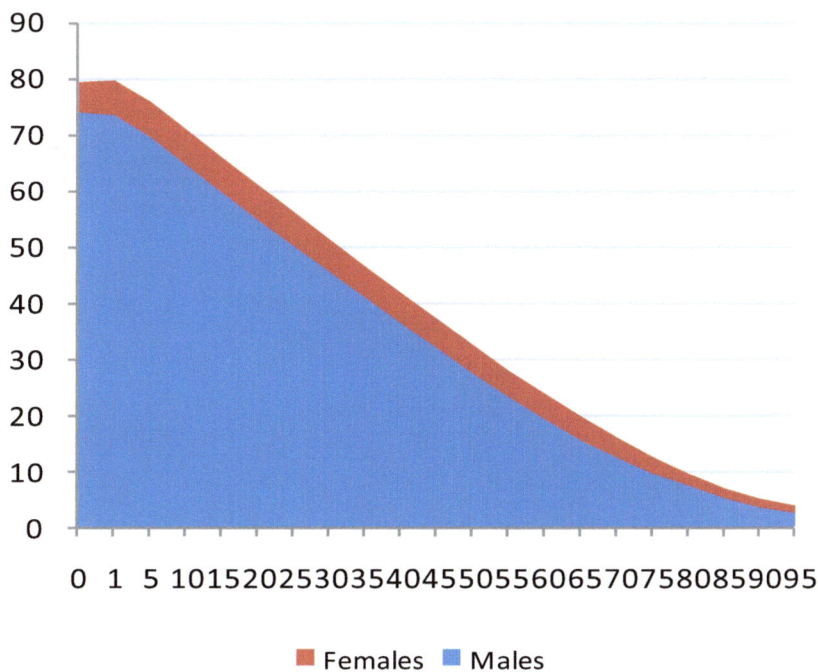

Figure 9. Life expectancy by age and sex, 2010.

Since the 1960's when the life expectancy was first computed for Aruba, it has known a steady increase until the end of the 20th century and the beginning of the 21st century, when the life expectancy in Aruba dropped with a year.

From 2005 to 2010, the life expectancy increased with nearly two years to 76.9 years. The life expectancy in Aruba is higher as compared to in the Caribbean and is comparable to the life expectancy in more developed regions of the world, see Figure 10.

2.1.2 Life Expectancy at 65 Years

The global population is aging at an unprecedented rate. According to the most recent estimations of the World Health Organization, within the next five years, the number of adults 65 years and older will outnumber the number of children under the age of 5. By 2050, these adults will outnumber all children under the age of 14.

Aruba, following the global trend, the life expectancy at 65 years has known a steep increase in the last decade. In 2010, persons aged 65 years had, on average, 17.6 more years to live, females having 4.4 more years to live than males. Compared to the year 2000, the life expectancy of males aged 65 years increased with 2.2 years (16.8 percent) and that of females with 3 years (18.0 percent). Compared to other regions

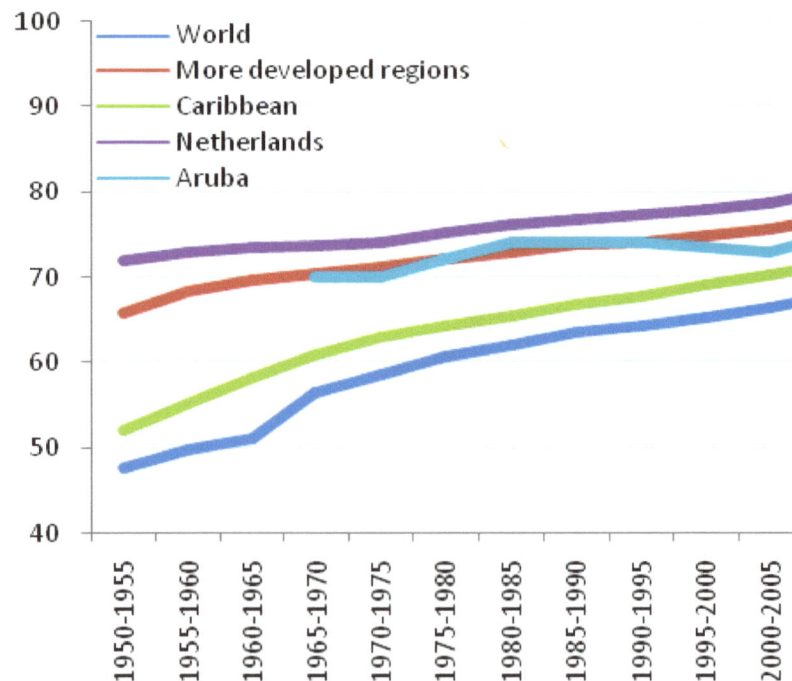

Figure 10. The life expectancy at birth in Aruba compared to other regions of the world.

in the world, the life expectancy at age 65 years in Aruba is comparable to 32 that in more developed regions.

A growing elderly population will inevitably be associated with higher costs of health care. Therefore it is important to take into account the health of the elderly population. In 2010, more than one third of the males and females older than 65 years were expected to continue living were to be spent in poor health see Figure 11.

2.2 Potential Years of Life Lost

Potential Years of Life Lost (PYLL) occurs when individuals die at an early age with the consequence of a greater loss of individuals' productivity. The PYLL per 100.000 population is calculated as stated below:

$$\frac{(\text{Estimated life expectancy-mean age death for premature deaths}) \times \text{Number of premature deaths}}{\text{Population under estimated life expectancy}} \times 100,000$$

Premature deaths are deaths which have occurred before the estimated life expectancy.

The graph in Figure 12 illustrates the different causes of death that are under surveillance with their respective PYLL per 100,000. On average the different causes of death have a PYLL lower or around 400 years. Cancer of the digestive system followed by cerebral vascular disease (CVD) have PYLL's higher than 400 years, 511 and 417 respectively. Not to mention external causes with a PYLL of 1,965 years.

External causes include for example transport accidents (land transport accidents), intentional self-harm (suicide), assault (homicide) and drowning. A total of 1,965 of potential healthy life years were lost due to external causes, this is mainly due to land

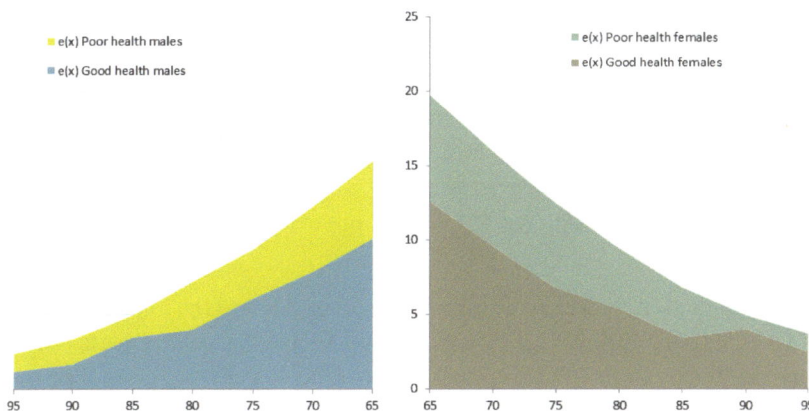

Figure 11. Number of years spent in good health and in poor health by sex and age, 2010.

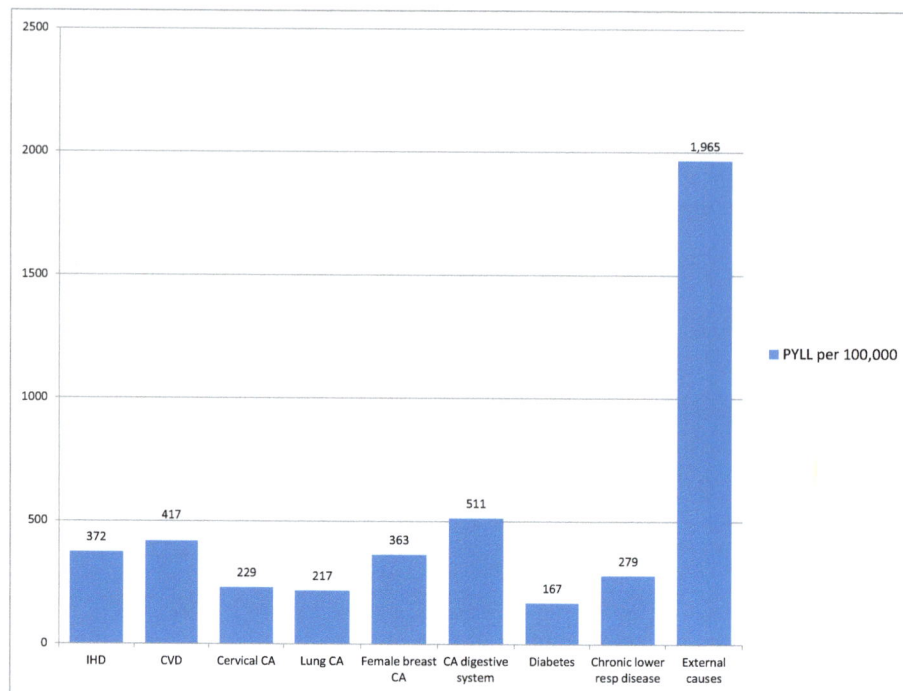

Figure 12. Potential years of life lost per 100,000, Aruba 2010.

transport accidents where young adults are mostly involved. Death at a young age increases the PYLL. These causes are responsible for most of the premature deaths on Aruba.

Further analysis of the external causes shows that land transport accidents claims for the highest PYLL in this category, see Figure 13.

Land transport accidents claims the highest PYLL in the Aruban male population. This means that males die at a very young age due to land transport accidents. In 2010 the PYLL for land transport accidents claimed 1077.7 years in the male population. If we compare this PYLL to Ischemic Heart Disease for the male population (PYLL=559.3), land transport accidents claimed almost double the PYLL. Cancer of the digestive system claimed 481.7 PYLL in the male population, see Figure 14.

For the female population, cancer of the digestive system claimed the highest number of PYLL in 2010 (PYLL = 629.9) followed by cerebral vascular disease (PYLL = 440.9), female breast cancer (PYLL = 363.0) and chronic lower respiratory diseases (PYLL = 361.2).

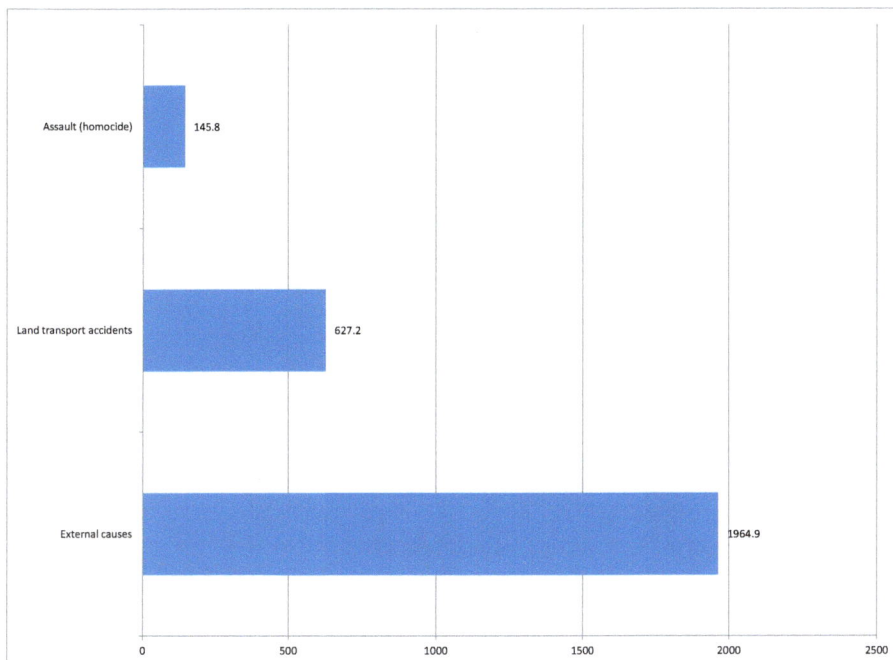

Figure 13. PYLL external causes of death, 2010.

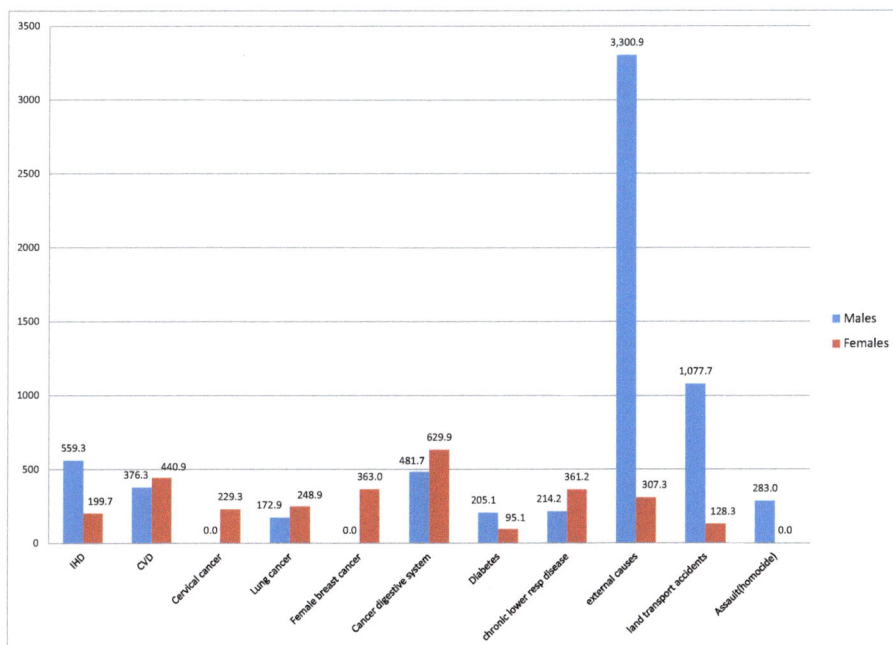

Figure 14. PYLL by gender, Aruba, 2010.

2.3 Causes of Death

Mortality is an index of the severity of a problem from both clinical and public health standpoints (Gordis, L. 2009). Mortality trends show the leading cause of death in a population. This information is used for development of prevention and intervention programs on a public health level. However mortality data relies directly on the quality of data received on the death certificate. The International Classification of Diseases, ICD-10 coding system by the WHO is used to code the different causes of death.

For the period from 2000 up to 2010, the leading causes of death for the Aruban population are diseases of the circulatory system, which covers 33 percent of the total deaths during the above mentioned period (see Figure 15). Diseases in this category include ischemic heart disease (IHD), cerebral vascular disease (CVD) and pulmonary heart diseases among others. The second leading cause of death is neoplasm, which covers 25 percent of the total registered deaths during the reported period. Malignant neoplasm of the trachea, bronchus and lung, of the digestive organs and peritoneum (excluding stomach and colon cancer) and of the female breast are among the most causes of death due to neoplasm in Aruba.

Figure 16 presents the leading causes of death for the age category 25 to 44 years. As this figure shows the trend for mortality due to land transport accidents has decreased from 2004 to present. The highest death rate registered for land transport accidents during this period was in 2003 of 37 per 100,000, while this rate has decreased to 21 per 100,000 deaths in 2010. Even though the overall death rate has decreased since 2004, there has been an increase from 2007-2010.

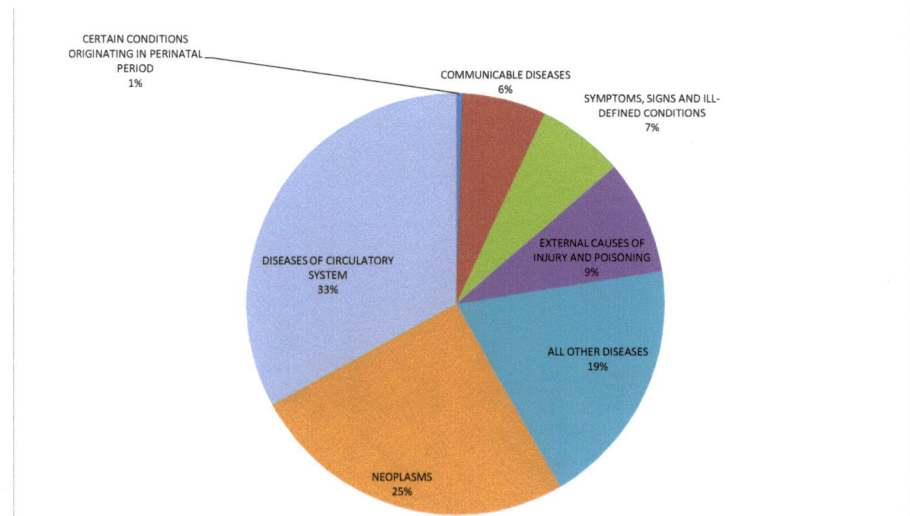

Figure 15. Mortality by Causes of death (iCd-67), Aruba Period 2000–2010.

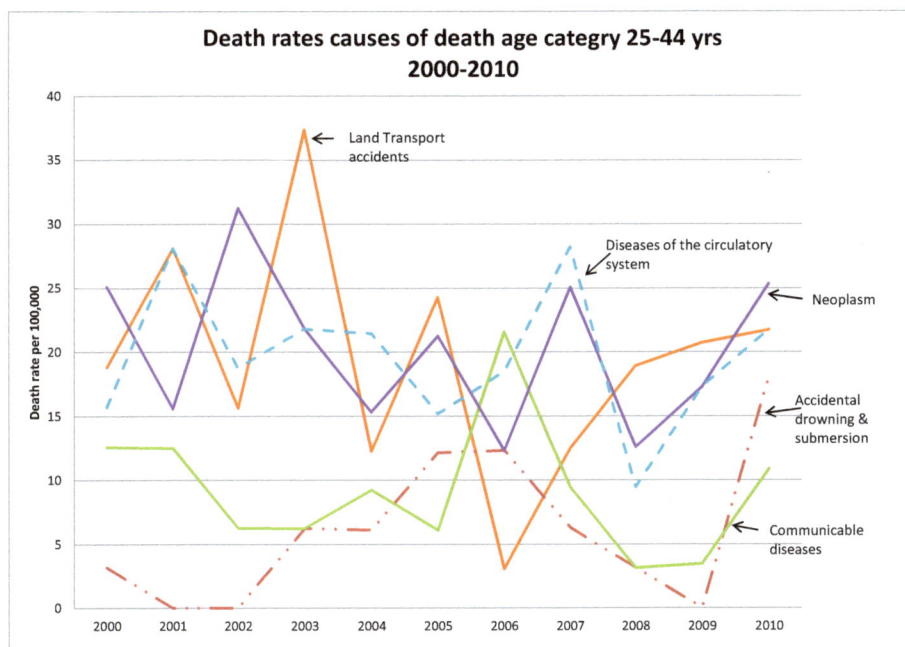

Death rates causes of death age categry 25-44 yrs 2000-2010

Figure 16. Death rates, causes of death by age categories, Aruba, period 2000–2010.

Death rates, due to diseases of the circulatory system, have been almost steady for the 25–44 years age category during this period of time. The death rate varies between 10 and 30 deaths per 100,000.

The trend for mortality due to Neoplasm is almost similar to diseases of the circulatory system, where the death rates vary between 10 and 30 deaths per 100,000 during this period of time.

Land transport accidents together with diseases of the circulatory system and neoplasm remain the three highest causes of death in this productive age category of the Aruban population.

2.4 Perinatal Death

Perinatal death is the total number of fetal deaths (stillbirths after at least 22 weeks of gestation) and early neonatal death (death of a live birth within 1 week of life).

As stated by the WHO in the Neonatal and Stillbirths World report, neonatal deaths and stillbirths stem from poor maternal health, inadequate care during pregnancy, inappropriate management of complications during pregnancy and delivery, poor hygiene during delivery and the first critical hours after birth, and lack of newborn care.

Several factors such as women's status in society, their nutritional status at the time of conception, early childbearing, too many closely spaced pregnancies and harmful practices are deeply rooted in the cultural fabric of societies and interact in ways that are not always clearly understood. (WHO, 2006)

A perinatal death rate is also used as a summary statistic for evaluating the effectiveness of perinatal care. The perinatal death rate for Aruba fluctuates between 7 and 10 fetal deaths per 1,000 live births per year, see Figure 17. However, from 2006 to 2010 there is a tendency of increase in this rate per year. In 2010 the perinatal death rate increased to 10 per 1,000 live births. This is the highest registered rate in the past 5 years in Aruba.

Aruba accounts yearly with an average of 1,200 live births. The number of deaths per specific cause of death is small, resulting in very small death rates per specific cause. However, the trend in specific cause of death will give an overview of the different causes of perinatal deaths. Causes of perinatal deaths can be various but the most common cause of perinatal deaths registered worldwide are complications during birth, such as obstructed labour and fetal malpresentation, however these are in the absence of obstetric care. Birth asphyxia and trauma often occur together and therefore it is difficult to obtain separate estimates. In the most severe cases, the baby dies during birth or soon after, due to damage to the brain and/or other organs. Less severe asphyxia and trauma will cause disability. Modern obstetric practices have almost eliminated birth trauma. (WHO, 2006)

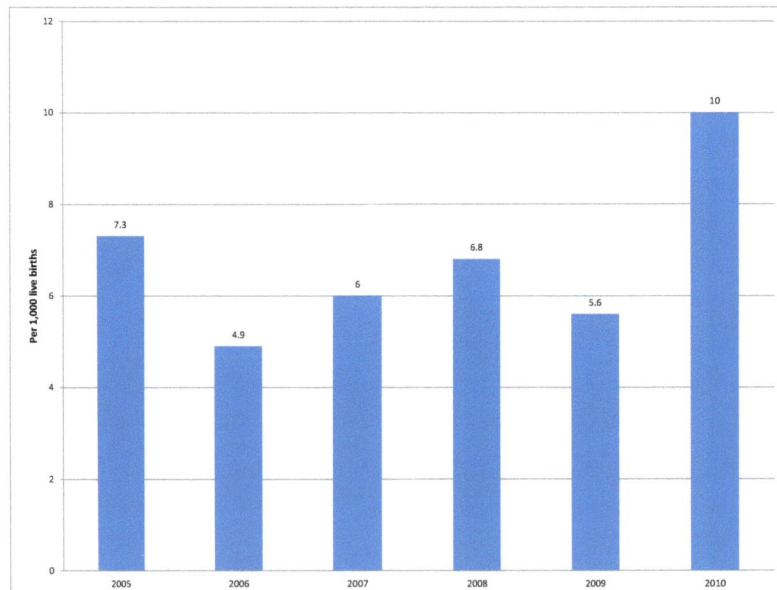

Figure 17. Perinatal death rate per 1,000 live births, Aruba 2005–2010.

Conversely, where modern obstetric care is not available, intra partum or early postnatal deaths are very frequent. It is estimated that in developing countries asphyxia causes around seven deaths per 1000 births, whereas in developed countries this proportion is less than one death per 1000 births. The majority of deaths occur soon after birth, some just before birth. (WHO, 2006)

The causes for perinatal deaths in Aruba are various and there is no clear trend of the specific cause, due to the small number of cases per specific cause, see Figure 18. However the group "Remainder of certain condition originating in the perinatal period" has known an exponential increase from 2006 until 2010.

'Slow fetal growth', 'fetal malnutrition', 'short gestation or low birth weight' and 'congenital malformations, deformations' and 'chromosomal abnormalities' are the two most common specific cause of perinatal death in Aruba.

2.4.1 Birth Weight

Low birth weight has long been debated as one of the causes of neonatal deaths. It is associated with the death of many newborn infants, but is not considered a direct cause. Around 15 percent of newborn infants weigh less than 2500 g, the proportion ranging from 6 percent in developed countries to more than 30 percent in other parts of the world. The main "culprit" is preterm birth and the complications stemming from it, rather than low birth weight itself.

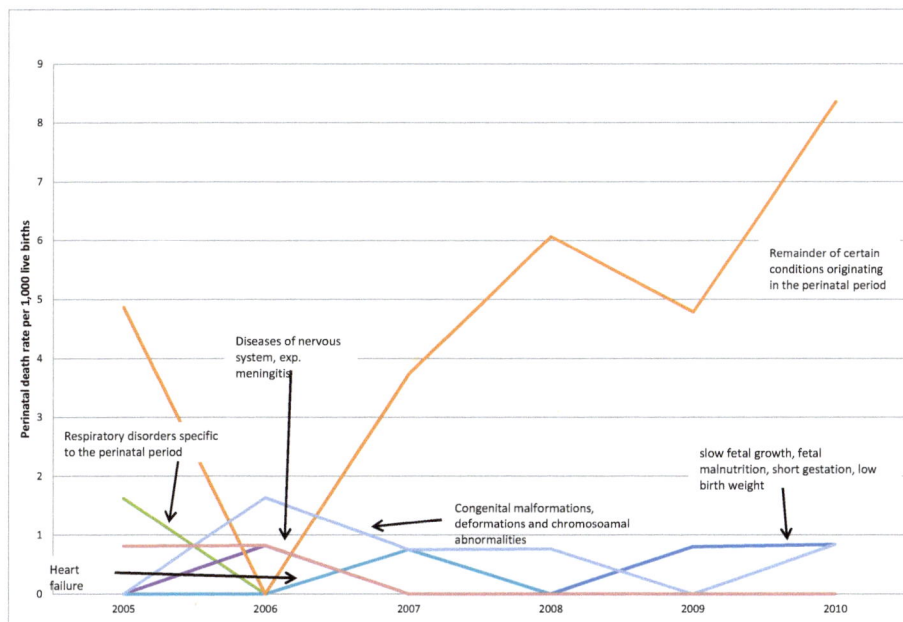

Figure 18. Perinatal death rates by causes per 1,000 live births.

Important determinants of weight at birth are maternal health and nutrition at conception. (WHO, 2006)

Aruba accounts yearly with an average of 1,200 live births. The birth weight is further analyzed using the standard worldwide cut off points.

As Table 2 shows, Aruba is comparable with other developed countries in the world in birth weight. In 2010 6 percent of all births weighted less than 2500 grams. It has to be noted that these births include the stillbirths.

Table 2. Distribution of birth weights for Aruba, 2010.

Proportion of birth weight		Number of births	%
Low birth weight (LBW)	< 2500 gram	84	6.7
Very low birth weight (VLBW)	< 1500 gram	28	2.2
Ultra-low birth weight (ULBW)	< 1000 gram	21	1.7

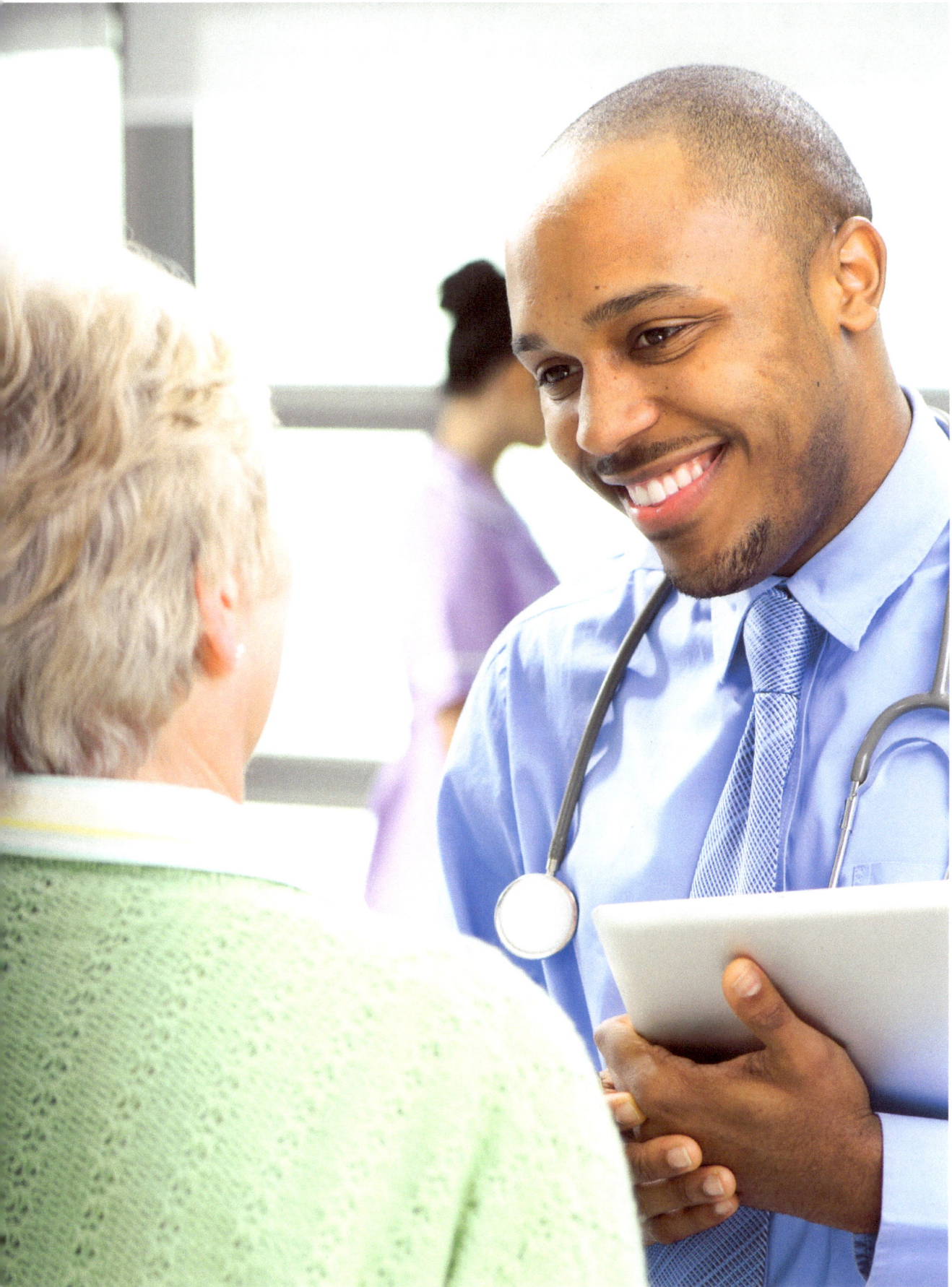

3. PHYSICAL HEALTH

Perceived health is a good indicator of actual health. Since the year 2000, a question on perceived health was included in the Population and Housing Census of Aruba, thus making important information available on the overall health of the population of Aruba.

Comparing data obtained from the 2010 Census to data from 2000 Census, the conclusion can be drawn that notwithstanding the rise in life expectancy observed in the last decade, the overall health of the population of Aruba has declined, (see Table 3). The decline was most prominent in young persons (between ages 15 and 24 years), in males and in persons not born in Aruba.

Table 3. Perceived health by age, sex level of education and country of birth, Aruba 2000–2010.

	Perceived health	
	2000	**2010**
	Good / Very Good	**Good / Very Good**
Total	88.2	85.8
Age		
0–14	98	96.3
15–24	96.3	93.8
25–44	92.3	90.6
44–64	78.4	78.2
65+	54.2	67
Sex		
Males	90.3	87
Females	86.2	84.8
Level of education		
Low level of education		79.3
Intermediate level of education		88.1
High level of education		91.3
Country of birth		
Aruba-born	87	85
Foreign-born	90.7	87.6

On the other hand, 2010 Census data revealed a slight improvement of the overall health of the middle aged and a substantial improvement of the overall health of the elderly relative to the year 2000.

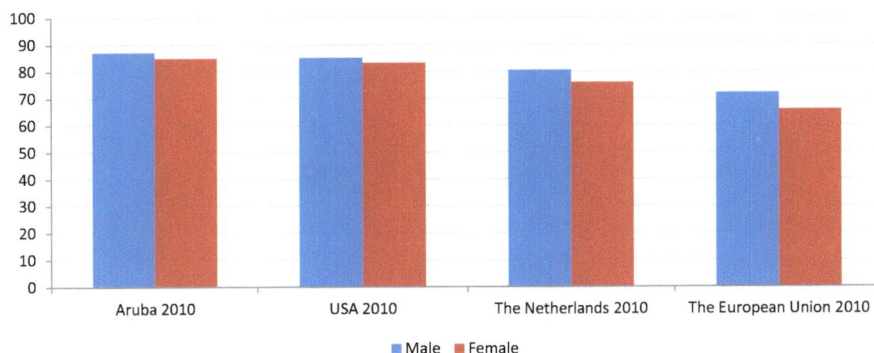

Figure 19. Perceived health for different countries/regions, 2010: Percentage of the Population Perceiving their health as being good/very good.

This is a valuable finding when taking into account the (financial) challenges to be met in the upcoming years as a result of the rapidly ageing of the population of Aruba. However, in 2010, still one third of the elderly population reported having bad or very bad health.

Overall, children, males, persons with a high level of education and foreign-born individuals experienced best health. As could be expected, the percentage of the population that reported being in good to very good health decreased with increasing age. Compared to other countries, the overall perceived health of the population of Aruba was relatively better (see Figure 19).

3.2 Self-Reported Diseases and Health Conditions

According to Census data, in 2010, 31.8 percent of the population of Aruba was suffering from at least one chronic health condition. With increasing age the prevalence of chronic health conditions increased substantially with almost half of all persons 65+ suffering from at least one chronic health condition. Women were significantly more affected by chronic health conditions than men, 35.6 percent of women suffering from chronic health conditions compared to 27.5 percent of men (see Figure 20 A).

Of the chronic health conditions included in the Census questionnaire, allergy was most often reported by both males and females, affecting 10.6 percent of males and 14.9 percent of females. In males, cardiovascular disease was the second most prevalent chronic health condition, reported by 7.0 percent of males, followed by chronic back problems (6.8 %) and migraine or severe headaches (4.1 %). In females on the other hand, migraine was the second most prevalent chronic health condition reported by 12.0 percent of females, followed by chronic back problems (9.3 percent) and cardiovascular disease (7.3 %).

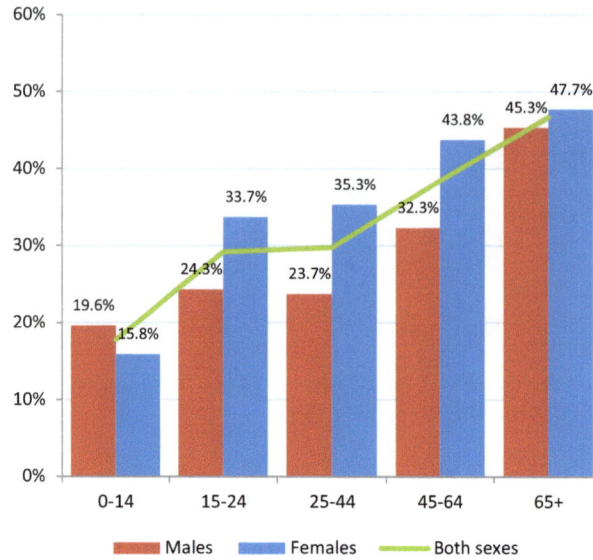

Figure 20 A. The prevalence of chronic health conditions in Aruba by age groups and sex.

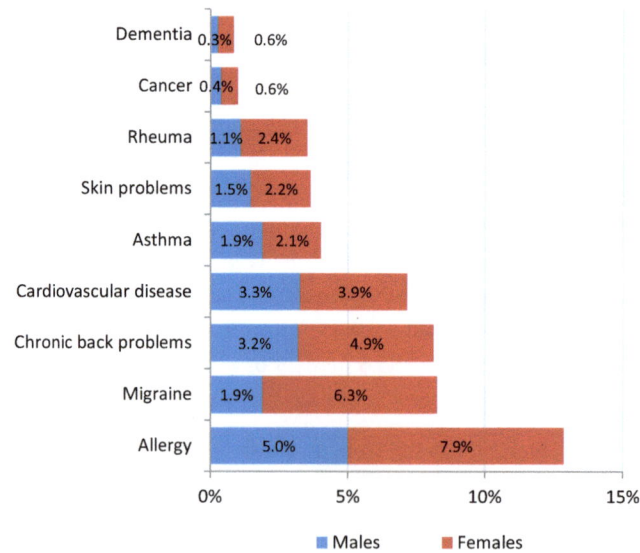

Figure 20 B. The prevalence of certain chronic health conditions in Aruba by sex.

In persons 65+, cardiovascular disease was the most prevalent chronic health condition, reported by 21.5 percent of persons 65+ (23.7 percent males and 19.9 percent females), followed by chronic back problems 14.2 percent (13.7 percent males and 14.6 percent females) and rheumatoid arthritis 12.1 percent (7.5 percent males and 15.4 percent females).

3.3 Cancer

Cancer is a term used for diseases in which abnormal cells divide without control and are able to invade other tissues. Cancer cells can spread to other parts of the body through the blood and lymph systems.

Cancer is the leading cause of death worldwide, accounting for 7.6 million deaths in 2008. The main types of cancer causing deaths are lung cancer with 18.2 % of the total deaths worldwide, followed by stomach cancer (9.7 % of total deaths worldwide) and liver cancer (9.2 % of total deaths worldwide). Figure 21 illustrates an overview of the total cancer cases worldwide for both sexes (age standardized incidence- and mortality rate)

In the Americas cancer is the second leading cause of death, with an estimated 2.5 million new cancer cases and 1.2 million deaths during 2008. The most common cancers in the American region include: prostate, lung, colorectal and stomach cancers in men. In women: breast, lung, colorectal and cervical cancers (see Figure 22).

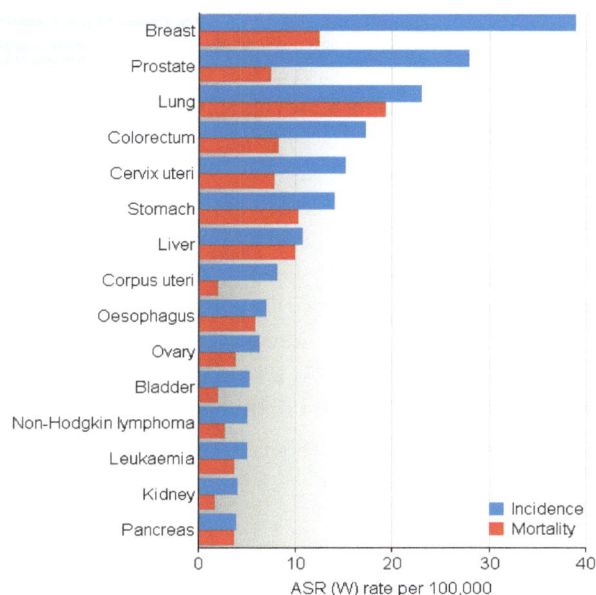

Figure 21. Overview of cancer incidence and mortality rates (age standardized).

Incidence

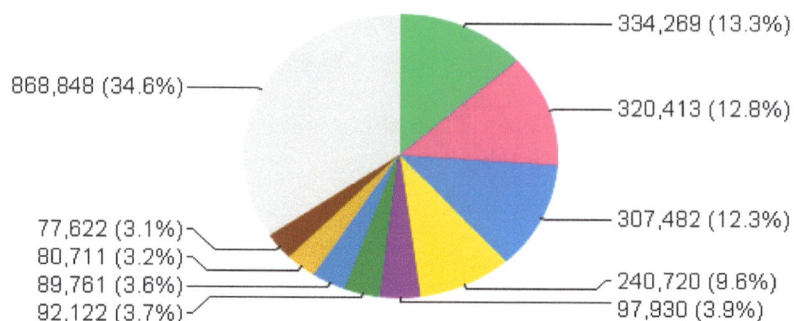

334,269 (13.3%)

320,413 (12.8%)

307,482 (12.3%)

240,720 (9.6%)

97,930 (3.9%)

868,848 (34.6%)

77,622 (3.1%)

80,711 (3.2%)

89,761 (3.6%)

92,122 (3.7%)

Figure 22. Overview of new cancer cases for the American region, 2008.

3.3.1 Cancer In Aruba

According to data received from the Pathology section of the National Laboratory of Aruba during the period of 2007 until 2010, skin cancer is the number one diagnosed cancer in Aruba for both sexes, with a total of 611 new diagnosed cases during the reported period (42.3% of the total primary diagnosed cancer in Aruba; see Figure 23).

The cancer dictionary of the International Agency for the Research on Cancer (IARC) only includes the malignant melanoma as skin cancer in their data base. During the period 2007–2010, there was a total of 12 malignant melanoma's diagnosed (2% of total skin cancer diagnosed), from which 5 males and 7 females (41.7% and 58.3% respectively).

3.3.2 Cancer in Both Sexes

There were a total of 832 newly diagnosed cancer cases for both sexes during the period of 2007–2010 (excluding the non-melanoma skin cancers). Of this total, 54.8% of these cases are female and 45.2% are male. As shown in the Figure 24, most of the new cancer cases in women are diagnosed in the age category of 15-59 years ($n = 219$), whereas in men this is in the age category of 60-74 years ($n = 270$). When added together, 73.6% of all the primary diagnosed cancer types are in the age category of 55–75+ years.

For both sexes, the number one diagnosed type of cancer is breast cancer in women with 212 new cases, followed by prostate cancer in men with 151 cases. Colorectal cancer is in the third place with a total of 119 cases (see Table 4).

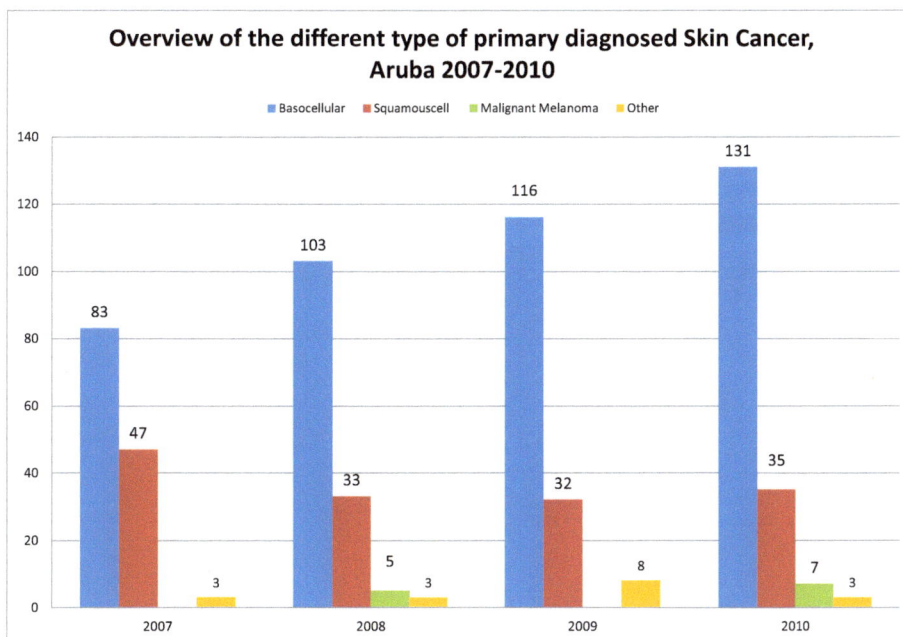

Figure 23. Overview of the total primary diagnosed skin cancer in Aruba.

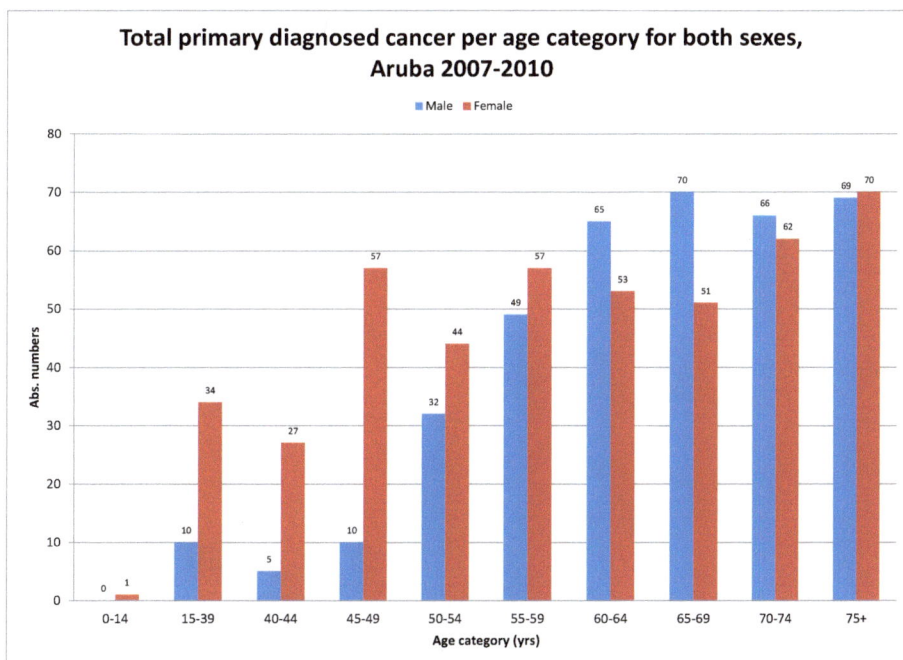

Figure 24. Primary diagnosed Cancer by age Category for both sexes, Aruba 2007-2010.

Figure 25 shows the trend of the top 10 diagnosed cancers in Aruba for the years 2007–2010.

There is a steep increase in both breast and prostate cancer cases. In addition, there is also an increase in primary cases of trachea/bronchus and lung cancer.

Table 4. Overview of the top 10 diagnosed types of cancer for both sexes, Aruba 2007–2010.

Type of cancer	n
Breast	212
Prostate	151
Colorectum	119
Cervix uteri	37
Stomach	36
Trachea/bronchus/lung	34
Corpus uteri	32
Bladder	25
Oesaphagus	19
Thyroid	18

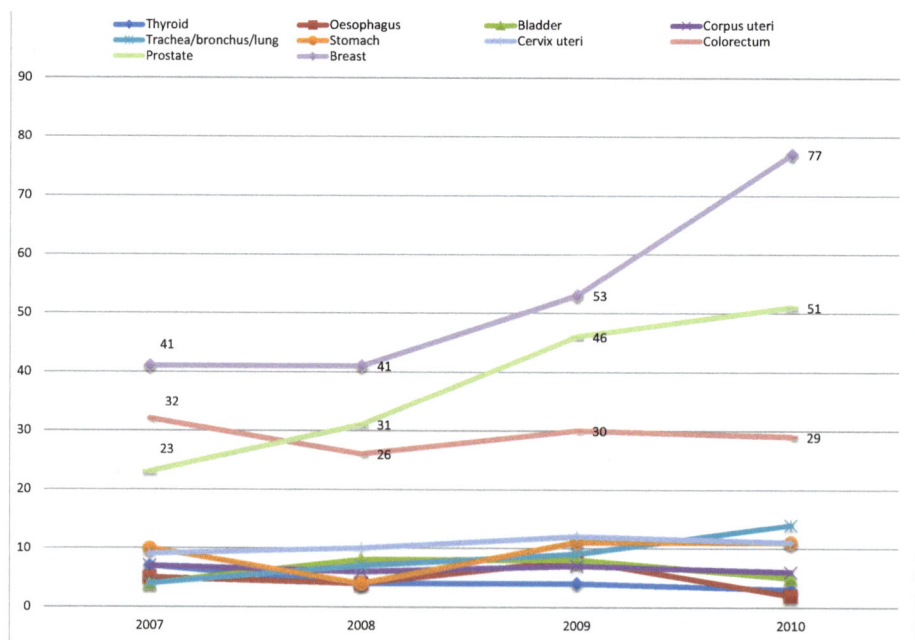

Figure 25. Trends in top 10 new diagnosed cancers for both sexes, Aruba 2007–2010.

3.3.3 Cancer in Males

Prostate cancer is the most diagnosed type of cancer in males on Aruba, with 18.1 percent of the total male cancers and with an average of almost 38 new cases diagnosed each year. In 2010, there were 51 new prostate cancer cases diagnosed, a two-fold increase as compared to 2007 (23 new cases).

The age standardized rate has also increased, from 44 cases per 100.000 in 2007 to 87.1 cases per 100.000 in 2010. This type of cancer concentrates itself in males starting at the age of 50 years, with an average age of 75 years at time of diagnosis and with a median age of 68 years.

Colorectal cancer is the second most diagnosed type of cancer in males on the island, with a total of 65 new cases during 2007–2010 (7.8 % of the total new cancer cases during the reported period).

Stomach cancer is the third most diagnosed type of cancer in males, with an average of 6 new cases during the reported year. The average age is 66.4 years and the median age for stomach cancer is 64 years. The minimum age at time of diagnosis was 35 years and the maximum age was 86 years old in 2009.

Figure 26 illustrates the incidence rate for the top 5 primary diagnosed type of cancer in males from 2007 till 2010 and Table 5 shows the minimum-maximum age per type of cancer and also the average and median age for each primary diagnosed cancer for males in Aruba.

Table 5. Overview of the minimum-maximum-median and average age for males at time of diagnosis for the top 5 cancers.

Type of cancer	Total new cases	Min age (yrs)	Max age (yrs)	Average age (yrs)	Median age (yrs)
Prostate	151	50	89	75	68
Colorectal	65	31	91	64.4	66
Stomach	24	35	86	66.4	64
Trachea/Bronchus/Lung	23	39	74	64	67
Bladder	18	55	87	69	70

3.3.4 Cancer in Females

The top 5 diagnosed cancers in females are skin cancer, breast cancer, colorectal cancer, cervical-endometrial cancer and ovarian cancer.

Breast cancer is, besides skin cancer, the most diagnosed type of cancer in females, with a total of 212 new cases from 2007–2010. This type of cancer comprises 46.5

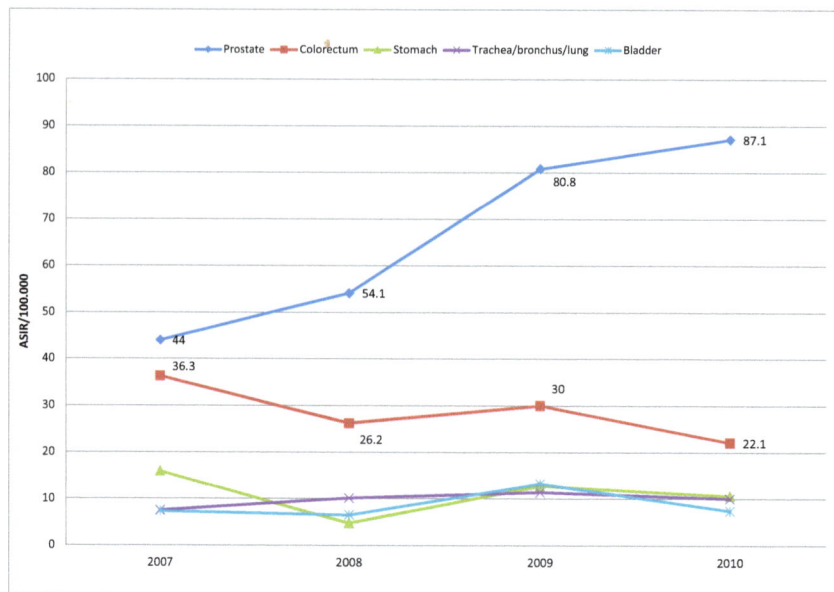

Figure 26. Incidence rate of the top 5 male cancer types in Aruba, 2007–2010.

percent of the total diagnosed new cancer cases in females. Of these 212 new cases, 75.9 percent are in the age category of 45-74 years ($n = 161$). The average age for females diagnosed with breast cancer is 59 years, while the median age of 60 years. This explains the concentration of the disease in women aged 60 years.

There is a steep increase in the number of new breast cancer cases from 2009 to 2010 due to the introduction of the Mamma Policlinic at the Dr. Horacio Oduber Hospital. The introduction of this clinic contributed to earlier detection of breast cancer in women. The minimum age a female was diagnosed with breast cancer was at the age of 24 years, while the oldest female with breast cancer was at the age of 98 years.

Colorectal cancer is also in the top 5 diagnosed cancers in females, with an average of 13 new cases per year, mostly in the age category of 55–74 years (67.3%), see Figure 27.

Ovarian cancer shows an exponential increase from 2007 to 2010, with an incidence rate in 2007 of 3.7 per 100,000 to an incidence rate of 15 cases per 100.000 in 2010, a fourfold increase. There is an increase in the number of cases in the age category of 45-49 years and in the age category of 70+ years.

Cervical-endometrial and ovarian cancer belong to the gynecological cancer. With a total of 37 new cases of cervical cancer during 4 years (8.1 % of the total female cancer cases), the youngest female diagnosed was at the age of 24 years, while the oldest female was diagnosed at the age of 92 years.

The average age is 48.8 years while the median age is 47 years, see Table 6.

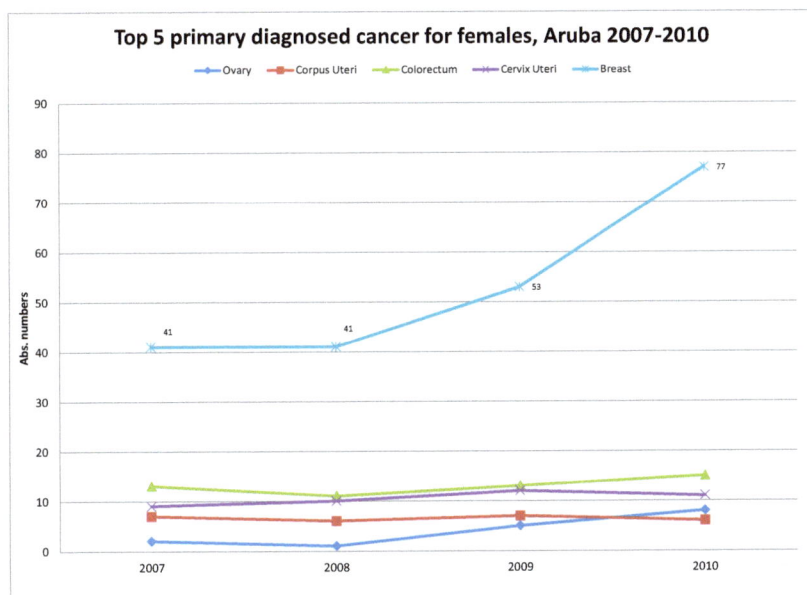

Top 5 primary diagnosed cancer for females, Aruba 2007-2010

Figure 27. Incidence rate of the top 5 female cancer types in Aruba, 2007–2010.

Table 6. Overview of the minimum-maximum-median and average age for females at time of diagnosis for the top 5 cancer.

Type of cancer	Total new cases	Min age (yrs)	Max age (yrs)	Average age (yrs)	Median age (yrs)
Breast	212	24	98	59	60
Colorectal	52	33	89	62.3	61
Cervix uteri	37	24	92	48.8	47
Corpus uteri	31	36	88	56	58
Ovary	16	41	82	61.3	59

During 2007 till 2010 there were a total of 31 endometrial (corpus uteri) cancer cases diagnosed (6.8 % of the total female cancer). Of the total registered cases, 80.6 % are in the age category of 45–74 years, with a minimum age at diagnosis of 36 years and a maximum age of 88 years.

3.4 Infectious Diseases

The Department of Public Health monitors infectious diseases which can be a threat to the Public Health of Aruba, using a surveillance system. This surveillance system is based on the National Ordinance for Infectious Diseases; this supports the mandatory notifications of infectious diseases. The surveillance system is based on a communication network consisting of public health authorities and care givers.

Together with the Caribbean Public Health Association (CARPHA) and the Pan American Health Organization (PAHO), Aruba is part of the Caribbean regional surveillance system.

3.4.1 Dengue

Dengue is one of the most prevalent infectious diseases in the Caribbean region. Dengue is prevalent from 1970 in Aruba. Also it is prevalent throughout the tropics and subtropics. Outbreaks have occurred frequently in the Caribbean, including Puerto Rico, the U.S. Virgin Islands, Cuba, Venezuela (South America), Paraguay (South America) and Costa Rica (Central America).

In 1986 Aruba experienced its first major Dengue outbreak. It has been calculated that during this epidemic more than 40,000 people were infected with the virus. Since 1986 Aruba has experienced more Dengue outbreaks during the rainy season. Such outbreaks became an annual event dating back to 2003, see Figure 28.

Dengue fever is a disease caused by a virus that is transmitted by the Aedes aegypti mosquito. The virus is transmitted to humans through the bites of infected female mosquitoes. After virus incubation of 4–10 days in the mosquito, this infected mosquito is capable of transmitting the virus for the rest of its life. Dengue is caused by one of four serotypes of Dengue fever virus(DEN-1, DEN-2, DEN-3 and DEN-4). Recovery from infection with one Dengue serotype provides lifelong immunity against that particular serotype to which the patient was exposed. Subsequent

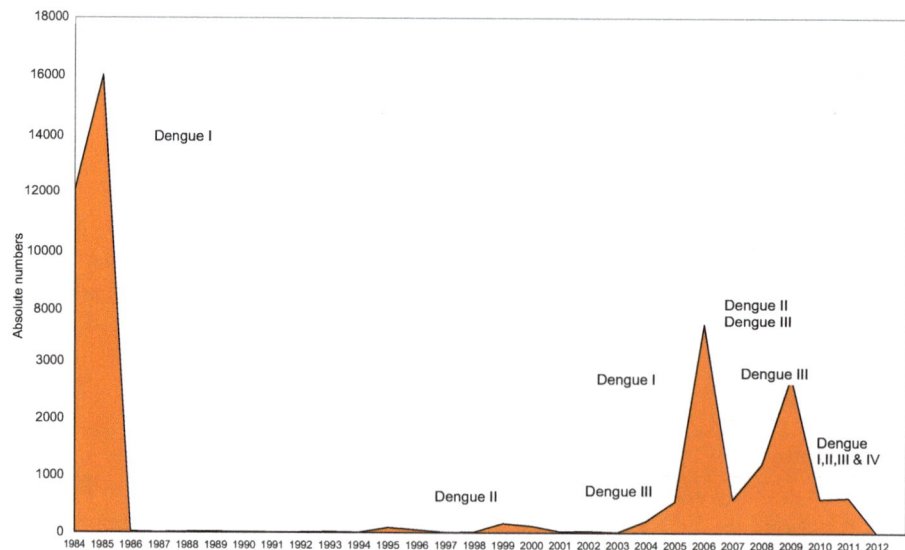

Figure 28. Dengue outbreaks Aruba, 1984–2012.

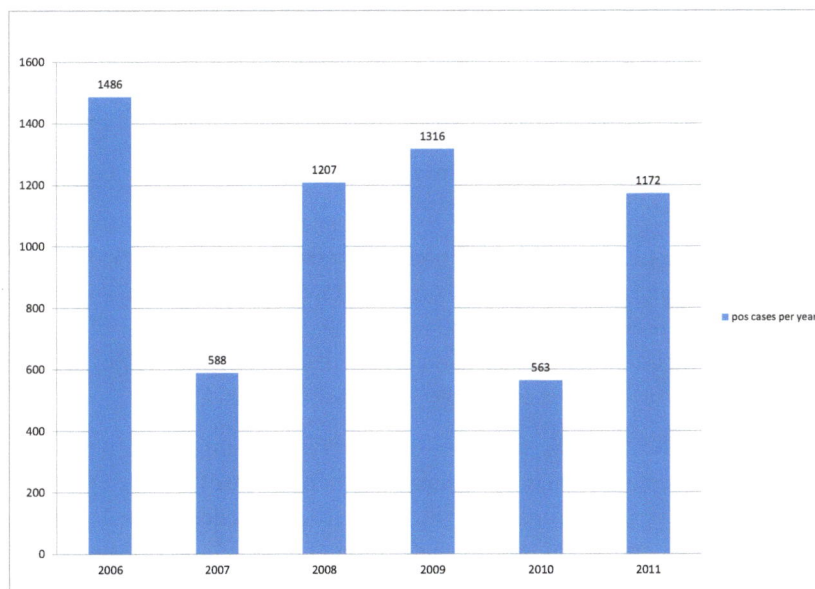

Figure 29. Number of laboratory confirmed cases per year Aruba, 2006–2011.

infections by other serotypes increase the risk of developing Severe Dengue (Dengue Hemorrhagic Fever and Dengue Shock Syndrome).

Dengue has become endemic on the island during the past 5 years, where viral activities are monitored even during the dry periods on the island.

In 2010 Aruba detected all 4 serotypes of the Dengue fever virus in circulation during the same period of time on the island. This increases the risk for developing severe Dengue. The most affected age category by the Dengue fever virus is the category of 25–64 years.

Figure 29 shows the number of laboratory confirmed Dengue cases per year. The number of cases per year exceeds 500 cases. Not to mention the high numbers during outbreaks, which are above not less than 1000 confirmed cases per year.

The Dengue surveillance system shows how Dengue manifests itself periodically through the years. As Figure 30 shows, Dengue has the highest prevalence during the end and beginning of the year. This specific period of time is considered as the rainy season of Aruba. This rain season runs from October through February the following year.

To maintain monitoring on the Dengue outbreaks on the island, the Epidemiology Unit maintains three curves the lower endemic curve, endemic curve and epidemic curve. These curves will give a weekly overview and gives the possibility to make projection of the Dengue situation on the island.

From 2010 to 2011 Dengue activities were observed during the dry periods, see Figure 30.

3.4.1.2 Aedes Aegypti Index

The Department of Public Health also monitors the indices of the vector transmitting the Dengue virus, the Aedes aegypti mosquito.

The three indices that are monitored throughout the year are the house index (Figure 31), the container index (32) and the breteau index. The house index is the percentage of houses infested with A. aegypti larve or pupae. The container index is the percentage of water holding containers infested with larvae and/or pupae. The Breteau Index provides the number of positive containers per 100 houses.

The Pan American Health Organization (PAHO) uses the standard limit of 4 percent of houses positive for containers being the maximum percentage of houses. When this limit is surpassed the area is considered high risk for prevalence of the *A. aegypti* mosquito. As Figures 31 and 32 show in the beginning of the year and at the end of the year the indices recorded in Aruba are above the PAHO limits.

3.4.2 Tuberculosis

Tuberculosis is a serious infectious disease caused by the Mycobacterium tuberculosis. Tuberculosis is considered worldwide one of the re-emerging diseases during the past 54 years.

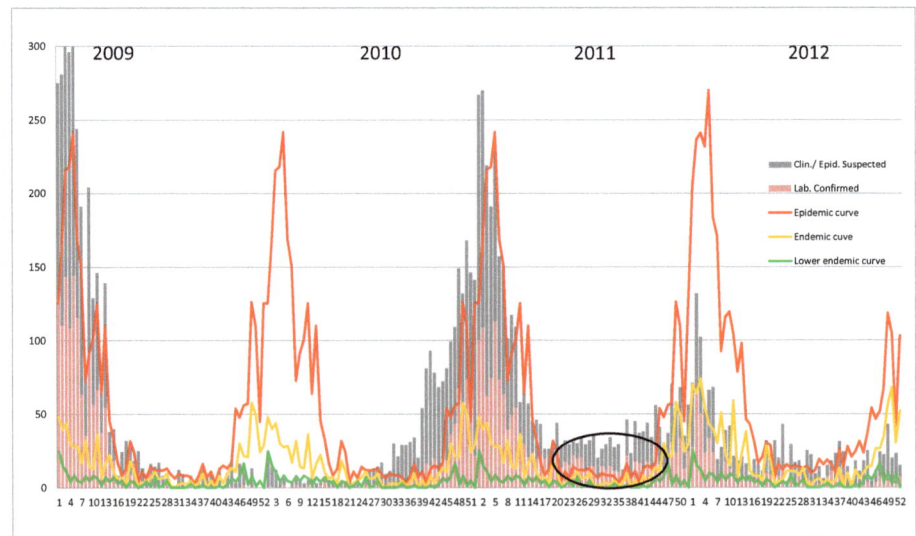

Figure 30. Epidemic and endemic dengue channels, Aruba, 2009–2011.

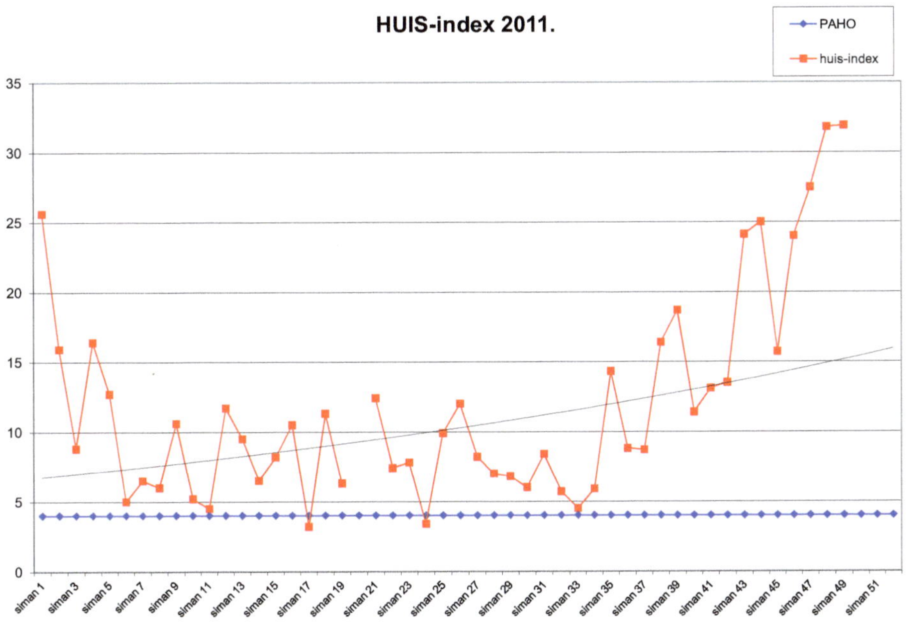

Figure 31. House index Aruba, 2011.

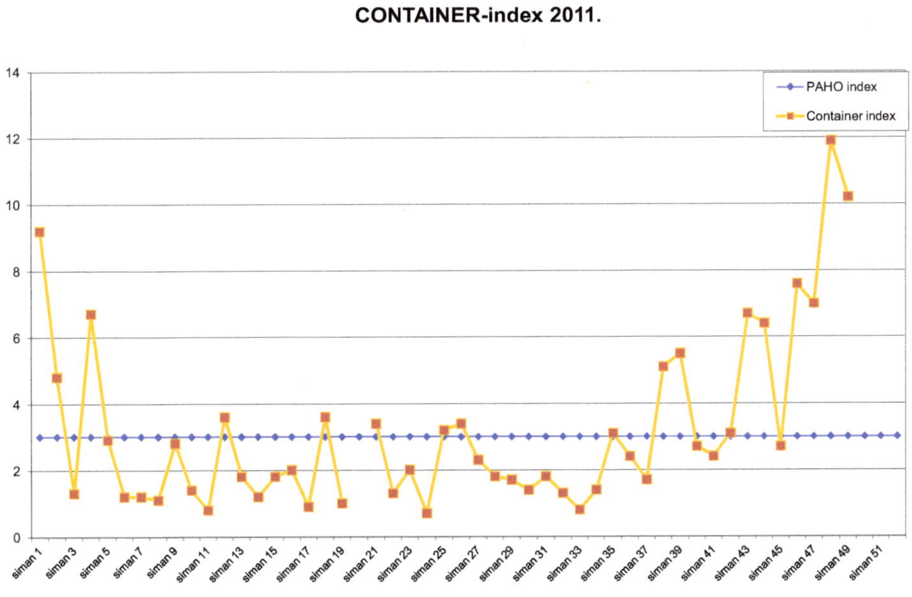

Figure 32. Container index Aruba, 2011.

Pulmonary tuberculosis is the most common form in Aruba. Open pulmonary tuberculosis is the most contagious form of tuberculosis. The bacterium is spread through the air by droplets formed during coughing or sneezing. The highest risk for contamination is in poorly ventilated or confined spaces. People with poorly functioning immune systems are more likely to get the disease.

Tuberculosis is seen in Aruba mainly in immigrants and travelers who come from endemic areas. Therefore it can be stated that tuberculosis is not an endemic but an imported disease in Aruba.

Figure 33 pointed that from 2003 to 2011 Aruba experienced an average 6.8 new cases of TB yearly; about 95 percent are imported cases. In Figure 34 confirmed cases and not confirmed cases are presented. The confirmed cases are confirmed by laboratory tests and chest X-rays, whereas the not confirmed cases are confirmed clinically by the pulmonologists. The clinically confirmed cases are also registered as TB this engaging the necessary close contact investigation.

3.4.3 Sexually Transmitted Infections

Sexually Transmitted Infections (STI's) are infectious diseases that are primarily transmitted through unprotected sexual contact by anal, oral or vaginal contact. In most cases, the organisms that cause STI's enter the body through the mucous Abs. numbers membranes. Some STI's can also be transmitted through other routes such

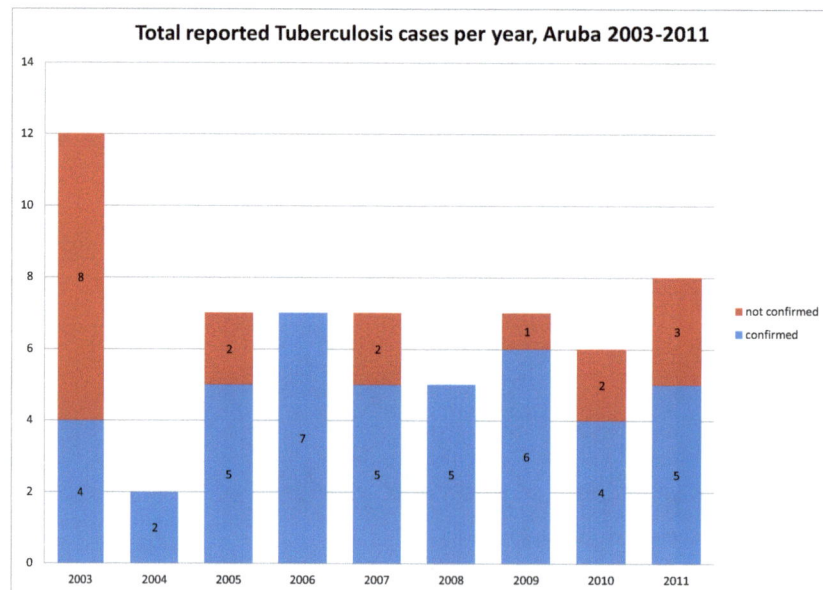

Figure 33. Tuberculosis cases per year Aruba, 2003–2011.

Total reported Tuberculosis cases per age category, Aruba 2003-2011

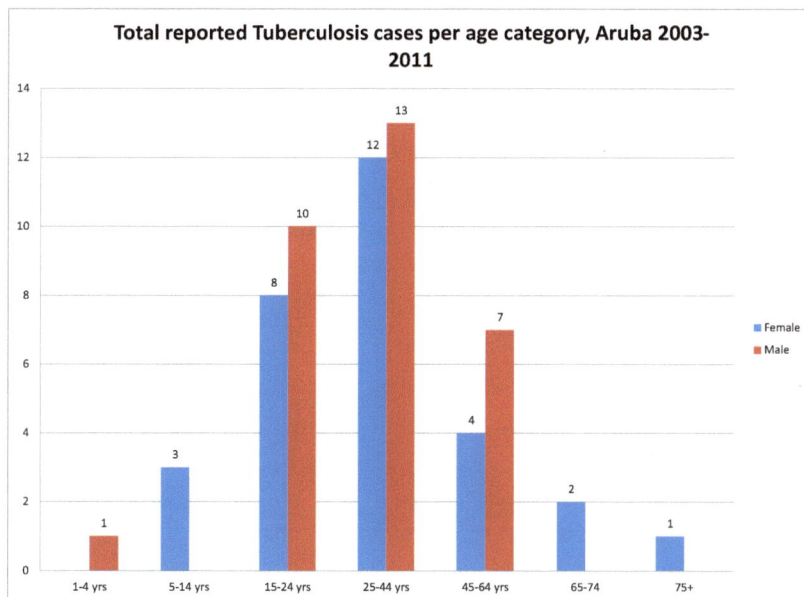

Figure 34. Tuberculosis cases by age category and gender in Aruba, 2003–2011.

as "from mother to child" during pregnancy or birth. STI's can also be transmitted through blood transfusions or the use of contaminated needles. Their effects are not always limited to the reproductive organs. STI's can cause serious complications, including infertility in women and men.

Reporting of STI's to the Service of Contagious Diseases is not optimal. Data presented in this chapter are indicative because of underreporting. It gives an indication of the different risk groups in the Aruban population exposed to STI's. International indicators consider the age category 15 to 24 year as the most sexually active age category. STI's are detected in the very early age of sexual activities, overall females are infected at an earlier age compared to males (WHO, 2011).

Figure 35 illustrates the absolute numbers of reported STI's per year in the age category 15 to 19 years. Syphilis is the most reported STI followed by Chlamydia. Overall, Syphilis, Gonorrhea and Chlamydia are the most common reported STI's at the Service for Infectious Diseases.

3.4.3.1 Syphilis

Syphilis is one of the oldest STI's known worldwide. In 2005 syphilis accounted for a global prevalence of 36 million cases (WHO, 2011). Although the global incidence for syphilis has been declining from 12.2 million new cases in 1995 to 10.6 million new cases in 2005, for the American region this is not the case. Instead the incidence for

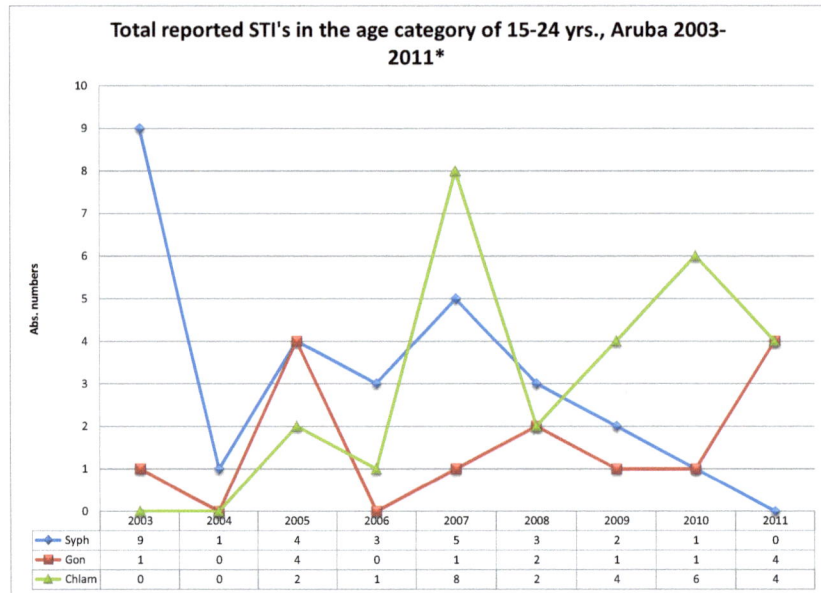

Total reported STI's in the age category of 15-24 yrs., Aruba 2003-2011*

	2003	2004	2005	2006	2007	2008	2009	2010	2011
Syph	9	1	4	3	5	3	2	1	0
Gon	1	0	4	0	1	2	1	1	4
Chlam	0	0	2	1	8	2	4	6	4

Figure 35. Absolute numbers of reported STI's by year in the age category 15–19 years Aruba, 2003–2011.

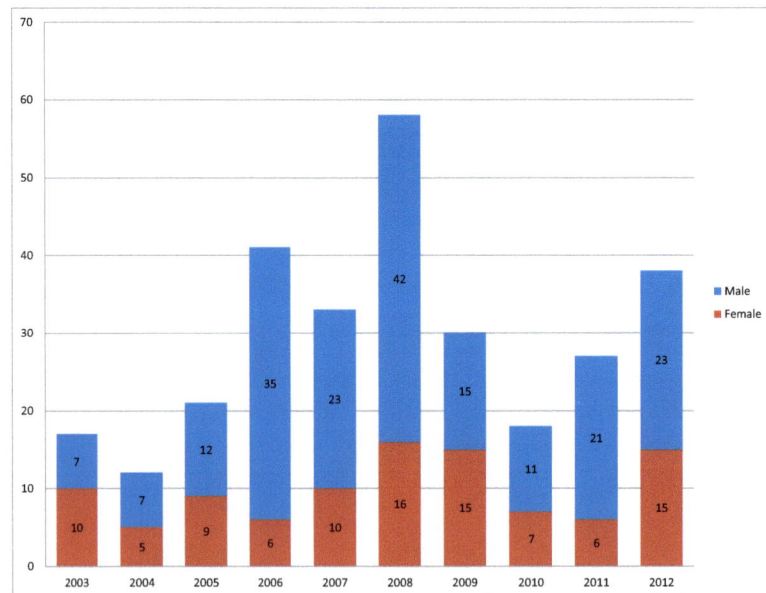

Figure 36. Absolute number of new syphilis cases by gender per year, Aruba 2003–2012.

syphilis has been on a rise from 1.26 million cases in 1995 to 2.39 million new cases in 2005 for the Latin American Region and the Caribbean (WHO,2001; WHO; 2011).

Yearly there is an average of 30 new cases of syphilis reported to the Service for Infectious Diseases in all age categories. The male gender is the most affected by this STI, see Figure 36.

The males in the age group 25 to 44 years are the most affected by syphilis followed by the age category 45 to 64 years. It is also important to notice that young female adults in the age category of 15–24 years are the most affected by syphilis compared to the males, see Figure 37.

3.4.3.2 Chlamydia

The second most common STI in Aruba is Chlamydia. In 2005 the global incidence for Chlamydia was 101.5 million cases; the American continent had the highest incidence (22.5 million). Women are the most affected by Chlamydia, see Figure 38.

In Aruba, from 2003 to 2011 there was an average of 7 new cases of Chlamydia per year. Similar to the worldwide incidence, the female gender is the most affected by this STI, see Figure 39.

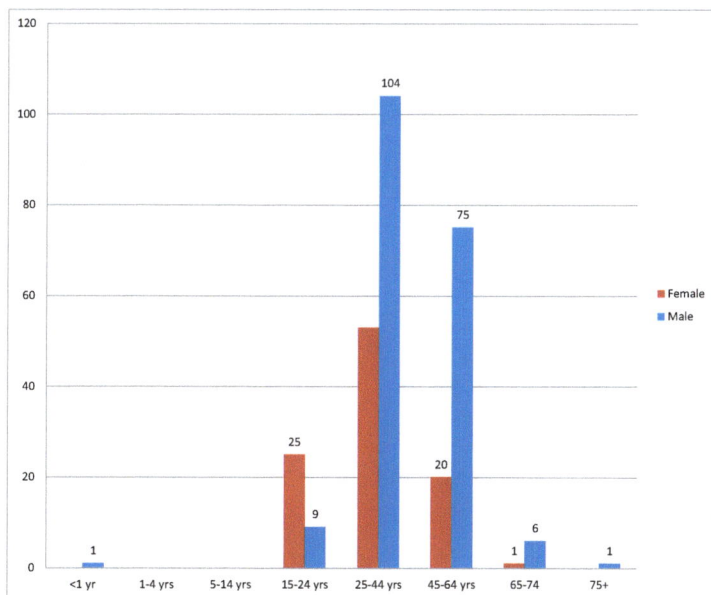

Figure 37. New syphilis cases per age category, Aruba 2003–2012.

Global estimated incidence of chlamydia, 2005

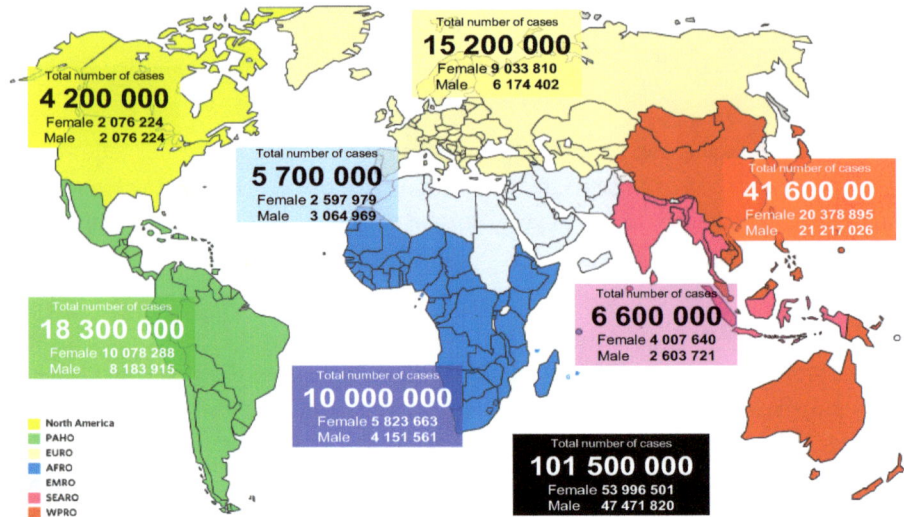

Figure 38. Global estimated common Chlamydia incidence, 2005.

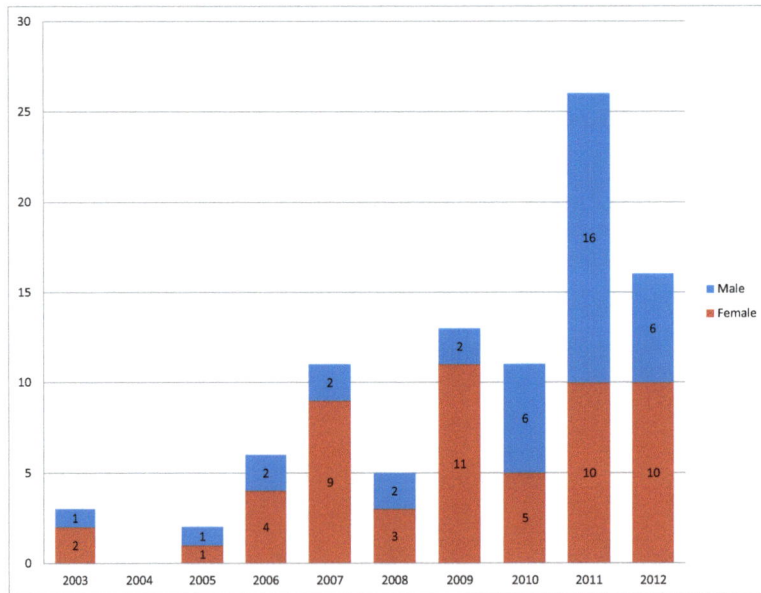

Figure 39. Chlamydia incidence by gender per year, Aruba 2003–2011.

3.4.3.3 Gonorrhea

WHO stated that Gonorrhea is a common STI, however up to 80% of women and 10% of the men are asymptomatic. Complications of Gonorrhea infections may lead to infertility in women, even blindness in the new born infant.

Worldwide the incidence of Gonorrhea has dropped during the 1980 to 1990 down to less than 20 per 100,000 cases worldwide. However from 1990's up till 2011 the incidence has been increasing in many different countries of the world and reached a global incidence of 62 million new cases in 1999 (WHO, 2001).

In Aruba, Gonorrhea is the least reported STI at the Service for Infectious Diseases, with an average of only 4.6 new cases per year during the past 10 years. Males accounted for the most reported cases of gonorrhea, see Figure 40.

During this same period the most affected population with Gonorrhea were in the age category 15 to 44 years. It is important to notice that during this period only 1 case in the age category of 5-14 years was reported. However one need to take into account the underreporting of Gonorrhea, see Figure 41.

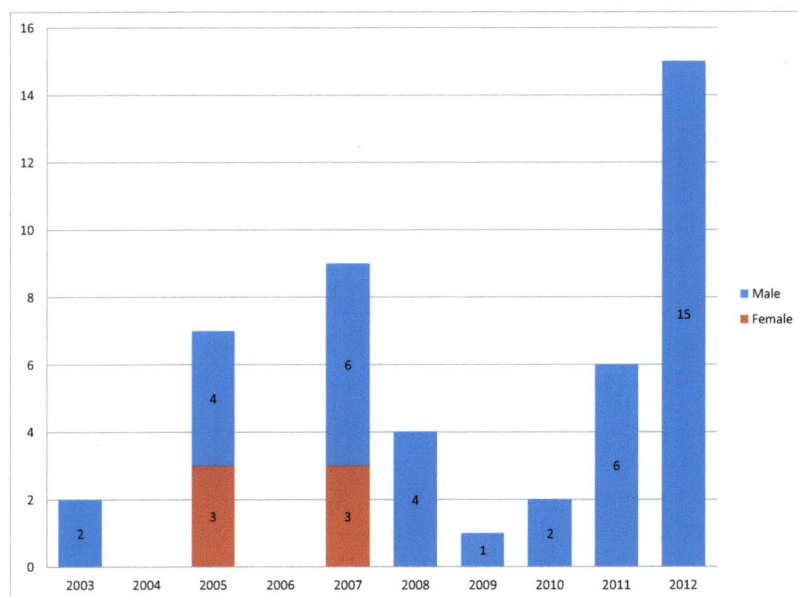

Figure 40. Absolute number of new cases of gonorrhea by gender, Aruba 2003–2011.

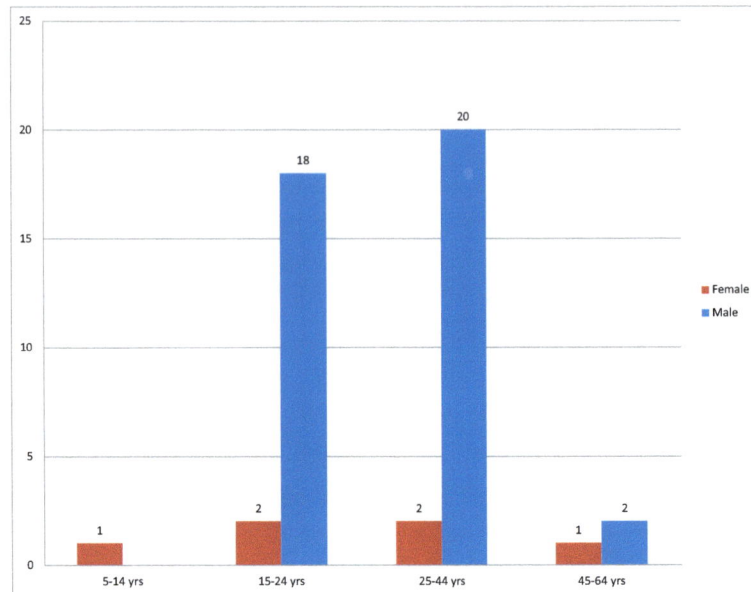

Figure 41. Total number of new cases of gonorrhea by age category, Aruba 2003–2011.

3.4.3.4 HIV/AIDS

Acquired immunodeficiency syndrome (AIDS) is caused by human immunodeficiency virus (HIV). HIV is transmitted through unprotected sexual contact, but also through blood contact, blood products and also from mother to child during pregnancy and lactation.

HIV/AIDS is not curable but treatable. There are medications available that inhibits multiplication of the HIV-virus in the body. This leads to less often HIV infection or delayed progression to AIDS.

The trend of cumulative cases of HIV, AIDS and death unknown related to HIV and People Living with HIV (PLHIV) per year is presented in Figure 42. Each year there is an average of 26 75+ new cases per year, with a minimum of 12 new cases and a 65-74 maximum of 28 new cases in a year. As this trend illustrates the incidence for HIV is on a rise together with the incidence for PLHIV. In addition, the AIDS cases have been stable over stable over the past 5 years.

More than 30 percent of the registered cases from 2000 to 2010 are born in Aruba and 70 percent of the cases are male and 27 percent are female. This information indicates that the epidemic in Aruba manifests itself mainly in the male gender. This finding is opposite to the rest of the Caribbean. In the Caribbean HIV cases are mostly in women. However, it is important to mention that these numbers represent only the HIV cases that are registered.

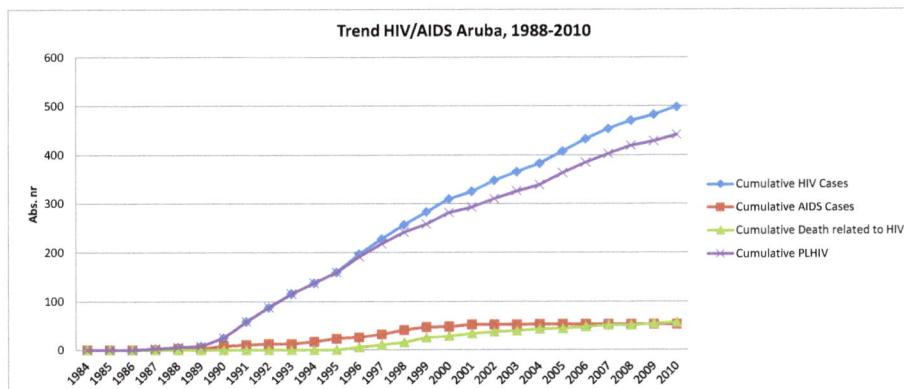

Figure 42. Cumulative HIV cases, AIDS cases, HIV deaths & PHIV in Aruba, 1984–2010.

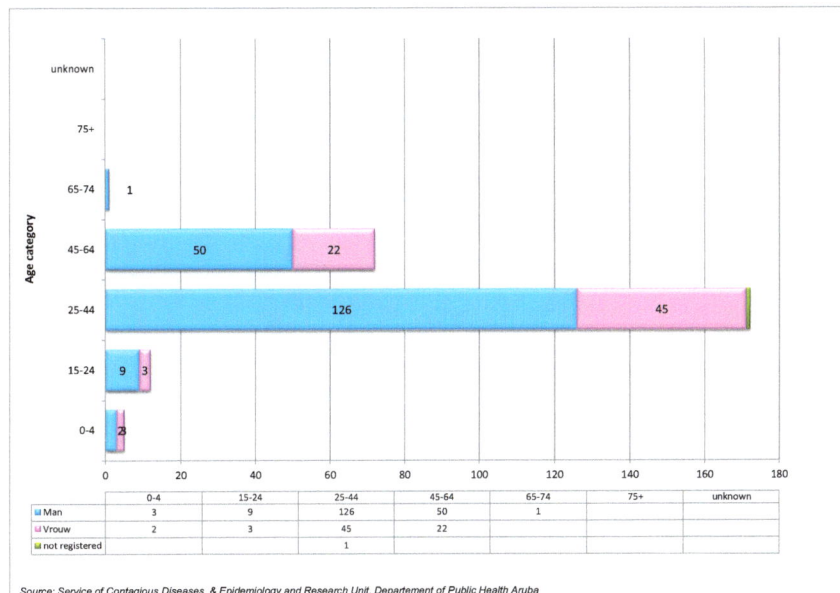

	0-4	15-24	25-44	45-64	65-74	75+	unknown
Man	3	9	126	50	1		
Vrouw	2	3	45	22			
not registered			1				

Source: Service of Contagious Diseases & Epidemiology and Research Unit, Departement of Public Health Aruba

Figure 43. HIV cases by age category, Aruba 2000–2010.

The most common mode of transmission of the HIV virus reported was heterosexual contact (59 percent) followed by men having sex with men (MSM) (29 percent). HIV affects mostly the young productive population between 25 to 44 years.

3.4.4 Hepatitis B

Hepatitis B is an infection of the liver caused by the hepatitis B virus (HBV). The virus is primarily found in the liver but is also present in the blood and certain body fluids. It is estimated that 350 million individuals worldwide are infected with the virus, which causes 620,000 deaths worldwide each year.

In Aruba an average of 35 new cases of Hepatitis B are registered yearly. Most cases are in males. During the past 5 years the most Hepatitis B cases were detected in the year 2009, see Figure 44 A and 44 B.

Most of the cases are imported cases and are in the age category of 25–44 years. In Aruba Hepatitis B vaccination is offered to all infants born after 2004.

The Services of Infectious Diseases handle the vaccination for:

- people working in risk groups; health care and public safety (police, ambulance personnel, firefighters, prison guards)
- household contact
- students who are going to study abroad
- sexual partners of carrier of HBV
- HIV patients

The Service of Infectious Diseases is also in charge of the Post-exposure prophylaxis (PEP) treatment. This treatment is used after possible exposure to the hepatitis B virus through sex, drug injection or injury such as needle stick injury. PEP is given to decrease the risk of infection with the hepatitis B virus. Stick needle injury PEP

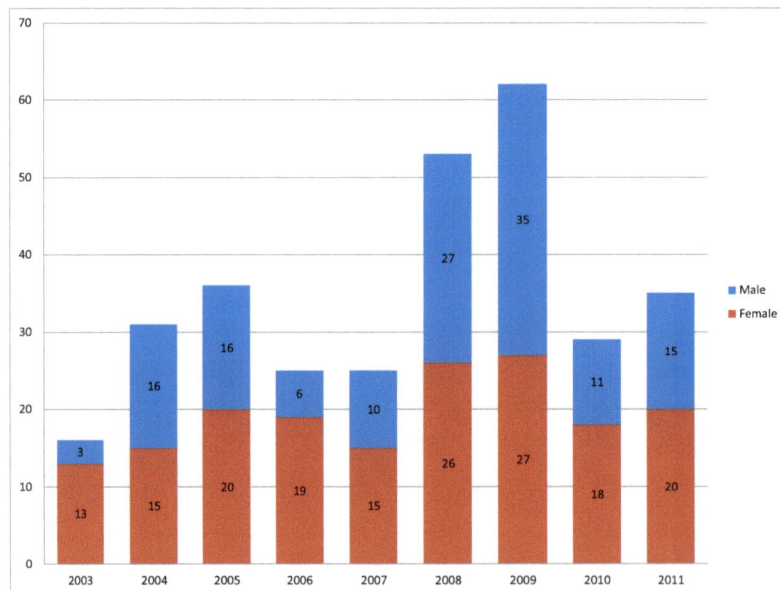

Figure 44 A. Total number of Hepatitis B cases by gender years.

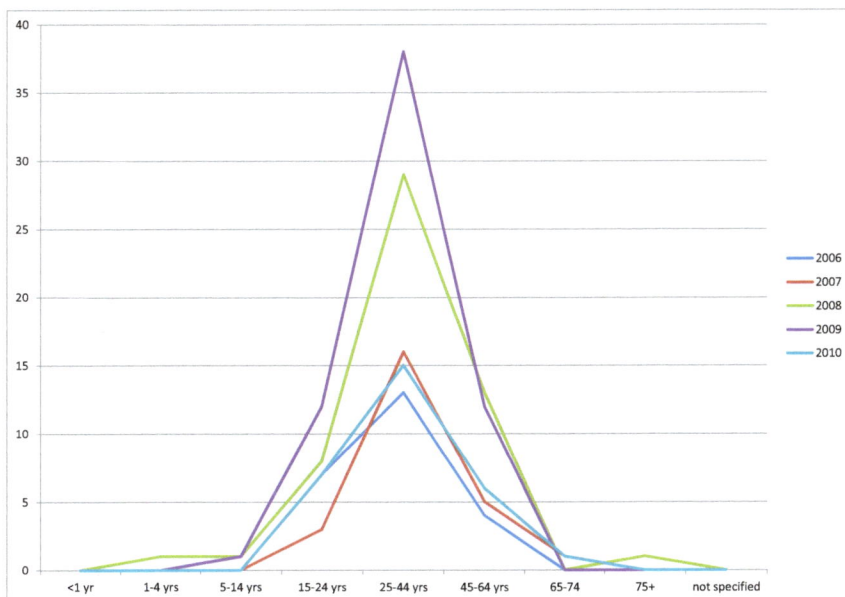

Figure 44 B. Hepatitis B cases by age categories, Aruba 2003–2011.

treatment is the most common type of HBV treatment requested at the Service for Infectious Diseases of the Department of Public Health.

3.4.5 Food Borne Diseases

3.4.5.1 Salmonellosis

Salmonellosis is a food borne illness caused by the Salmonella bacteria carried by some animals, which can be transmitted from kitchen surfaces and can be in water, soil, animal faeces, raw meats and eggs.

Salmonellosis, as with many other food borne diseases, is 60 also present on the island. To prevent transmission of these bacteria the Service of Infectious Diseases of the Department of Public Health carries out a yearly screening of the people working in the HORECA industry. This screening is under the regulation "PersoneelsBesluit en Waren Verordening GT2." Among the many tests included in this screening, a faeces smear on Salmonella, Shigella and Campylobacter is also included. Only HORECA personnel with a "Health Certificate" are allowed to work.

Salmonellosis In Aruba

Yearly there are about an average of 30 notifications of Salmonella cases. As it is illustrated in Figure 45, 2005 had 60 the largest number of notifications of Salmonella infection, in this year Aruba experienced a Salmonella outbreak with the Salmonella Oranienburg bacteria at a local restaurant.

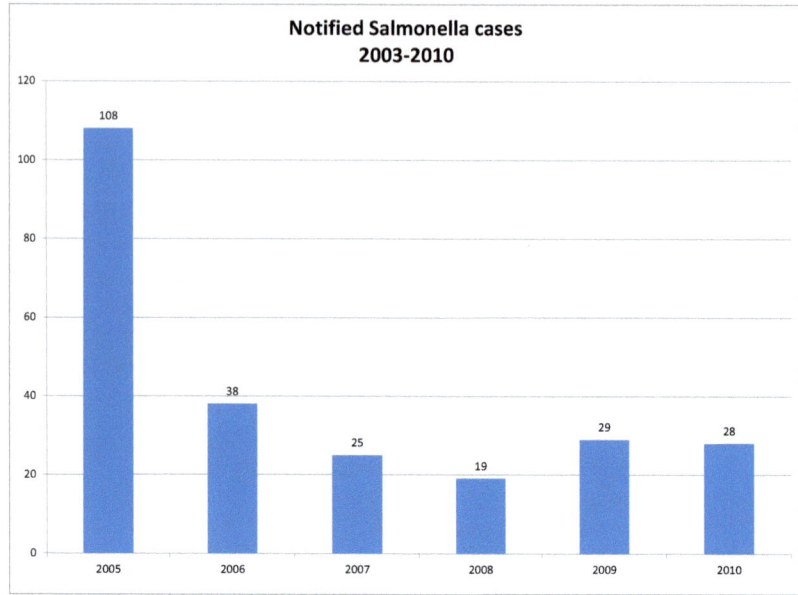

Figure 45. Notified salmonella cases, Aruba 2005–2010.

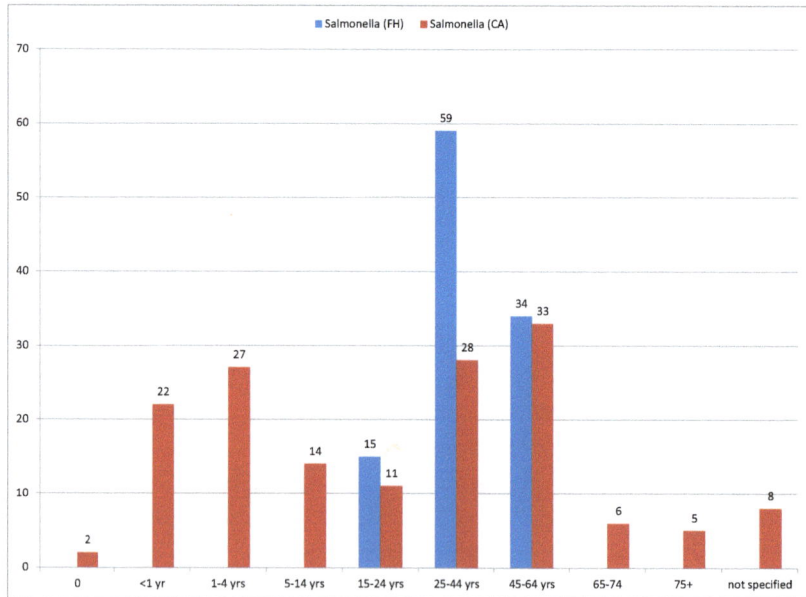

Figure 46. Notified salmonella cases by age category, Aruba 2005–2010.

From 2005 to 2010 a selection was made of the Salmonella cases which were detected in the regular community acquired, and food handlers. These cases were analyzed by 20 age categories. 10

As Figure 46 shows Salmonellosis notification from the community are present in each age category varying from babies to the elderly. As expected, the age category of Salmonella cases among food handlers varied between the ages of 15 to 64 years. During this same period notifications from the regular community were higher as compared to the food handlers, 59.1 percent and 40.9 percent respectively.

3.4.5.2 Shigellosis

Shigellosis is also a food borne disease but is caused by a group of bacteria called Shigella. Shigellosis presents itself with bloody diarrhea. Among the few symptoms present are fever and stomach cramps. Some individuals who are infected may not develop any symptoms, but may still infect others with the bacteria. Transmission occurs from person to person but also through contaminated food.

Yearly there is an average of 14 notifications of Shigellosis. Compared to Salmonellosis the prevalence of Shigellosis is lower.

Based on Figure 48 below, we conclude that the majority of the community acquired Shigellosis cases are between 1–14 years of age. Furthermore, the food handlers Shigellosis cases are all between the ages of 15–64 years, with a peak occurrence of Shigellosis cases in the 25–44 age categories.

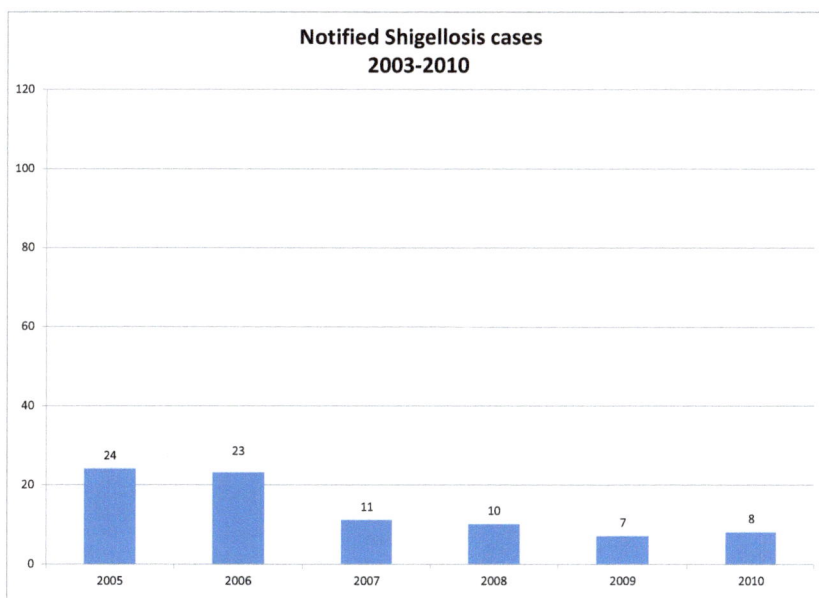

Figure 47. Shigellosis notifications per year.

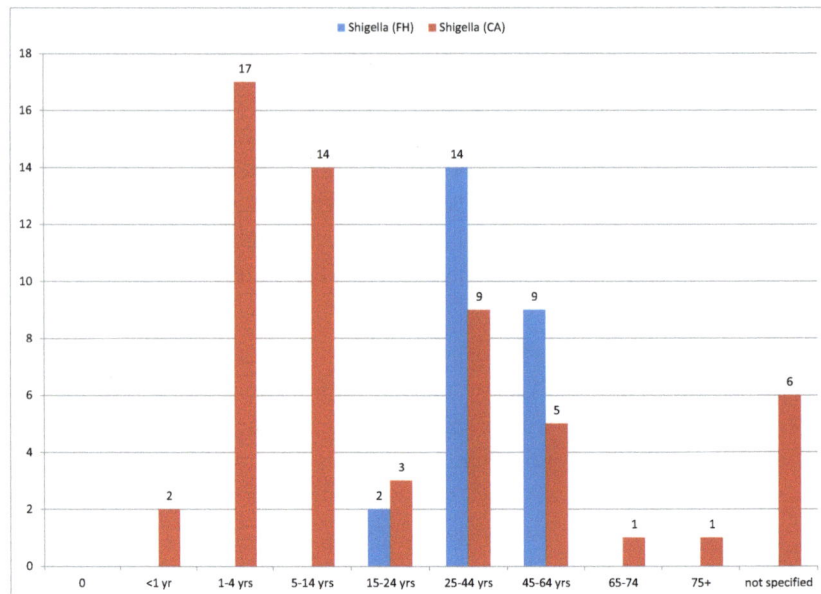

Figure 48. Shigellosis notifications by age category, Aruba 2005–2010.

However the percentages of Shigellosis notifications between food handlers and community acquired differ from the Salmonellosis percentages. Food handlers accounted for only one third of the notifications during 2005 to 2010, while the regular community acquired accounted for about 70 percent of the notifications.

3.5 Vaccinations

3.5.1 Vaccinations Infants

Through the years, vaccination has proven to be among the most cost-effective, cost-beneficial, high-impact action most widely accepted by society for the improvement of the people's health. More than half of the gains in reducing child mortality in Latin America and the Caribbean in recent years are attributable to immunization.

Basic vaccination services are free in Aruba. The Youth Health Care Unit of the Department of Public Health vaccinates infants at the White and Yellow Cross clinics located at the six different districts on the island. Even though these vaccinations at the clinics are also available to the four year olds, only 70% are actually vaccinated here. The remaining 30% receive their vaccines through the yearly school vaccination-campaigns which are also managed by the Youth Health Care Unit of the Department of Public Health.

Children are vaccinated against the following diseases; Diphtheria, Pertussis, Tetanus, Poliomyelitis (DPTP), Hepatitis B, Pneumococcal disease, Heamophilus influenza type b infections (Hib), Measles, Mumps and Rubella (MMR). Table 7 shows the different vaccine phases by age and vaccine.

Table 7. Vaccination program Youth Health Care of the Department of Public Health.

Phase	Age	Vaccine 1	Vaccine 2
Phase 1	1 month	Hep B	
	2 months	DPT/IPV/HIB	PCV
	3 months	Hep B	
	4 months	DPT/IPV/HIB	PCV
	6 months	DPT/IPV/HIB	
	9 months	Hep B	
	12 months	PCV	MMR
	15 months	DPT/IPV/HIB	
Phase 2	4 years	DP/IPV	
Phase 3	10 years	MMR	DP/IPV

Basic vaccinations consist of three DPTP Hib and Hepatitis B vaccinations, and one MMR vaccination. This basic vaccination should be completed by the age of 2. In the fifth year of life the DP/IPV booster should be administered.

Table 8. Vaccination coverage 2 year olds.

2 years	2007	2008	2009	2010	2011
DPTP HiB3 (basic coverage)	98,9%	98,7%	98,7%	98,8%	96,8%
DPTP HiB 4	96,1%	96,2%	96,0%	94,9%	92,4%
MMR1	94,8%	95,2%	96,0%	92,7%	93,4%
HEP B3	97,2%	97,2%	96,7%	96,6%	93,9%

Coverage of babies/toddlers registered at WYC (undocumented children excluded)*

A 95 percent vaccine coverage is considered a high density of immunized persons in a population, which offers sufficient protection for the unvaccinated, this is called herd immunity. This high coverage has been maintained in Aruba throughout the past years except during 2010/2011 for the Measles, Mumps and Rubella vaccine and in 2011 for the Hepatitis B vaccine.

3.5.1.1 Vaccination Preschool And Primary School Children

Pre-school and primary school children are vaccinated during the school-based vaccination campaign which is held yearly. This campaign targets children in the second year of preschool, and in the first and fifth grade of primary school. The coverage of MMR and DP/IPV of the school population after school vaccination campaign is illustrated in Tables 9 and 10.

Table 9. Vaccine coverage in 5 year old by type vaccine per school year.

5 years	2007-2008	2008-2009	2009-2010	2010-2011
DP/IPV	97,4%	98,5%	97,1%	96,5%
MMR	98.3	97.8	98.2	98.5

Table 10. Vaccine coverage in 10 year old by type vaccine per school year.

10 years	2007-2008	2008-2009	2009-2010	2010-2011
DP/IPV	98,1%	97,8%	95,8%	97,0%
MMR	98,2%	97,8%	96,0%	97,4%

Children with learning-difficulties attending special schools in Aruba are vaccinated at the age of 10.

3.5.2 Vaccination Risk Groups

Vaccination of risk groups such as international travelers and work related high risk group is a highly effective method of preventing certain infectious diseases. In terms of public health, prevention is better and more cost-effective than cure. These vaccinations not only protect against many travel-related infections, such as yellow fever, tetanus and hepatitis A, but also prevent the importation of these rare diseases onto the island.

Protection against work related risk infections, such as Hepatitis B and Tetanus is also achieved with vaccination of this risk group.

International travel is overwhelmed by a large and increasing number of individuals for professional, social recreational and humanitarian purposes. Travelers are as such exposed to a variety of health risk in unfamiliar environments.

Healthcare workers, law enforcement and other type of personnel may be exposed to risks of contracting infections with certain vaccine preventable diseases. The Services of Infectious Diseases of the Department of Public Health sells vaccinations to travelers, work related risk groups and individuals.

In Aruba the most common reason for the request of a vaccination amongst the adult population are international Travel vaccinations for students, USA Visa requests and travels for vacation purposes.

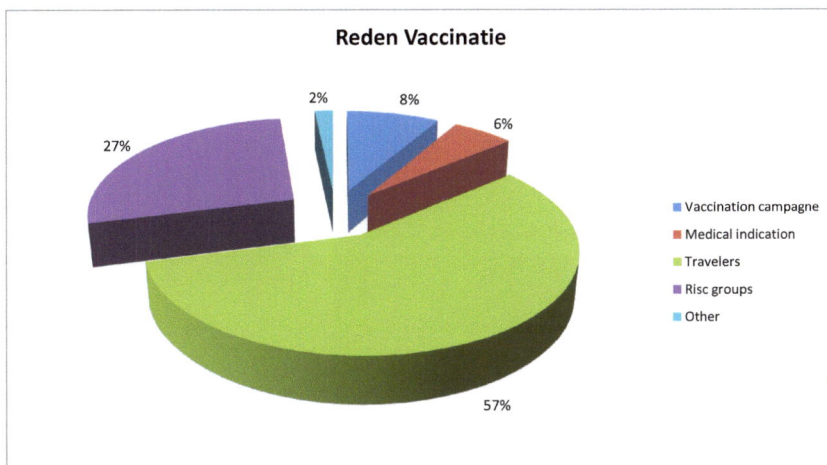

Reden Vaccinatie

- 2%
- 8%
- 6%
- 27%
- 57%

Legend:
- Vaccination campagne
- Medical indication
- Travelers
- Risc groups
- Other

Figure 49. Different reasons for vaccination request, Aruba 2010.

Figure 50 shows the many different types of vaccines sold during 2010 by the Service of Infectious Diseases. The most common vaccine sold is against Yellow Fever followed by DTP, Hep B and Vaxigrip.

As mentioned above, the Service of Infectious Diseases sells to and vaccinates work groups who are at risk. These include governmental organizations as well as nongovernmental organizations.

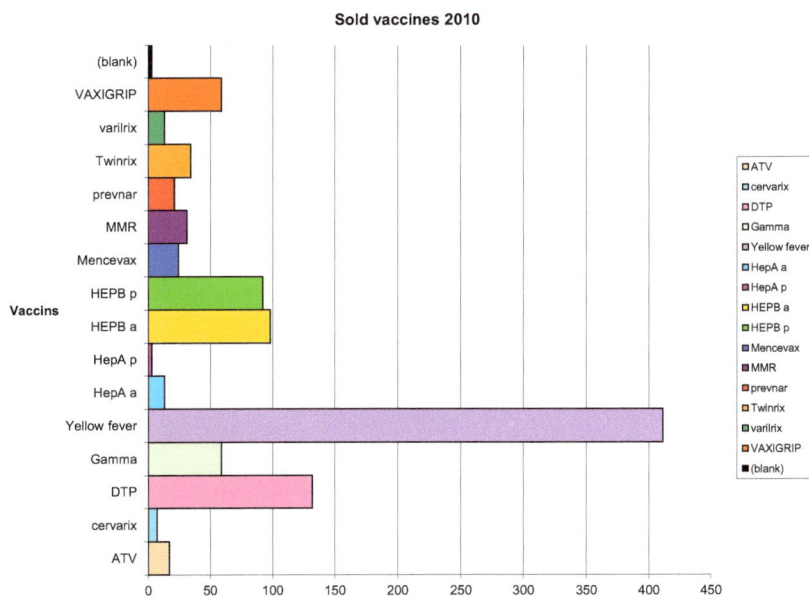

Sold vaccines 2010

Vaccins: (blank), VAXIGRIP, varilrix, Twinrix, prevnar, MMR, Mencevax, HEPB p, HEPB a, HepA p, HepA a, Yellow fever, Gamma, DTP, cervarix, ATV

Legend:
- ATV
- cervarix
- DTP
- Gamma
- Yellow fever
- HepA a
- HepA p
- HEPB a
- HEPB p
- Mencevax
- MMR
- prevnar
- Twinrix
- varilrix
- VAXIGRIP
- (blank)

Figure 50. Solid vaccine during 2010.

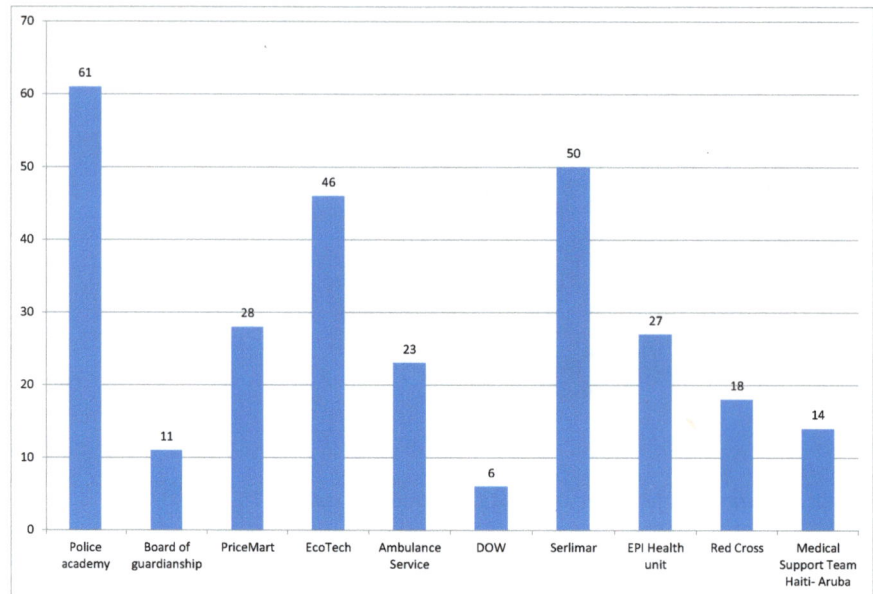

Figure 51. Different sectors receiving vaccinations, Aruba 2010.

Figure 51 illustrates the different sectors receiving vaccinations on a routine basis. To make vaccines accessible to the population of Aruba, the Department of Public Health purchases vaccines through the revolving funds of PAHO. This purchase through PAHO makes vaccines more accessible because of the attractive price offered.

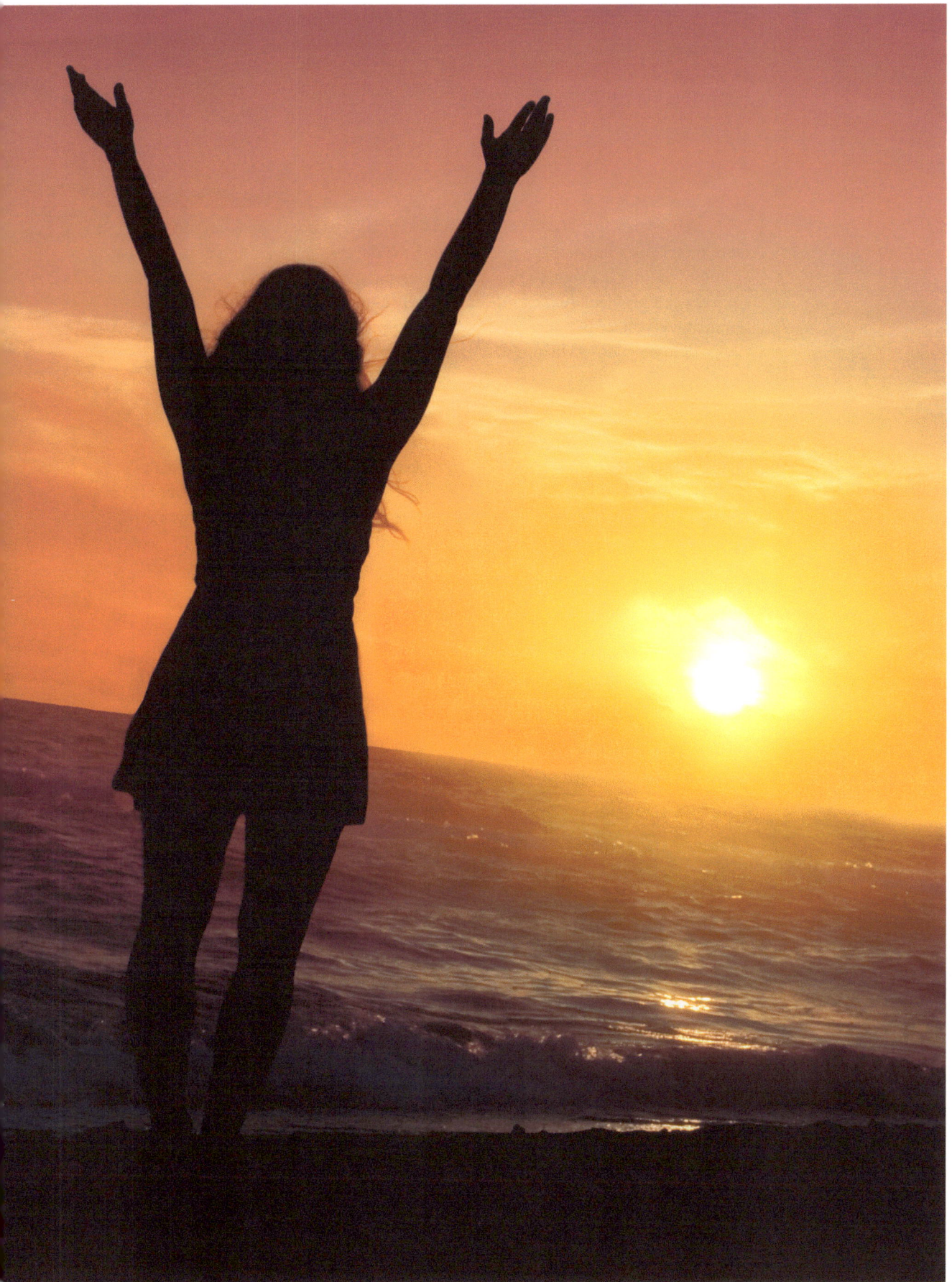

4. MENTAL HEALTH

According to World Health Organization, the burden of mental health illnesses is continuously growing. Mental and behavioral health disorders are common, affecting more than 25 percent of all people at some time during their lives and are present at any point in time in about 10 percent of the population. Depression is an important global health problem due to both its relatively high lifetime prevalence and the significant disability that it causes. By 2030, depression will be one of the leading causes of disease along with HIV/AIDS and heart disease (VicHealth, 2012).

4.1 Psychiatric Care

The only authorized organizations in Aruba that provide specialized psychiatric care are the Psychiatrische Afdeling Algemeen Ziekenhuis (Psychiatric department of the General Hospital / PAAZ), Sociaal Psychiatrische Dienst (Social Psychiatric Unit/ SPD of the Department of Public Health), Vrijgevestigde psychiaters (Independent Psychiatric Practitioners/ Balance) and the Coördinatie Bureau Drugs Bestrijding (Drug Prevention Coordination Bureau/ CBDB). The SPD and Balance are the two organizations that provide specialized service to the majority of the population in need of mental health care. Balance has the highest absolute number of patients (Staring, 2010).

According to the study by J. Staring the two major diagnoses, amongst the participant population (excluding PAAZ patients) 18 years and older, are schizophrenia and have other psychotic disorders and mood disorders as can be seen in Table 11. Together these two general diagnoses are responsible for 61.3 percent of the top ten diagnoses studied in the population. Other disorders that follow are bipolar disorders (7 %), anxiety disorders (6 %) and opioid disorders (4 %).

Table 11. Frequency and percentage of top 10 diagnoses.

Grouped Diagnoses	n	%
Schizophrenia and other psychotic disorders	284	34.2
Mood disorders	225	27.1
Bipolar disorders	56	6.7
Anxiety disorders	49	5.9
Other/unknown	40	4.8
Opioid-related disorders	34	4.1
Personality disorders	32	3.9
Adjustment disorders	22	2.6
Sleep disorders	13	1.6
Impulse-control disorders (Not elsewhere classified)	13	1.6

In the table above, approximately 284 persons were diagnosed with schizophrenia (excluding PAAZ) in the Aruban population. About one in five of the participant population who suffered from schizophrenia and other psychotic disorders was between 50 and 55 years of age (Figure 52).

As shown in Figure 53 schizophrenia was more common among men than women. When compared to the United States of America (USA Schizophrenia affects men and women with equal frequency (NHIMH, n.d.). In the Netherlands it is more common among men than women; however this was reversed for the ages 60 years and older.

As for mood disorders, these disorders may involve depression only (also referred to as "unipolar depression") or they may include manic episodes (as in bipolar disorder, which is classically known as "manic depressive illness"). Individuals with mood disorders suffer significant distress or impairment in social, occupational, educational or other important areas of functioning. Worldwide, major depression is the leading cause of years lived with disability, and the fourth cause of disability-adjusted life years (DALY's) (PHAC, 2002).

As depicted in Table 11 approximately 225 persons have mood disorders representing 27 percent of the total diagnoses studied in the Aruban population. As seen in Figure 54 these disorders are more frequent in the age group 45–49 years of age. Furthermore, mood disorders are by far more common among the female population than the male population (Figure 53).

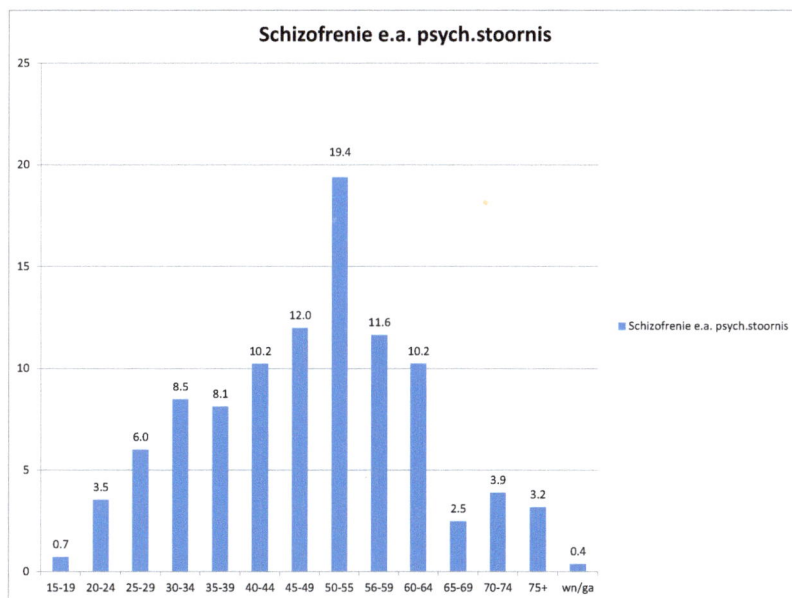

Figure 52. Schizophrenia and other psychotic disorders by age category in percentage, Aruba 2010.

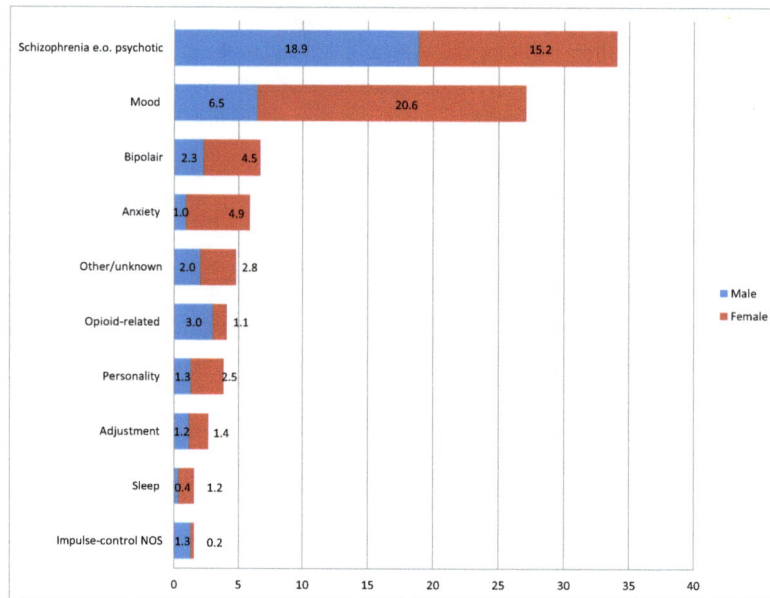

Figure 53. Percentage diagnoses DSMV-IV by sex, Aruba 2010.

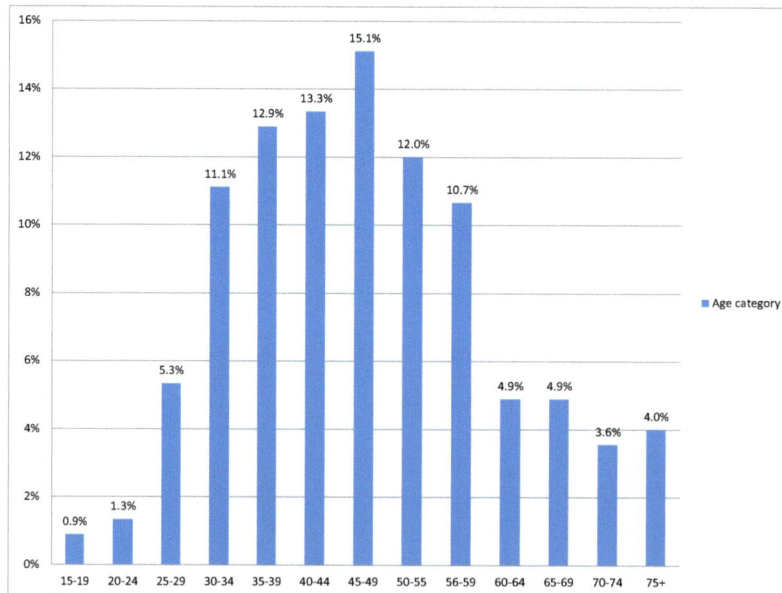

Figure 54. Mood disorders per age category.

As mentioned before mood disorders include Major Depressive Disorder. According to the National Institute of Mental Health this disorder is the leading cause of disability in the United States of America for ages 15–44. Major Depressive Disorder affects approximately 14.8 million American adults, or about 6.7 percent of the U.S. population age 18 and older in a given year.

4.2 Self-Reported Mental Health

According to the STEPS survey conducted in 2006 there was an increase recorded in 2006 of number of persons with psychological issues including, loneliness, sleep problems, and anger compared to 2001. The respondents scored particularly high on sleeplessness (18 %), loneliness (19.3 %) and anger (18.6 %). Typically, women have higher rates of depression and anxiety disorders. On the other hand men have higher levels of substance abuse or anti-social disorders.

Self-reported psychological problems STEPS investigation 2006:

- 1 in 4 persons aged 25–64 years complained about psychological problems(stress, depression and fear).

- Women have more complaints about their mental well-being than men; and younger adults more than persons 55–64 years of age.

- People with lower education are twice more likely to indicate they have mental problems than persons with VWO or higher.

- People who think of themselves as being fat have twice the likelihood of complaining about psychological problems.

- Psychological complaints are closely related to high blood pressure and cholesterol.

- Psychological well-being and physical health proved to be connected. Psychological problems were found to be closely related to headaches/migraines and stomach ailment.

- 1 in 5 persons have problems with sleeping.

- 1 in 5 persons often feel lonely.

4.3 Suicidal Behavior

Every year, almost one million people die from suicide; a "global" mortality rate of 16 per 100,000 or one death every 40 seconds. Although traditionally suicide rates have been highest among the elderly male, rates among young people have been increasing to such an extent that they are now the group at highest risk worldwide.

The countries with the highest suicide rates are those in Eastern Europe such as Estonia, Latvia, and Lithuania.

Mental disorders (particularly depression and alcohol abuse disorders) are a major risk factor for suicide in Europe and North America. Suicide is complexed with psychological, social, biological, cultural and environmental factors involved. The World Health Organization estimates for the year 2020, 1.53 million people will die from suicide, and 10–20 times more people will attempt suicide worldwide. This represents an average of one death every 20 seconds and one attempt every 1–2 seconds, making suicide a serious public health issue.

4.3.1 Suicide

According to mortality data from the Department of Public Health of Aruba from 2000 through 2009 a total of 61 persons died as a result of suicide, an average of 6 persons per year, see Figure 55.

It was exceptionally more frequent among men than women, on average 5 males versus 1 female per year. Mortality due to suicide occurred mostly among the age group of 30–39 years. The prevalence of suicide in Aruba in 2009 was of 3.6 per 100,000 inhabitants, see Figure 56.

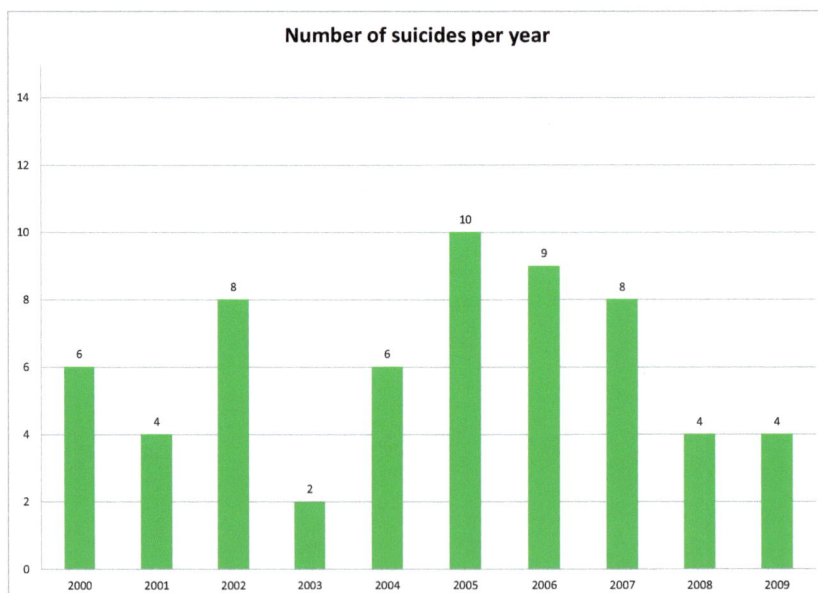

Figure 55. Number of suicides per year, Aruba 2000–2009.

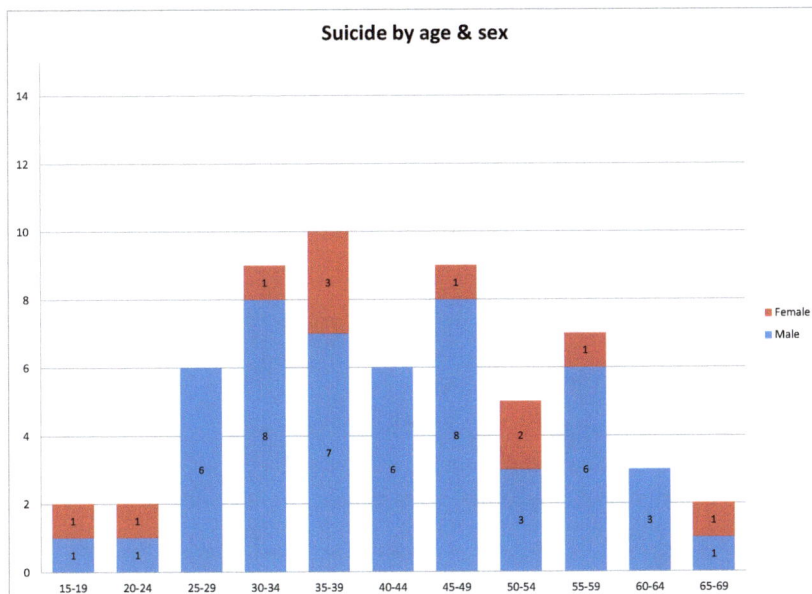

Figure 56. Suicides by age and sex Aruba, 2000–2010.

In the Netherlands during the period of 2003–2007 an average of 1000 men and 470 women committed suicide. In 2011 the suicide rate was 9.9 per 100.000 inhabitants. Suicide was more frequent among men, mainly between the ages of 40–60 years.

In the U.S. the overall rate was 11.3 suicide deaths per 100,000 people. Almost four times as many males as females die by suicide. In 2007, it was also the third leading cause of death for young people ages 15 to 24.

4.4 Para Suicide (Attempted Suicide)

As many studies done worldwide showed that parasuicide is an apparent attempt at suicide, commonly called a suicidal gesture, in which the aim is not death. For example, a sub lethal drug overdose or wrists slash. Parasuicidal behavior refers to suicidal attempts or other deliberate self-inflicted injuries with or without suicide intent. Parasuicide behavior is considered as a risk factor for suicide. Borderline personality disorder (BPD) is highly associated with parasuicidal behavior.

Para suicide is more common among women, particularly women younger than 45 years, and to be more specific those women between the ages of 15 and 25 years. This is in contrast with suicide, where men are the majority. The highest rates of parasuicide are found in divorced women, single, or teenage wives, and is often linked to poverty. Most cases of parasuicide are associated with mental health problems, particularly: depression, alcoholism and personality disorder.

Other factors that make an act of parasuicide more likely include:

- Relationship Problems
- Being Unemployed
- Being Physically ill, particularly epileptic
- Being Mentally Handicapped
- Being Neglected or Abused by Parents
- Having a Parent deceased at a young age
- Coping with a loved one's illness

According to data obtained from the H. Oduber Hospital 38 persons were hospitalized in 2009 for attempted suicide of which 21 were female and 17 were male. In 2010 this number increased to 53 persons, of whom 31 were female and 22 male (Figure 57).

During 2009 most of the cases of attempted suicide, 23.6%, occurred in the age category of 25–29 years. In 2010 the age category in which most of the cases occurred, 26.4%, was 15–19 years, see Figure 58.

The most frequent means used to attempt suicide in 2009 was by ingesting analgesics, antipyretics and antirheumatics. In 2010 the most frequent means were other specified drugs and medicinal substances, see Figure 59.

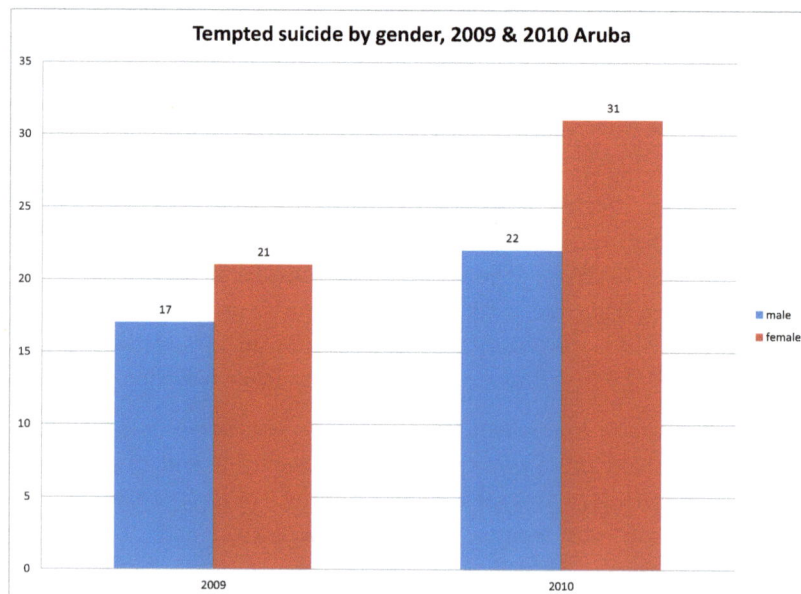

Figure 57. Attempted suicides by gender, Aruba 2009.

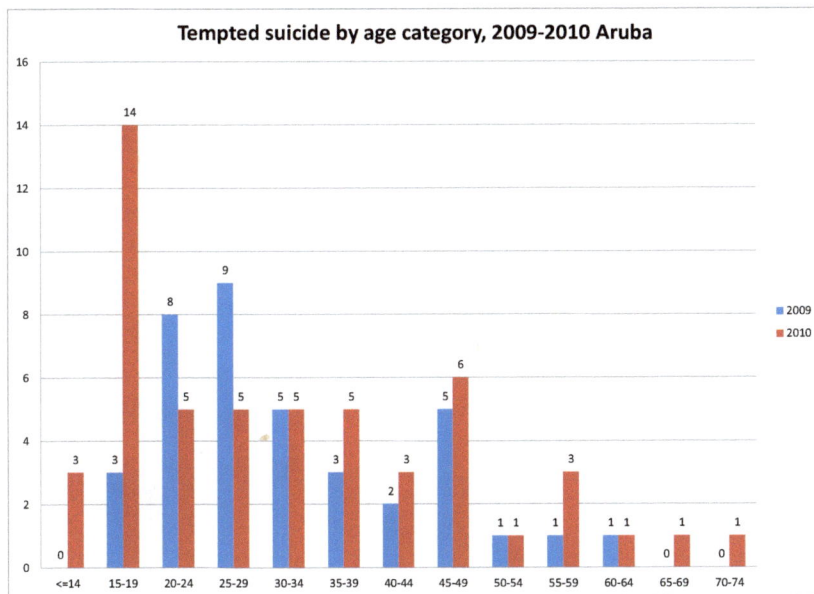

Figure 58. Tempted suicide by age category, Aruba 2009–2010.

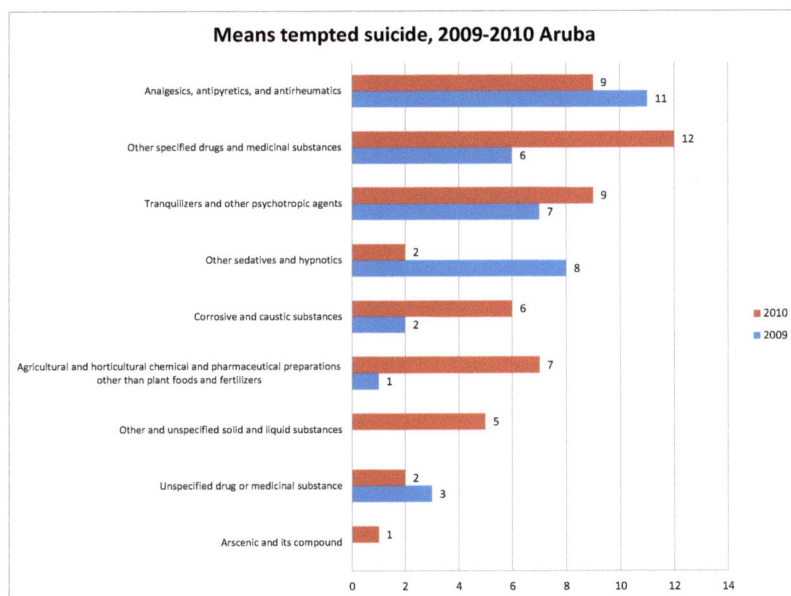

Figure 59. Means tempted suicide, Aruba 2009–2010.

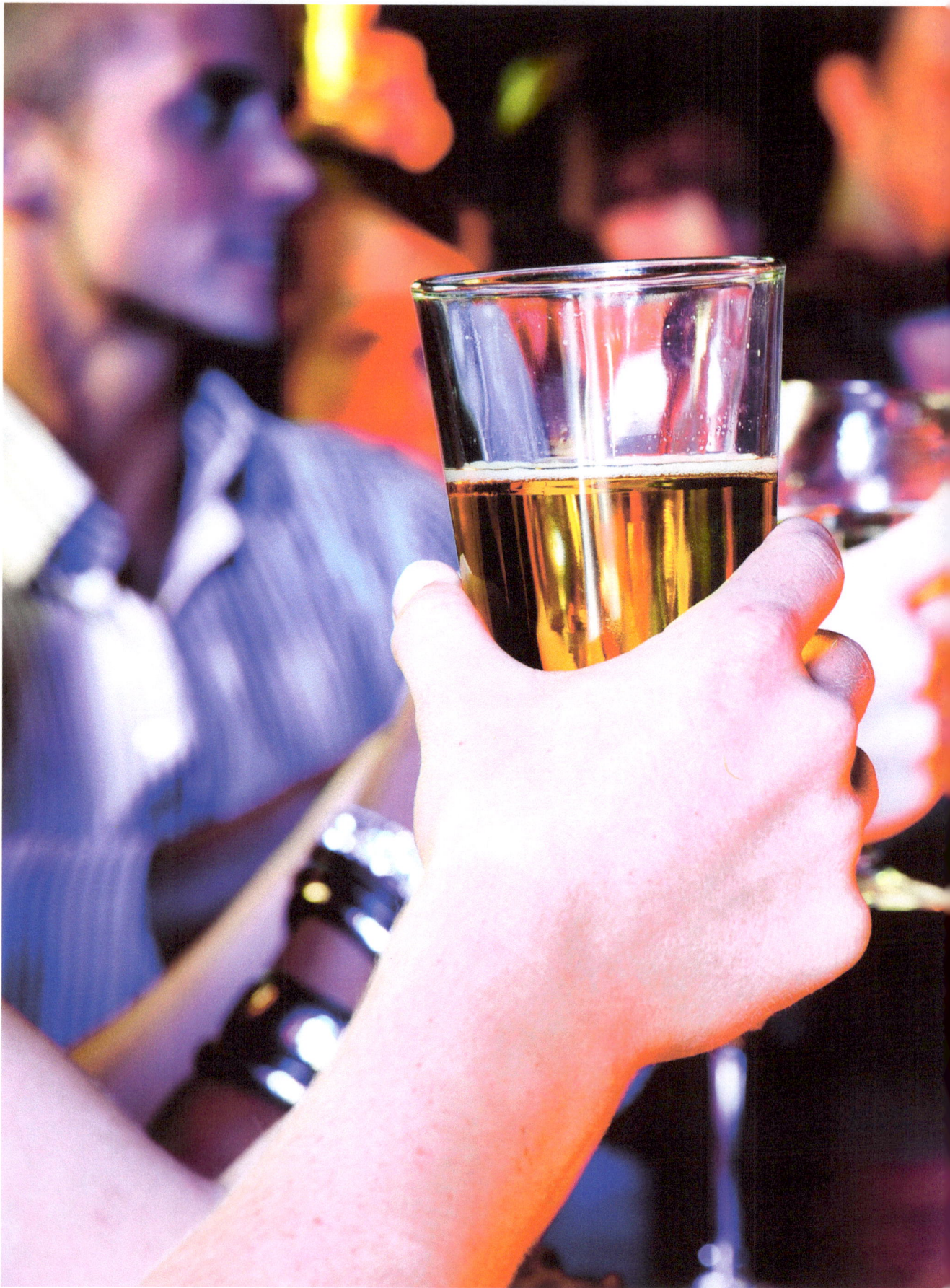

5. LIFESTYLE

5.1 Physical Activity

Lack of physical activity is a major risk factor for developing chronic non-communicable diseases. According to estimations of the WHO, physical inactivity is the direct cause of 10 to 16 percent of all cases of breast cancer, colon cancers, and diabetes and of 22 percent of all cases of ischemic heart disease (WHO, 2003). On the other hand, regular physical activity is associated with a wide range of physical, social, economic, and mental health benefits.

In Aruba, the most recent figures on the physical activity of the population were obtained via the 2006 STEPS Aruba Risk factor & Behavior Survey which assessed the risk factors associated with the development of chronic non-communicable diseases in persons between 25 and 64 years of age. The data obtained indicated that these individuals spent, on average, 2 hours and 17.7 minutes per day on physical activity, which included time spent doing physical activity at work, travelling from one place to another and recreating. The majority of this time was spent on low and moderate levels of physical activity. Only 9.5 minutes per day were spent on high levels of physical activity (see Figure 60 A).

On the other hand, more than 4 hours and 58.6 minutes per day were spent on sedentary activities, including sitting and reclining at home, sitting at a desk,

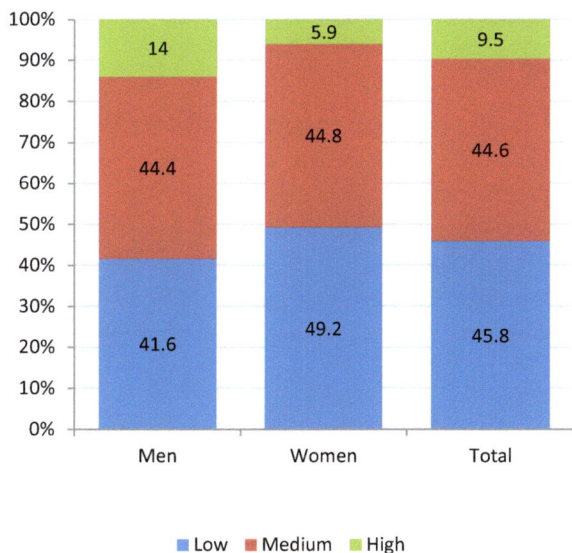

Figure 60A. The proportion of time spent per day on low, moderate and high levels of physical activity.

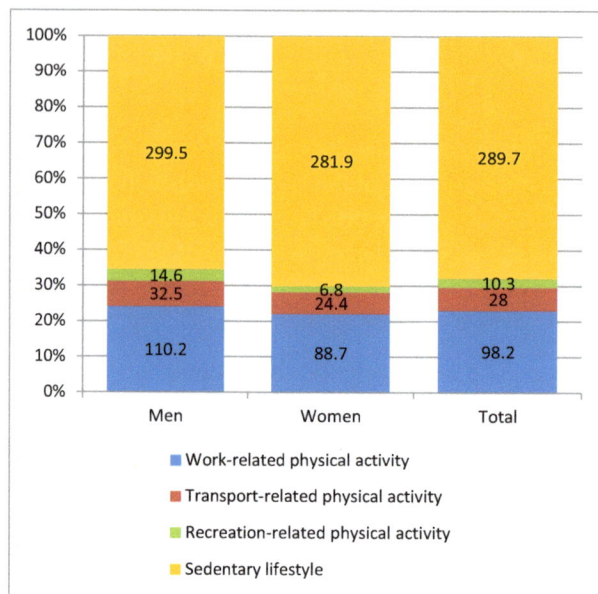

Figure 60B. The proportion of time spent per day on different types of physical activity.

travelling in a car, watching television (see Figure 60 B). Overall, those who reported spending significantly less time on physical activities were: women, persons born in Aruba, persons between 55 and 64 years of age and persons who were not employed.

5.1.1 Work-Related Physical Activity

In a typical week, persons between 25 and 64 years of age reported spending 1 hour and 38.2 minutes per day on work-related physical activity. The time spent on work-related physical activity was primarily related to occupation, skilled agricultural workers and fishery workers, craft and related trade workers and persons with elementary occupations reported spending significantly more time per day on work-related physical activity. Those who reported spending significantly less time per day on work-related physical activities were: professionals, associate professionals, technicians and clerks.

Overall, more time was spent per day on moderate levels of work-related physical activity (57.4 minutes per day) than on vigorous levels of work-related physical activity (40.4 minutes per day), women spending twice as much time on moderate levels of work-related physical activity than on vigorous levels of work-related physical activity.

5.1.2 Transport Related Physical Activity

For transport-related physical activity, persons between 25 and 64 years of age reported spending, in a typical week, 28.0 minutes per day on activities such as walking or using a bicycle to travel from one place to another. Overall, the results of the STEPS 2006 Risk Factor Behavior Survey showed that employed persons, persons living in the upper central area of Aruba (Santa Cruz), and persons with a low personal income reported spending significantly more time on transport-related physical activity.

5.1.3 Recreation Related Physical Activity

On average, the STEPS 2006 revealed that 10.3 minutes per day were spent on recreation-related (leisure) physical activities, such as walking, cycling, swimming, volleyball and football. Men reported spending significantly more time on recreation-related physical activities than women and younger persons reported spending more time on recreation-related activities compared to older persons.

5.1.4 Sedentary Activities

Overall, persons between 25 and 64 years of age reported spending the majority of their time on sedentary activities, such as sitting and reclining at home, or with friends, sitting at a desk at work, travelling in a car, reading, playing computer games, and watching television. In total, 4 hours and 49.7 minutes per day were spent on sedentary activities. Persons between 35 and 44 years of age, persons born in Aruba, and persons with a high level of education reported spending significantly more time on sedentary activities.

5.2 Nutrition

Unhealthy diet is clearly related to a range of risk factors that are directly or indirectly related to the development of chronic health conditions, such as cardiovascular disease, stroke, high blood pressure, high blood cholesterol, type 2 diabetes, bowel conditions, and certain types of cancer.

Overconsumption of foods in general and of energy-rich products in particular, is the root of the problem. Food products high in fats, salt and sugar, and low in dietary fibers, complex carbohydrates, and essential vitamins and minerals are nowadays in most westernized countries part of the daily menu.

5.2.1 The Consumption of Fruits And Vegetables

According to the World Health Organization, low fruit and vegetable intake is among the top 10 risk factors contributing to global mortality. Nutritional experts (WHO,

CDC) recommend consuming at least 400 grams (5 servings) of fruits and vegetables per day for the prevention of chronic diseases. In Aruba, the STEPS 2006 Health Survey revealed that persons between 25 and 64 years of age reported consuming fruits on an average 4 days per week and vegetables on an average of 6 days per week. Compared to data obtained during the 2001 Health Survey this indicates a slight decrease in the consumption frequency of fruits and a slight increase in the consumption frequency of vegetables (see Figure 61 A).

However, participants to STEPS 2006 reported consuming on average only 0.8 servings of fruit and 1 serving of vegetables per day. The majority reported consuming between 1 and 3 combined servings of fruits and vegetables per day. Only 2.4 percent reported adhering to the recommended 5 combined serving of fruits and vegetables per day. The results indicated furthermore that both the frequency and the number of fruits consumed were related to age, sex, country of birth, and level of education. Women, persons between 55 and 64 years of age, persons not born in Aruba and persons with a high level of education consumed fruits on a higher frequency and in larger amounts. Where the consumption of vegetables was concerned, the level of education was the sole variable related to both the frequency and the number of vegetables consumed. Persons with a higher level of education reported consuming vegetables on a higher frequency and in larger amounts.

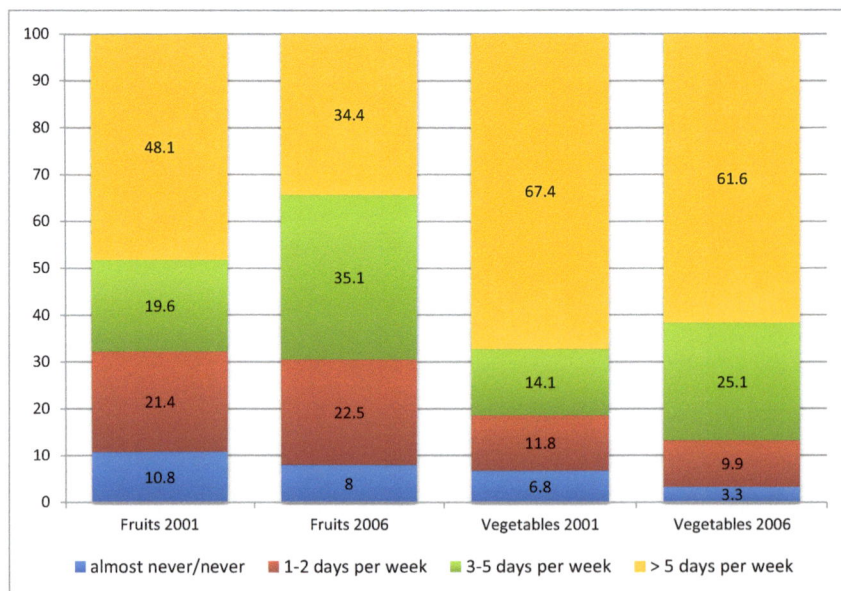

Figure 61A. The frequency of consumption of fruits and vegetables, Aruba 2001–2006.

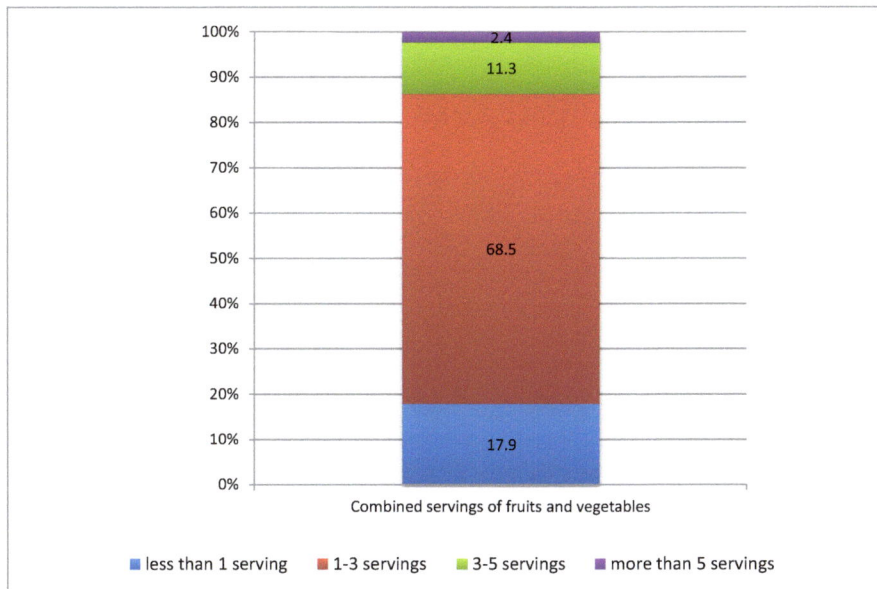

Figure 61B. The number of combined servings of fruits and vegetables, 2006

5.2.2 Use of Oil or Fat For Meal Preparation

The relationship between the intake of dietary fats and chronic non-communicable diseases has been extensively studied, particularly where cardiovascular disease is concerned. Research indicates that the intake of dietary fats strongly influences the risk of cardiovascular disease. The intake of saturated fatty acids, in particular, is directly related to cardiovascular risk. In addition, a high intake of saturated fats has been linked to a higher risk of impaired glucose tolerance, and higher fasting and insulin levels. The STEPS 2006 revealed that the majority (82.4 percent) of persons between 25 and 64 years of age used vegetable oil for meal preparation. Only 0.4 percent reported using mostly lard (see Figure 62).

5.3 Weight and Overweight

Since 1980 obesity has more than doubled worldwide. More than 1.4 billion adults (older than 20 years) were overweight in 2008. Of these, more women compared to men were overweight, 300 million and 200 million respectively (WHO, 2012). 65% of the world population lives in countries where obesity kills more people compared to underweight. Not forget to mention that more than 40 million children under the age of five are overweight (WHO, 2012).

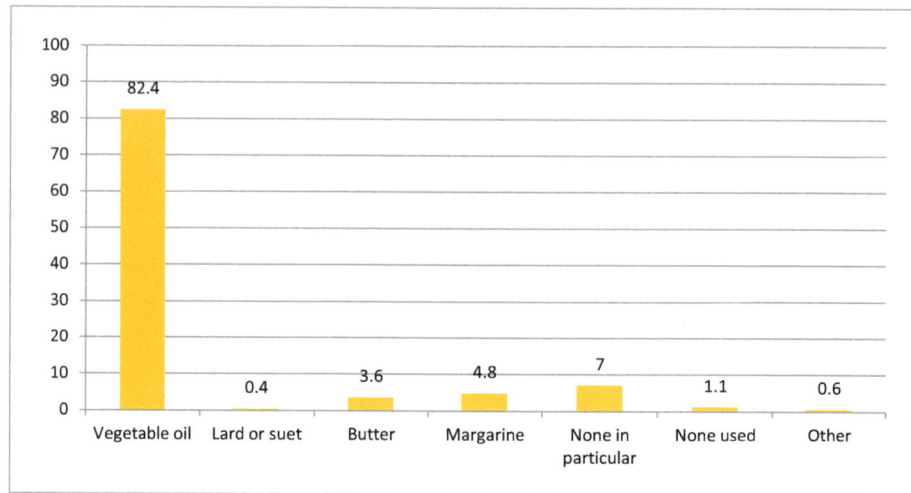

Figure 62. Percentage using certain types of oil or fat most often for meal preparation.

WHO defines overweight as the following:

- BMI greater than or equal to 25 is overweight

- BMI greater than or equal to 30 is obese.

The BMI or Body mass index is a simple index for weight-height used for classification of overweight and obesity.

$$BMI = \frac{\text{Weight in Kg}}{(\text{height in m})^2}$$

5.3.1 Overweight and Obesity — School Population

All school children in Aruba undergo a health-screening at school done by the Youth Health Care Unit of the DPH during the second year of pre-school and in the 5th grade of primary school. Part of this screening consists of weighing, measuring and calculating Body Mass Index (BMI).

Aruba has a high percentage of overweight and obesity among the adult population as showed by the STEPS Aruba Risk Factor & Behavior Survey. Among schoolchildren, the fifth graders, these percentages are also elevated.

Table 12 shows that from 2007 to 2010, the percentage of boys who are overweight has slowly decreased, this is the same for boys who are obese. However the decrease in the percentage of obese boys was more steadily as compared to the decrease in the percentage of overweight boys.

Table 12. Percentage weight status preschoolers by gender, Aruba 2007–2010.

	2007	2008	2009	2010				
	Girls	Boys	Girls	Boys	Girls	Boys	Girls	Boys
n	624	652	590	619	528	638	633	678
Underweight	10.9%	13.3%	13.4%	14.9%	11.9%	15.7%	10.4%	11.1%
Normal weight	64.4%	61.3%	63.4%	64.1%	65.3%	63.9%	64.0%	71.1%
Overweight	14.3%	12.0%	12.5%	10.2%	12.0%	11.6%	13.9%	9.4%
Obese	10.4%	13.3%	10.7%	10.8%	10.8%	8.8%	11.7%	8.4%

The percentage of girls in preschool who are overweight decreased slightly and was followed by an increase during this same period of time. The percentage for obese girls is showing a slight increase from 2007 to 2010, from 10.4 percent to 11.7 percent, see Figure 63.

The percentages of overweight and obese boys seem to decrease over the years contrary to the percentages of the girls which seem to be increasing. Overall the percentages of girls who are overweight and obese are higher than the boys. This is similar to the international findings of Markus and Hirasing 2010 (Markus & Hirasing, 2010).

Fifth graders have higher percentages of overweight and obesity as compared to the preschoolers. During 2008 to 2010, the percentage of overweight boys increased from 20.8 percent in 2008 to 27.5 percent in 2010. However the percentage of obese boys have decreased during this same period from 18.6 percent to 14.9 percent, see Table 13.

Again girls in the 5th grade show a different trend in overweight and obesity, where the percentage of overweight girls increased from 23.3 percent in 2008 to 26.6 percent in 2010, this is a 3.3 percent increase. Also the percentage of obese girls has also increased during this same period, from 15.6% to 16.4%, see Figure 64.

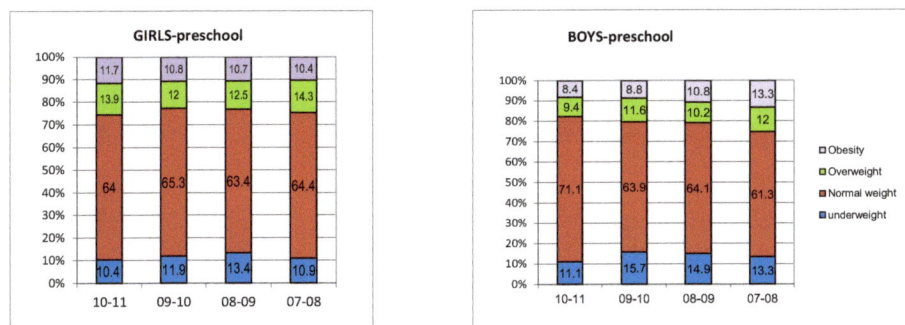

Figure 63. Percentage of obesity and overweight in preschool children, Aruba 2007–2010.

Table 13. Percentage weight status 5th graders by gender 2008–2010.

	2008		2009		2010	
	Girls	**Boys**	**Girls**	**Boys**	**Girls**	**Boys**
n	546	553	703	698	538	557
Underweight	7.3%	6.0%	8.1%	6.6%	6.1%	5.4%
Normal weight	53.8%	54.6%	53.3%	48.1%	50.9%	52.2%
Overweight	23.3%	20.8%	25.2%	26.9%	26.6%	27.5%
Obese	15.6%	18.6%	13.4%	18.3%	16.4%	14.9%

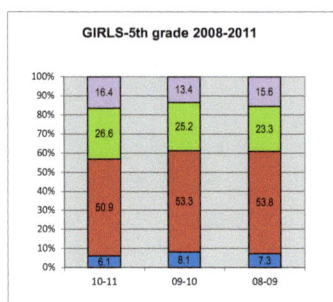

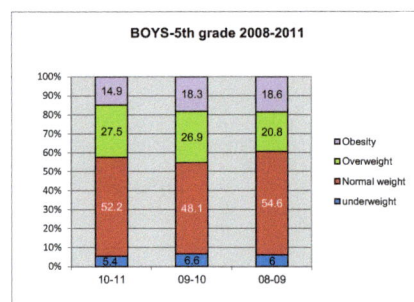

Figure 64. Percentages of obesity and overweight in 5th grade school children, Aruba 2008–2010.

It is noted overall that preschoolers have a higher percentage of boys and girls who have a normal weight. A proportion of about 10% becomes overweight in the 5th grade. This is showed in the high percentage of overweight boys and girls in the 5th grade.

5.3.2 Overweight Adults

In 2001, the Health Survey showed that Aruban men between 25 and 64 years old weighed on average 86.6 kg, while women weighed 74.3 kg. Their average lengths were respectively 1.73 and 1.61 meter. The STEPS-survey conducted in 2006 found exactly the same average length for men and women as in 2001. However, the mean weight of men had increased to 90.4 kg. Women remained more or less at the same weight (74.6 kg).

Table 14 presents the average BMI-values for persons by age and sex. The STEPS research shows that in 2006 Aruba has reached the point where the average adult male is obese. The average BMI-value for males aged 25-64 years is currently 30, for females this is 28.8. In 2001, the Health Survey found an average BMI of 29.0 for men and 28.9 for women. From a young age on, the average male is seriously overweight.

In age-group 25–34 years, the mean BMI is already 29.8. At that age women are also overweight, but to a lesser extent than men (BMI 27.0).

Table 14. Average BMI values by age and sex, STEPS Aruba 2006.

Men	Women	Total
29.8	27	28.3
30.5	28.4	29.3
29	30.3	29.7
31.4	30.2	30.7
30	28.8	29.3

5.3.2.1 The Super Obese

The International Classification of adult underweight, overweight and obesity according to BMI of the World Health Organization further divides the obesity group into the following categories:

- Category I with BMI 30–34.9
- Category II with BMI 35–39.9
- Category III with BMI > 40

Table 15. BMI categories including subcategories obesity, by sex.

	Men	Women	Total
	%	%	%
BMI < 20	1.1	4.2	2.8
BMI < 20–24.99	16.1	23.8	20.5
BMI <25–29.99	36.1	36	36.1
BMI <30–34.99	30.8	21.6	25.5
BMI <35–39.99	11.7	7.7	9.4
BMI 40+	4.2	6.8	5.7
Total	100.0	100.0	100.0
No of cases	326	488	814

The above table shows the percentage of males and females by BMI categories, including the three obesity subcategories. It is very worrisome that no less than 15.1 percent of Aruba's adult population between 25 and 65 years fall within the categories of obesity with very high or extreme high health risks. A higher proportion of men than women fall within the category of obesity with high health risk (30.8 percent against 21.6 percent). At the very high levels of obesity (Cat. II and III) the total proportion of both sexes is almost equal. Although the percentage with a BMI above 40 is higher for women, the difference is so small that it can easily be attributed to small sample variability.

Although in the Netherlands six in ten men and nearly half of the women are overweight, obesity is more common in other EU countries (Blokstra et al., 2011, IOTF-Prevalence Data, 2012). The most unfavorable situation is in Spain, England, Scotland, and Ireland, with an approximate 70 percent of overweight males.

In the Netherlands 13 percent of men and 14 percent of women are seriously overweight (obese). As in other EU countries this percentage is higher in men (16.4 percent) and women (15.9 percent) with a relatively low educational level (Blokstra et al., 2011). In most other EU countries, obesity is more common than in the Netherlands. England and Scotland have the highest percentages: one in four adults is obese.

5.4 Tobacco and Alcohol Use

According to the World Health Organization, smoking and other forms of tobacco use are the second major cause of death in the world, given that they are the major cause of many of the world's top killer diseases, such as heart and vascular diseases, different types of cancer, and respiratory diseases. Tobacco is also linked to huge economic costs, given high public and private expenses to treat tobacco-caused diseases, decreased productivity of ill tobacco users, and untimely death of tobacco users.

On the other hand, the consumption of alcohol has been demonstrated in numerous studies to have both beneficial and detrimental effects on health and well-being. The detrimental effects of alcohol consumption appear with start with the 88 use of 2 to 3 alcoholic beverages per day. However, not only the volume of alcohol consumed is relevant when investigating the effect of alcohol on health, but also the pattern of consumption of alcohol is important. Binge drinking in particular has been linked with a number of negative health outcomes, including alcohol-related accidents, mental distress, higher odds of overweight and obesity and worse health-related quality of life.

5.4.1 Tobacco Use Among Adults

According to data collected during the STEPS 2006 Health Survey, 16.2 percent of persons between 25 and 64 years of age smoked tobacco, of which the majority smoked daily (77.8 percent). The prevalence of smoking and of daily smoking was twice as high among men (22.4 percent, and 17.2 percent) as among women (11.2 percent, and 8.9 percent). In addition, men started smoking earlier in life (at 18 years of age) when compared to women (at 21 years of age). Men also reported having smoked for a longer period of time than women (26 years and 22 years, respectively) and smoking more manufactured cigarettes per day than women (18 cigarettes and 10 cigarettes, respectively).

Overall, the prevalence of current smokers in Aruba was relatively low when compared to that in the United States and the Netherlands, especially where women were concerned. In total, 11.2 percent of women reported being current smokers during the STEPS 2006 Health Survey, compared to 18.4 percent of women in the United States and 25.3 percent in the Netherlands (see Figure 65).

5.4.2 Tobacco Use Among Youth

Tobacco use is one of the main risk factors for a number of chronic diseases, including cancer, lung diseases, and cardiovascular diseases (WHO, 2012). According to the Youth Health Survey 2012, 27.9 percent ($n = 1330$) of the youth attending secondary school have ever tried a cigarette.

Most of them (38.5 percent; $n = 512$) tried their first cigarette when they were between 13 and 15 years of age. It is remarkable that 48.1 percent of the youth were younger than 12 years when they tried a cigarette for the first time. More than half of the youth, who ever smoked, were males (51.5 percent). Of these secondary school going youth between 12 and 19 years of age, the majority who ever smoked are between 15–17 years of age (56.5 percent; $n = 751$), whereas 25.3 percent of them are 14 years or younger.

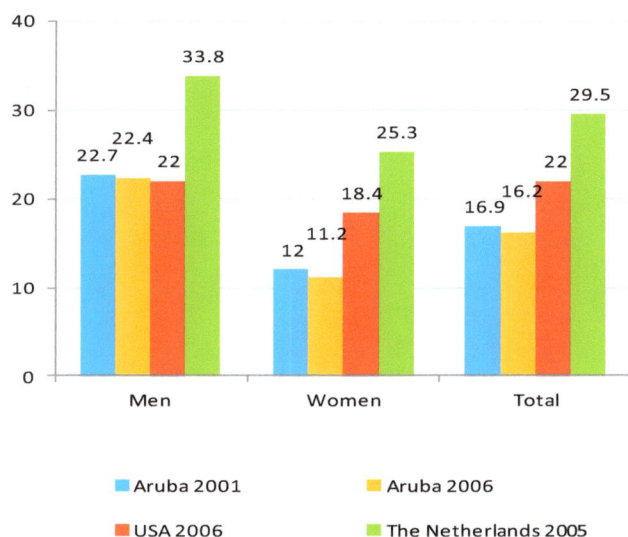

Figure 65. Youth who ever smoked by age category and gender, YHS Aruba 2012.

According to data collected, 4 percent ($n = 123$) of the youth stated that they smoked one cigarette or more per day during the last 30 days and 2 percent ($n = 93$) have stated to have smoked less than one cigarette per day during the last month. The majority of the youth stated that they have been smoking for 1–5 days during the last month (3.9 percent; $n = 184$). Only 0.7 percent of the youth who ever smoked stated that during the last 30 days they were smoking more than 20 days ($n = 33$).

5.4.3 Alcohol Use Among Adults

During the STEPS 2006 Health Survey, 52.9 percent of men and 26.6 percent of women between 25 and 64 years of age reported consuming alcohol in the month prior to the survey and were categorized as current drinkers. On the other hand, 21.9 percent of men and 38.5 percent of women reported never having used alcohol (see Figure 66).

The majority of persons, who reported having consumed alcohol in the year prior to the survey, reported consuming alcohol less than once a month (61.1 percent). Only 4.1 percent reported using alcohol on a daily basis. However, it is important to mention that there was again a significant difference between men and women in the frequency of alcohol consumption (see Figure 67). For example, whilst 0.6 percent of women reported consuming alcohol on a daily basis, 7.1 percent of men did.

When consuming alcohol, men reported consuming, on average, as many as 6.9 standard alcoholic beverages a day, nearly twice as many as women who reported

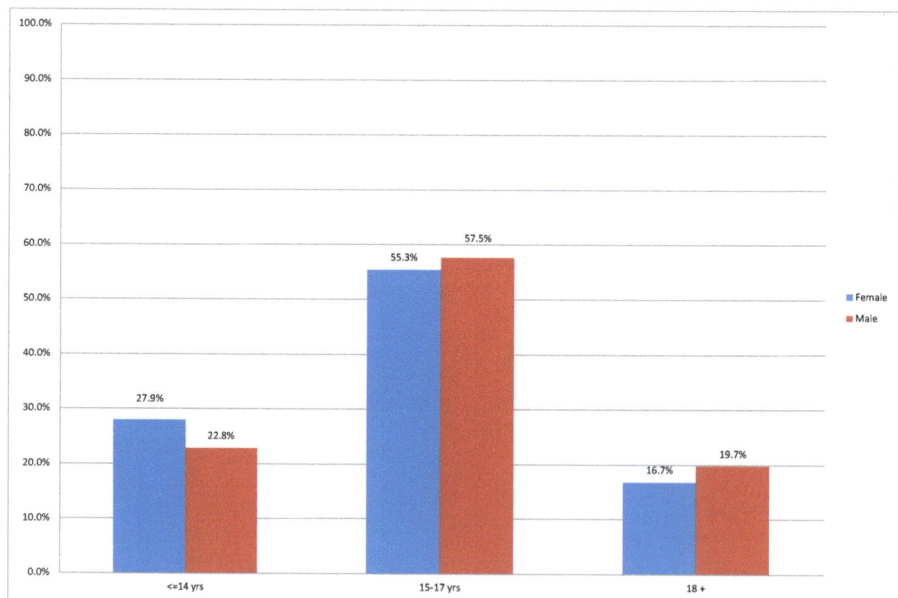

Figure 66. Youth who ever drank alcohol by age category and gender, YHS Aruba 2012.

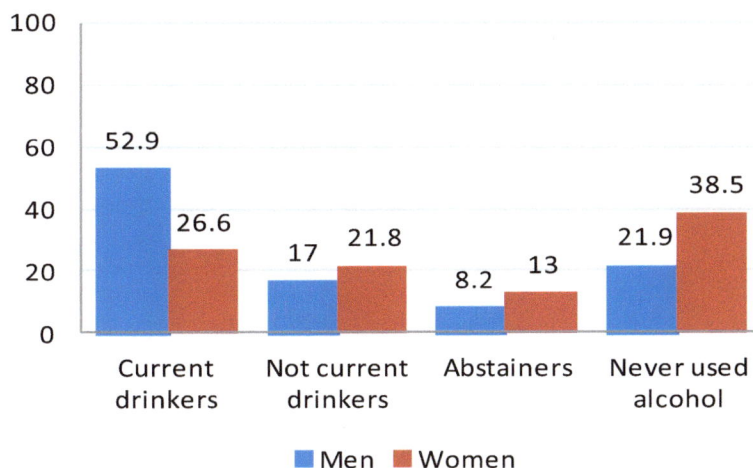

Figure 67. Men and women categorized according to their alcohol use, Steps 2006 Health Survey

consuming 3.6 alcoholic beverages a day. Moreover, 50.2 percent of men reported consuming 6 or more standard alcoholic beverages a day when consuming alcohol, compared to 17.8 percent of women. Particularly during the weekend, relatively more alcoholic beverages were consumed per day, especially where men were concerned.

Further analysis of the number of alcoholic beverages men and women reported consuming on a single occasion revealed that 15.0 percent of men and 7.8 percent of women could be categorized as binge drinkers given that they reported consuming respectively 5 or more (men), and 4 or more (women) alcoholic beverages on a single occasion. However, when taking into account the group of men and women who reported having consumed alcohol in the month prior to the survey, 73.7 percent of these men and 55.0 percent of these women could be categorized as binge drinkers.

It is also important to mention that the age at which young people start using alcohol is a powerful predictor of alcohol-related harm, abusive consumption of alcohol, and the development of alcohol-related disorders. During the STEPS 2006 Health Survey, men reported having started consuming alcohol at age 18 and women at age 21, which is relatively later in life when compared to the United States and the Netherlands, where persons start using alcohol at the mean age of 14 years and 16.5 years, respectively.

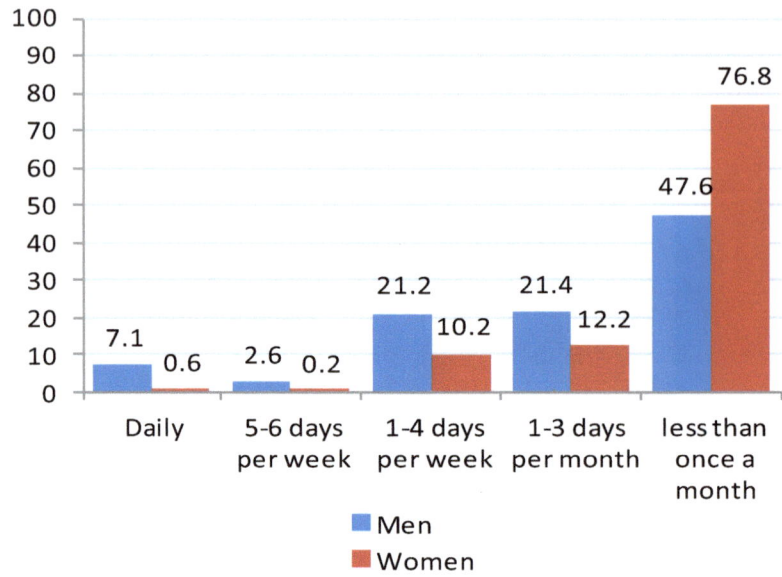

Figure 68. The frequency of alcohol consumption in the year prior to the Steps 2006 Health Survey, by gender.

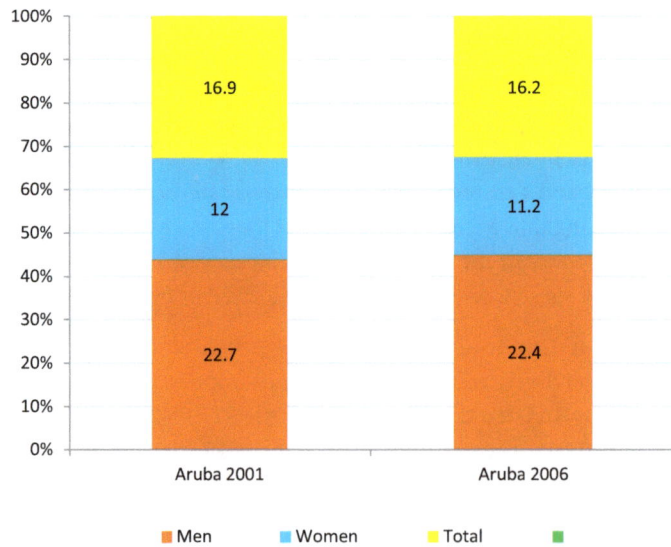

Figure 69. Amount of alcoholic beverages consumed per day when consuming alcohol, by gender.

5.4.4 Alcohol Use Among Youth

The harmful use of alcohol results in 2.5 million deaths each year. According to the WHO, 320 000 young people between the age of 15 and 29 die from alcohol-related causes, resulting in 9 percent of all deaths in that age group (WHO, 2012).

In Aruba, 70.2 percent (n = 3283) of the youth between 12-19 years stated that they tried alcohol, whereas 29.8 percent stated that they never drank alcohol.

Most of the teenagers who tried alcohol for the first time were 13 to 15 years of age, from which 52.5 percent were female and 47.5 percent were males. It has to be mentioned that more than 50 percent (56.1 percent) of the ones who ever tried alcohol were males who were less than 10 years old.

Analyzing the data in more detail, we see that females in the age category equal or less than 14 years old ever drank alcohol more than males in that same age category (31.5 percent compared to 29.6 percent). Both genders in the age category of 15–17 years old have stated that they have drunk alcohol (57.5 percent males versus 55.3 percent females; see Figure 70).

Furthermore, more than 60 percent of the youth between 15–17 years of age have been drinking at least one drink containing alcohol for 5 to 10 days during the last month. During the last 30 days, when they had been drinking alcohol, 63.5 percent (n = 99) of the females in the age category of 15–17 years said that they had drunk 5 or more drinks on the days they drank, whereas 64.7 percent of the males in the same age category drank only 3 drinks on the days they had been drinking.

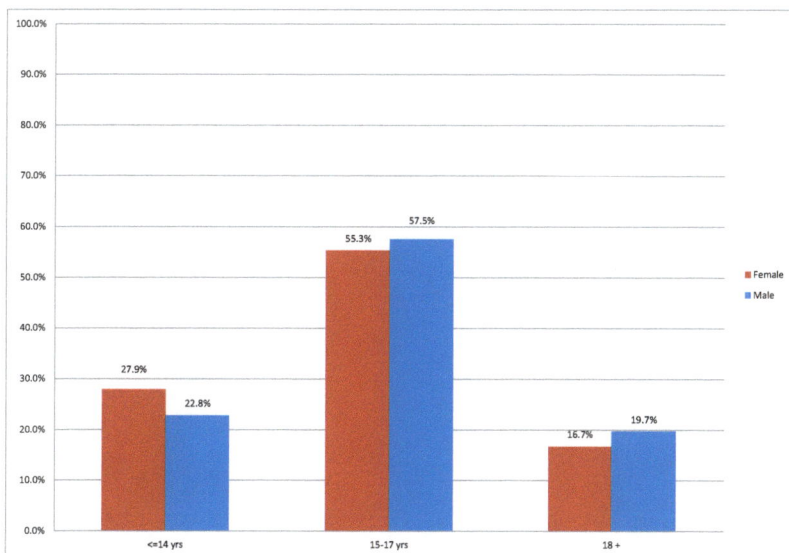

Figure 70. Youth who ever drank alcohol by age category and gender, YHS Aruba 2012.

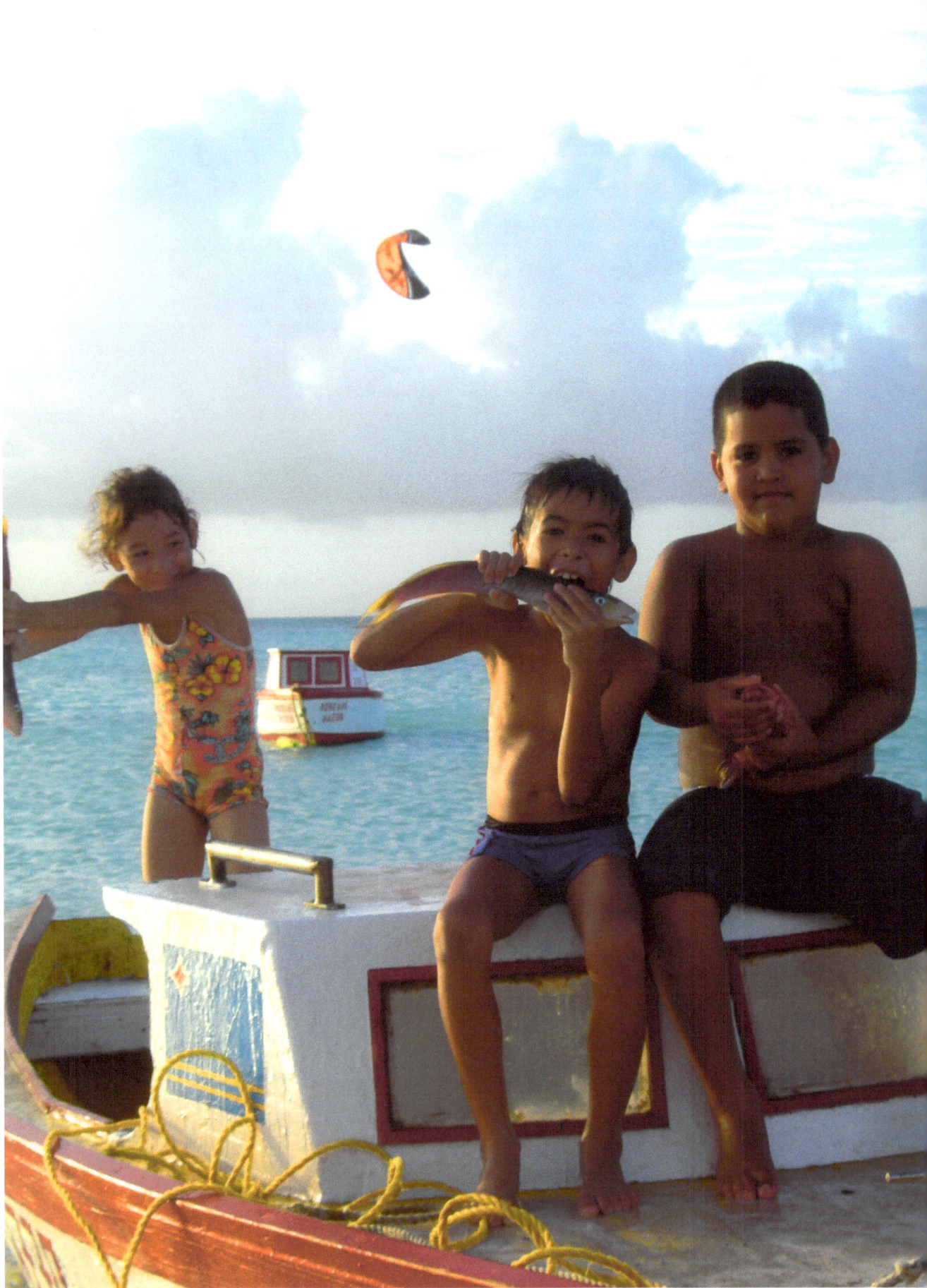

6. YOUTH HEALTH

In 2012, the Department of Public Health conducted a health survey among secondary school going youth between 12 and 19 years. A total of 4765 students participated and completed the questionnaire.

6.1 Drug Use

6.1.1 Cannabis

According to data from the Youth Health Survey, 15.5 percent of the respondents ($n = 724$) stated that they smoke marihuana, from which 46.5 percent are female ($n = 337$) and 53.5 percent are male ($n = 387$).

Further analysis shows that almost two thirds (59.5 percent, $n = 431$) of the studied population, who do smoke marihuana, are in the age category of 15–17 years. Besides more than half of the females (52.6 percent) in the age category younger than 14 years do smoke marihuana. In the older age categories 15–17 years and 18 + years, males have the highest percentages of smoking marihuana, 52.0 percent and 62.5 percent respectively.

When asked the age when they first tried marihuana, more than half, 51.4 percent, were between 13–15 years old when they first tried marihuana. A third (30.7 percent) was between 16 and 18 years. It is particular to mention that 5.4 percent of the studied youth had tried marihuana when they were less than 10 years old, see Table 16.

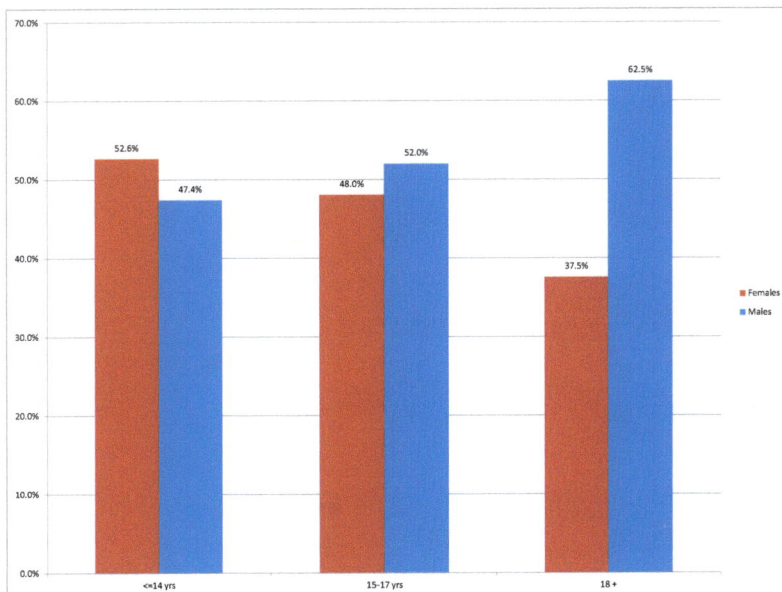

Figure 71. Marihuana use per age category by sex, YHS Aruba 2012.

However the fact that males have overall a higher percentage of marihuana use, a higher percentage of the females as compared to the males have tried marihuana once they are older than 18 years (58.3 percent), see Figure 72.

Table 16. Age category first tried marihuana.

Age first tried marihuana	Number	Percent
less than 10 years old	39	5.4
11 or 12 years old	79	10.9
13–15 years old	372	51.4
16–18 years old	222	30.7
older than 18 years	12	1.7
Total	724	100.0

The frequency of use during the life time is the highest at 1–2 times, 40.7 percent of the population who uses marihuana. More than one fifth of the ones who use marihuana, 23.3 percent has stated to have used marihuana more than 20 times during their lifetime. Figure 73 analyzed the frequency of use by gender. As this figure shows, males have a higher frequency of use as compared to the males, 50.6 percent have used 10–19 times and 68.3 percent more than 20 times during their live. Overall the boys between 12–19 years have the highest percentage of marihuana use and also the highest frequency of use.

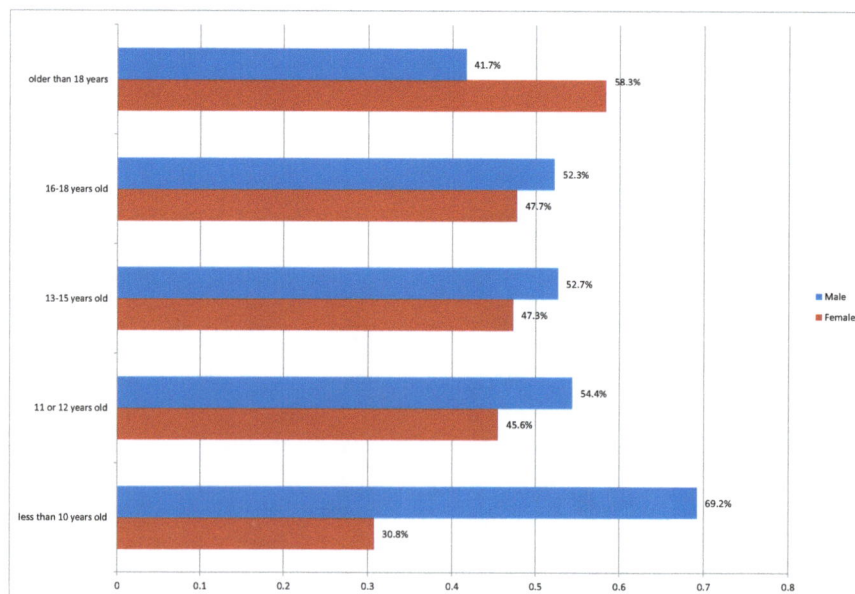

Figure 72. Age first tried marihuana by age and sex, YHS Aruba 2012.

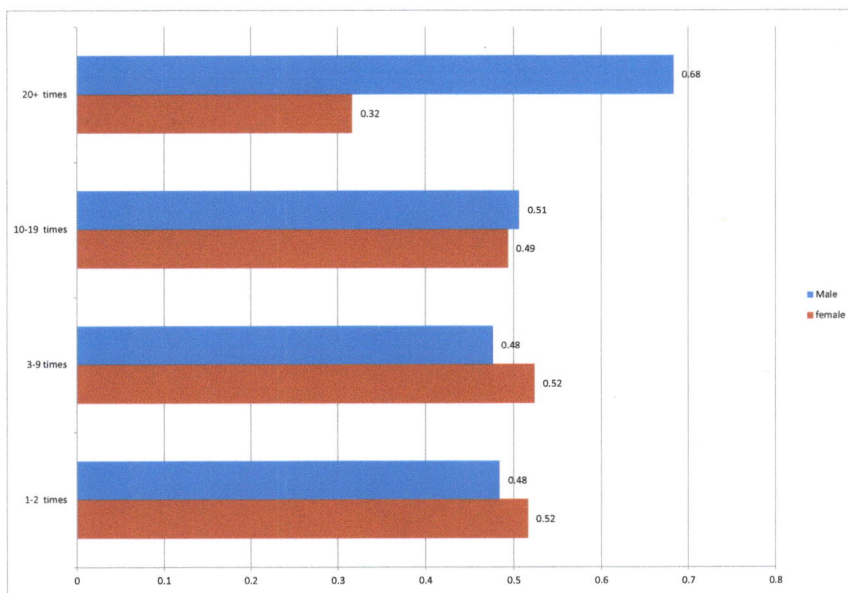

Figure 73. Frequency marihuana use by gender, YHS Aruba 2012.

6.1.2. Hard Drugs

Besides marihuana the use of hard drugs was also prevalent among the youth, 2.6 percent ($n = 120$) of the studied population has stated to have used hard drugs during their life. The frequency of hard drug use by gender is illustrated in Figure 74.

However the number of hard drug users is low as compared to the users of marihuana, we see a tendency of hard drug is higher among the females as compared to the males. Further analysis by age category shows that 29.2 percent of the youth between 12–19 years have used hard drugs in their live.

6.2 Sexuality

Many young people engage in risky sexual risk behaviors that can result in unintended health outcomes.

The results of the Youth Health Survey 2012 showed that 38.1 percent of both male and female between 12–19 years 50.0% have ever had sexual intercourse.

Most of them had their first sexual experience at an average 46.5% age of 14.4 years. More than three quarters (78.8 percent) have 46.0% had their first sexual intercourse when they were between 15 and 17 years, 10.5 percent were between 12 and 14 years 44.0% and only 6.3 percent were older than 18 years. It is important to mention that 4.4 percent of the studied population stated to have had their first sexual intercourse at 11 years or younger.

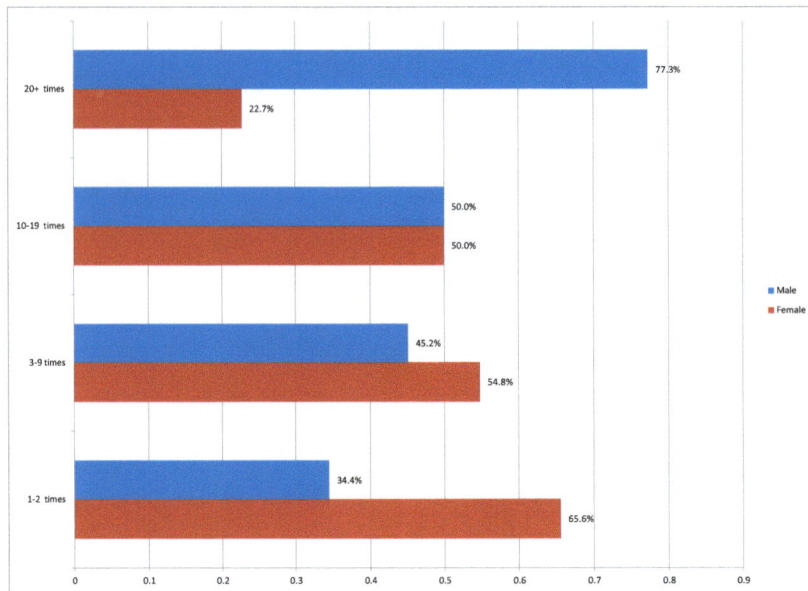

Figure 74. Frequency of hard drug use during life by gender, YHS Aruba 2012.

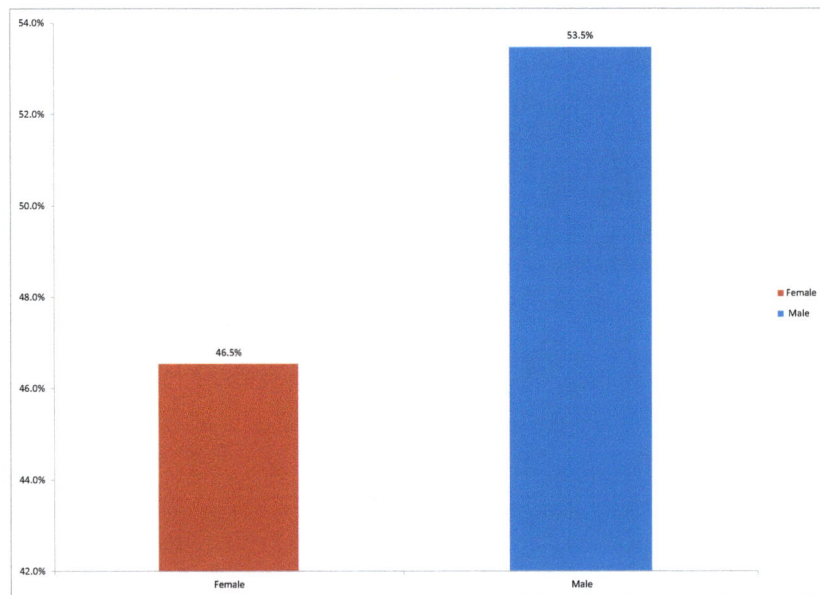

Figure 75. Sexually active youth by gender, YHS Aruba 2012.

Of the ones who ever had sexual intercourse, 46.5 percent were females ($n = 838$) and 53.5 percent were males ($n = 963$), see Figure 75. The majority of these teenagers, who have stated to have had sexual intercourse, were in the age category of 15–17 years (61.1 percent females and 61.0 percent males). There are no large difference in percentages between the female and males who have had sexual intercourse.

6.2.1 Sexual Preferences and Attraction

More than half of the males, 50.8 percent have stated to have had sex with females and 43.9 percent of the females had sex with males. Also 60.7 percent of both males and females stated to be attracted to the opposite sex. However 2.9 percent of the females and 3.2 percent of the males stated to be attracted to the same sex, while 28.8 percent did not understand the question.

More than half of the school going youth between 12 and 19 years never had sexual intercourse, 61.9 percent, more females than males have never had sexual intercourse (54.0 percent female & 46.0 percent males). The main reason for not having sexual intercourse were mainly, 'wait until older' and 'don't want to risk to get an STI, see the following table for detailed results.

Table 17. Main reason for not having sex, YHS Aruba 2012.

Reason for not having sexual intercourse	Females	Males
Wait until older	24%	40.3%
Don't want to risk an STI	11.7%	8.2%

For both males and females the percentage was higher for these answers in the age category of younger than 14 years. Of the female respondents in this age category, 60.5 percent ($n = 208$) want to wait until older and 59.6 percent ($n = 56$) in this same age category stated not wanting to risk an STI. For the males in this same age category these same reasons were stated with 62.8 percent ($n = 309$) and 69.0 percent ($n = 69$) respectively.

6.3 Youth Mental Health

Adolescence is a time of dramatic change. The journey from child to adult can be complex and challenging. Young people often feel tremendous pressure to succeed at school, at home and in social groups. At the same time, they may lack the life experience that lets them know that difficult situations will not last forever.

According to the Youth Health Survey Aruba 2012 conducted under the school attending population aged 12–19 years different factors were measured such as loneliness, feeling of hopelessness, suicidal thoughts and even attempts. These are factors that form a view of the mental and emotional state under the Aruban youth.

The study showed that during the past 12 months about 16 percent (15.9 percent) of the youth between 12–19 years felt lonely most of the time. More females compared to males felt lonely, 70.5 percent and 29.5 percent respectively.

More than half (53.3 percent) belong to the age category between 15 and 17 years, while more than a third (33.2 percent) were younger than 14 years of age, and 13.5 percent were older than 18 years, see Table 18.

Table 18. Frequency experience loneliness.

Loneliness	Age category		
	<=14 yrs	15–17 yrs	18 +
Rarely	38.6	48.1	13.4
Sometimes	33.9	49.9	16.2
Most of the time	33.2	53.3	13.5
Always	38.5	51.5	10

Trouble with sleeping was another factor asked, almost 5 percent (4.5 percent) had trouble sleeping most of the time at night because of worries. Again more females compared to males had troubles sleeping, 69.8 percent and 30.2 percent respectively.

More than half (51.9 percent) belong to the age category between 15 and 17 years, while more than one third (34.0 percent) were between 12 and 14 years of age, and 14.1 percent were 18 years and higher.

The feeling of sadness and hopelessness during the past 12 months was the most common experienced feeling compared to all other feelings. During the past 12 months almost half, 42.2 percent, experienced this feeling. Two third (66.3 percent) of those who experienced this feeling where female, only one third (33.7 percent) were male. When further analyzed by age, more than half (51.8 percent) belong to the age category between 15 and 17 years, while a third (33.3 percent) were between 12 and 14 years of age, and 14.9 percent were older than 18 years.

Suicidal thoughts were also prevalent among the population studied. Almost 15 percent (14.6 percent) thought about suicide during the past 12 months. Again the females had the highest percentage, almost 70 percent (69.1 percent). Among the males, this percentage was much lower than 30.9 percent. The youth between the ages 15 and 17 had the highest percentage of individuals having thought about committing suicide, 52.7 percent, followed by the youth aged 12-14 years, see Table 19.

To think about suicide is one thing, but to actually plan a suicide is considered a more serious matter. When asked if the respondents made a plan about killing themselves during the past year almost 15 percent (14.6 percent) of the students answered yes, from which 69.1 percent were female and 30.9 percent were male.

More than half (52.7 percent) belong to the age category between 15 and 17 years, 36.8 percent were between 12 and 14 years of age, and 10.5 percent were 18 years and higher. Moreover, it is to be taken more seriously when suicide is attempted. Almost 10 percent (9.3 percent) have tried to commit suicide at least once before.

Table 19. Risk factors suicide school going youth.

Risk factors for suicide

Total	Male	Female	12–14 yrs	15–17 yrs	18 + yrs
14.6%	30.9%	69.1%	36.8%	52.7%	10.5%
14.6%	30.9%	69.1%	36.8%	52.7%	10.5%
9.3%	28.9%	71.1%	39.5%	50.9%	9.6%

However more than a quarter, 26.1 percent, of the ones who have suicidal thought have tried to kill themselves 2–3 times, see Figure 76. Again females had the highest percentage as compared to the males, 71.1 percent and 28.9 percent respectively. This is 2.5 times higher compared to the males.

More than a quarter (26.1 percent) tried 2 or 3 times to attempt suicide without having any previous suicidal thoughts. From this 26.1 percent, again females (79.8 percent) had the highest percentage compared to the males (20.2 percent). As Figure 77 illustrates, overall females have attempted suicide more often than males.

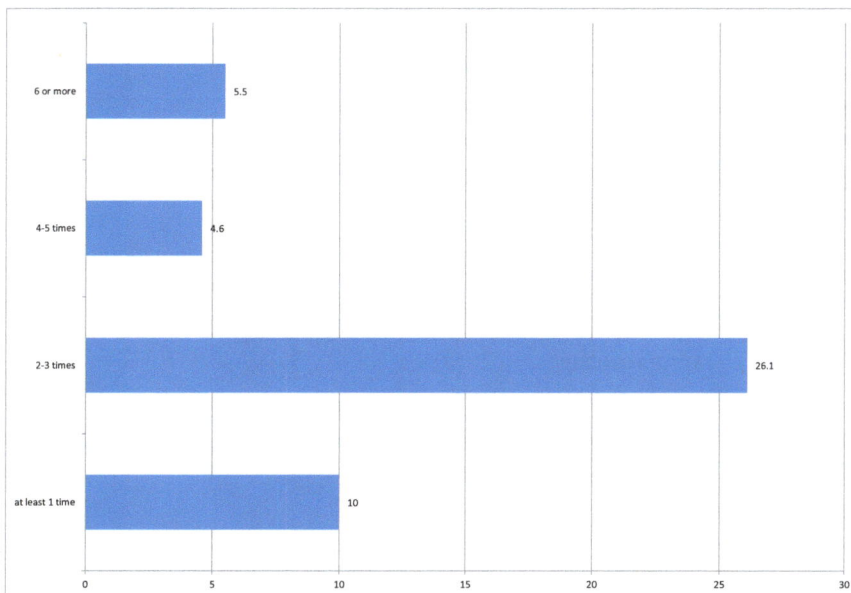

Figure 76. Frequency attempted suicide of youth having suicidal thoughts, YHS Aruba 2012.

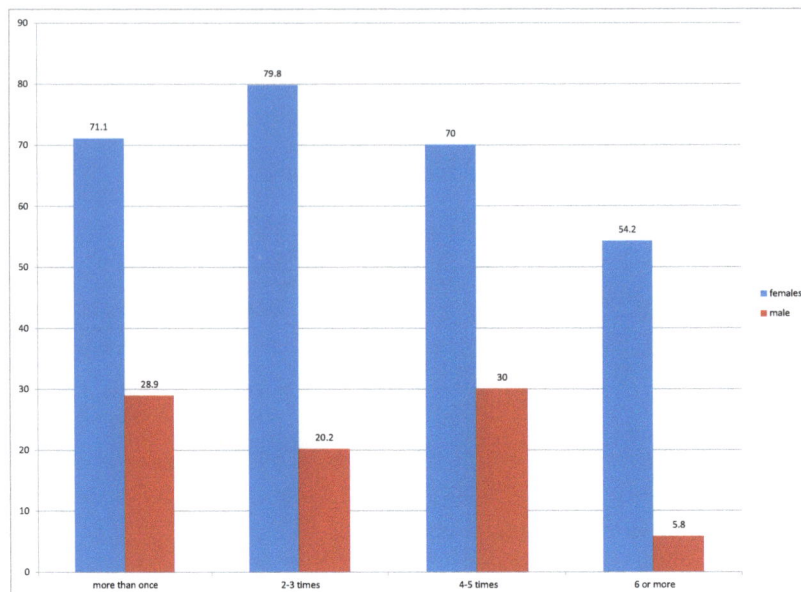

Figure 77. Frequency of attempted suicides by gender, YHS Aruba 2012.

Almost fifty-one percent (50.9 percent) of those who tried to kill themselves at least once during the past year belong to the age category between 15 and 17 years, 39.5 percent were between 12 and 14 years of age and 9.6 percent were 18 years and older.

These data are similar to data from the U.S. where females attempt suicide more often than males. However the percentages are higher among the youth. In the U.S. in 2009, 6.3 percent of high school students (grades 9–12) attempted suicide. Of those, 8.1 percent were female, 4.6 percent were male. For Aruba this percentage is 9.2 percent from the total population high school going youth, from which 6.6 percent are female and 2.6 percent are male.

According to the Central Bureau for Statistics in the Netherlands from 2000 to 2008, 3752 suicides took place among people between the ages of 10–19. Most of the cases occurred among persons aged 15–19 with a total of 2584, and 1168 cases occurred among persons 10–14 years of age.

However according to mortality data obtained from the Department of Public Health Aruba, for the years 2000–2009 only one case of suicide was registered for the age group 15–19 years.

6.4 Breastfeeding

As stated by the WHO "Breastfeeding is the natural way of providing young infants with nutrients they need for healthy growth and development".

Breastfeeding provides bonding between mother and child as well as health benefits for both. Breast milk protects babies against common diseases in children such as atopic eczema, ear infections, respiratory tract infections and diarrhea.

Mothers who breastfeed have a lower risk of breast cancer and osteoporosis. Other advantages of breastfeeding are lower health care costs, including doctor's visits and hospitalization, and an increase in work productivity of the mothers since 100 infants who are breastfed are sick less often. Research shows that children who have been exclusively breastfed during the first 6 months of life have a lower risk of becoming obese in adulthood.

Obesity is a high risk factor for the development of chronic diseases such as cardiovascular diseases and diabetes during adulthood. Taking into consideration that chronic diseases are the number one cause of death in Aruba, breastfeeding has an important role in the decrease of chronic diseases.

In 2002 the prevalence of breastfeeding was measured for the first time in Aruba. Figure 78 shows the percentage of baby's receiving exclusive breastfeeding at the moment of birth was less than 10 percent. This percentage that declined to 0 during the first 6 months of the baby's life. Of the remaining 90 percent, 70 percent received breastfeeding in combination with formula and 17 percent received no breastfeeding at all.

The same investigation was repeated in 2010 and the results showed an increase in breastfeeding. The percentage of newborn babies exclusively breastfed increased from 10 percent in 2002 to 24 percent in 2010. Babies exclusively breastfed at the age of 6 months, increased from 0 percent in 2002 to 9.1 percent in 2010.

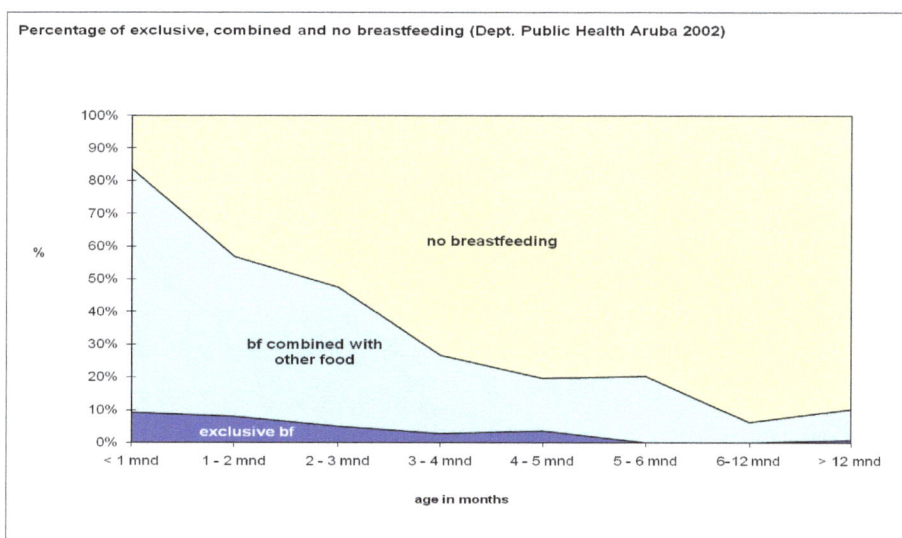

Figure 78. Percentage of exclusive, combined and no breastfeeding, Aruba 2002.

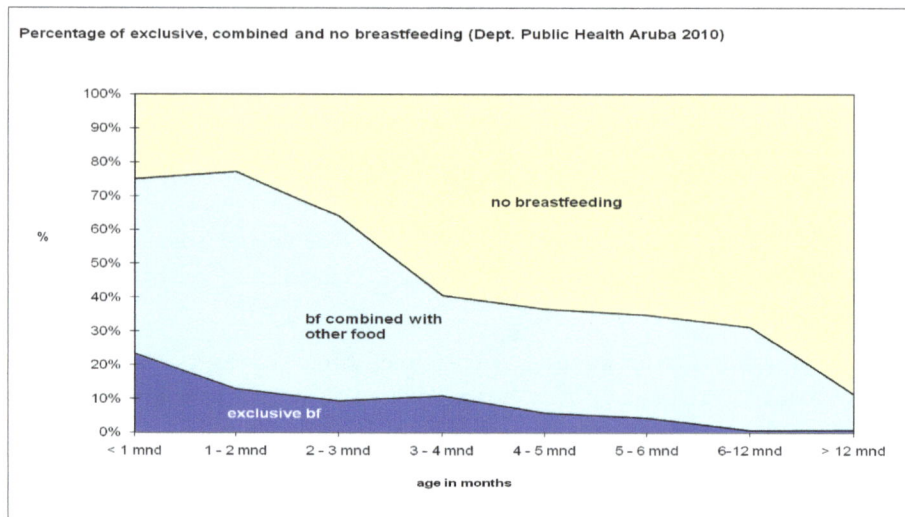

Figure 79. Percentage of exclusive, combined and no breastfeeding, Aruba 2010.

The remaining 90 percent in 2002 that were breastfed in combination with other food, and also those who were not breastfed, have also decreased in 2010.

The group of newborn babies who were breastfed in combination with other food, decreased from 70 percent in 2002 to 52 percent in 2010. Yet, the percentage of newborn babies who were not breastfed, has increased from 17 percent in 2002 to 23 percent in 2010, see Figure 79.

Exclusive breastfeeding has increased from 9.2 percent in 2002 to 24.8 percent in 2010.

Also the average week a baby was breastfed has increased from 13 weeks in 2002 to 15 weeks in 2010. Overall it can be concluded that breastfeeding, whether in combination or exclusively has increased in an 8 year period.

Breastfeeding is heading towards a positive direction for Aruba; however there is still room for improvement. Worldwide the percentage of exclusive breastfeeding is 38 percent, for Aruba this percentage is only 13 percent. Together with Trinidad & Tobago, the United States of America, Dominican Republic and Surinam, Aruba ranks in the top three of the lowest percentages where breastfeeding is exclusive during the first six months of life, see Figure 80.

Peru has the highest percentage (63%) of exclusive breastfeeding, followed by Bolivia, Colombia and Ecuador, for details see Figure 80.

In order to determine the reasons and contributing factors to the low prevalence of breastfeeding in Aruba a study about knowledge, beliefs and actions was done in 2003 among a group of mothers.

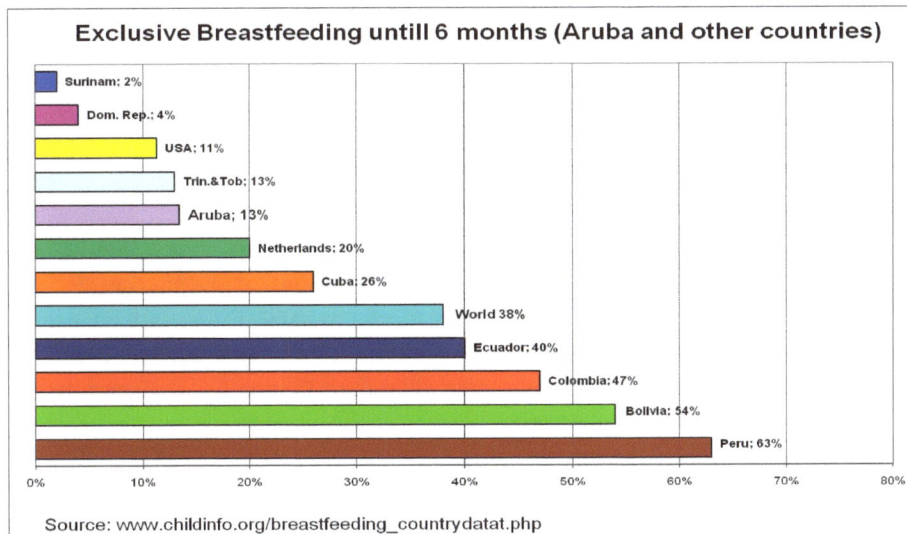

Exclusive Breastfeeding untill 6 months (Aruba and other countries)

Surinam: 2%
Dom. Rep.: 4%
USA: 11%
Trin.&Tob: 13%
Aruba; 13%
Netherlands: 20%
Cuba; 26%
World 38%
Ecuador; 40%
Colombia; 47%
Bolivia; 54%
Peru; 63%

Source: www.childinfo.org/breastfeeding_countrydatat.php

Figure 80. Exclusive breastfeeding until 6 months (Aruba and other countries).

The main reason for stopping early was that the mothers felt that the milk production decreased or that the baby refused breastfeeding. Also, returning to work was one of the most important factors stated by the mothers.

Analyzing these reasons, we can conclude that there is a lack of knowledge about the process of breastfeeding. External factors have its influence on breastfeeding such as work resumption, which play an important role in the period of breastfeeding the baby.

6.5 Dental Health

6.5.1 Toddlers

The White Yellow Cross Foundation offers services in the field of ambulatory care with the support of the Department of Public Health. The DPH offers the services of the dentists who give the dental consultations at the ambulatory care.

Since 2001 "Nutrition and Dental Care" for toddlers is also offered at ambulatory care of the WYC. The consultation includes a nutritionist and a dentist for the oral examination. The oral history and examination include oral habits, oral hygiene practices, growth and development (dental age), injury history, caries (Nursing Bottle Caries / Early Childhood Caries) and other potential problems.

Parents are informed about the importance of teaching their children good oral hygiene habits at an early stage. In addition to information about oral health care, parents are also informed about the dental coverage provided for by the AZV. All toddlers are referred afterwards to their dentists for regular check-ups. The dental check-up include observation of any abnormality in the oral cavity e.g.

- numbers of the teeth present according to the infant age
- oral manifestation due to bad habits (thumb sucking or pacifier)
- Nursing bottle syndrome
- Bad hygiene.

From 2004 to 2007 the attendance percentage of toddlers was approximately 50. From 2008 to 2010 the attendance percentage increased to 60. The low attendance to the "Nutrition and Dental Care" clinic is common for the clinics offered at the White Yellow Cross Foundation for children older than 15 months. At 15 months the infants complete their immunizations according to the schedule for that age group. Most parents take their babies to the White Yellow Cross Foundation primarily to be vaccinated. Attendances tend to increase when the initial appointment is followed up by a reminder.

The number of toddlers seen at the "Nutrition and Dental Care" clinic has increased from 578 in 2004 to 805 in 2010. The "Nutrition and Dental Care" clinic was held twice a week from 2001 to 2007, see Figure 81.

In 2008 an additional clinic was added which could explain the increase in attendance in that year. Aruba has an average of 1144.5 live births per year. The

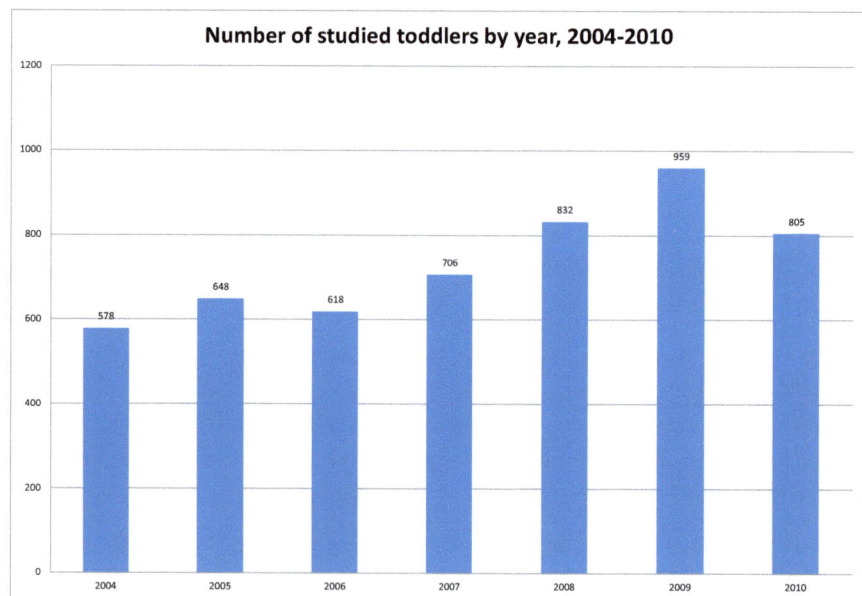

Figure 81. Number of toddlers attending "Nutrition and Dental Care" Per year, YDC Aruba.

majority of these babies used the services of the White Yellow Cross Foundation. The "Nutrition and Dental Care" clinic sees approximately about 60 percent of the children born each year.

6.5.2 Habits Toddlers

There has been a steady decline in the prevalence of oral habits in the children studied in this same period, see Figure 82. The prevalence of the oral habit "thumb (digital) sucking" was 22.3 percent in 2004 and decreased to 18 percent in 2010. The prevalence of the "use of a pacifier" was 21.1 percent in 2004 and decreased to 19 percent in 2010. The decline in the prevalence of oral habits could be attributed to the increase in the prevalence of breastfeeding in Aruba. Studies have shown 104 that breast-fed children tend to develop non-nutritive sucking habits less frequently. The percentage of children who slept with the baby bottle doubled from 2004 to 2008, from 2.4 percent to 4.0 percent. From 2008 to 2010 the percentage of children who slept with the baby bottle decreased and has stayed below 5 percent.

6.5.3 Percentage Toddlers with Dental Caries by Year 2004-2010

The percentage of toddlers with dental caries increased steadily from 3.2 percent in 2004 to 5.3 percent in 2010, see Figure 83. The increase in the prevalence of dental caries in the primary dentition is a global trend. The increase of the prevalence of

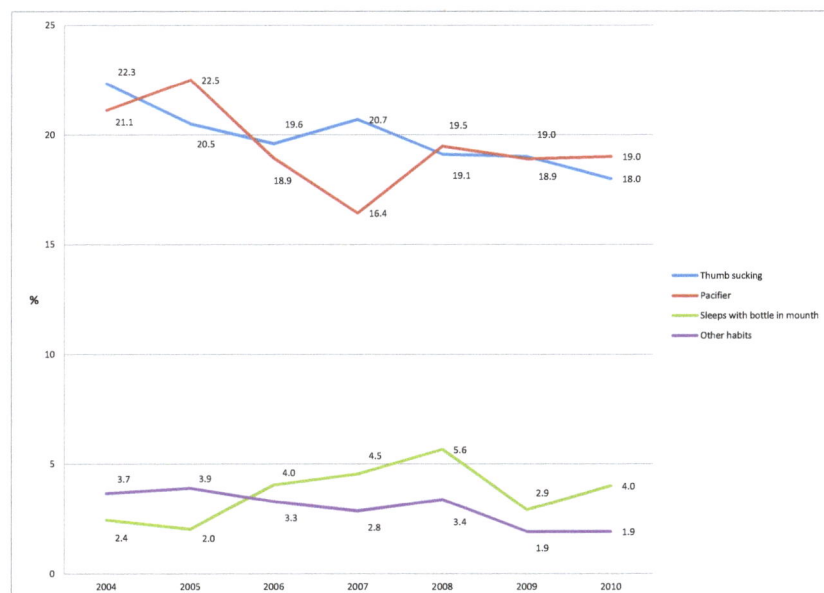

Figure 82. Habits toddlers in percentage, Aruba 2004–2010.

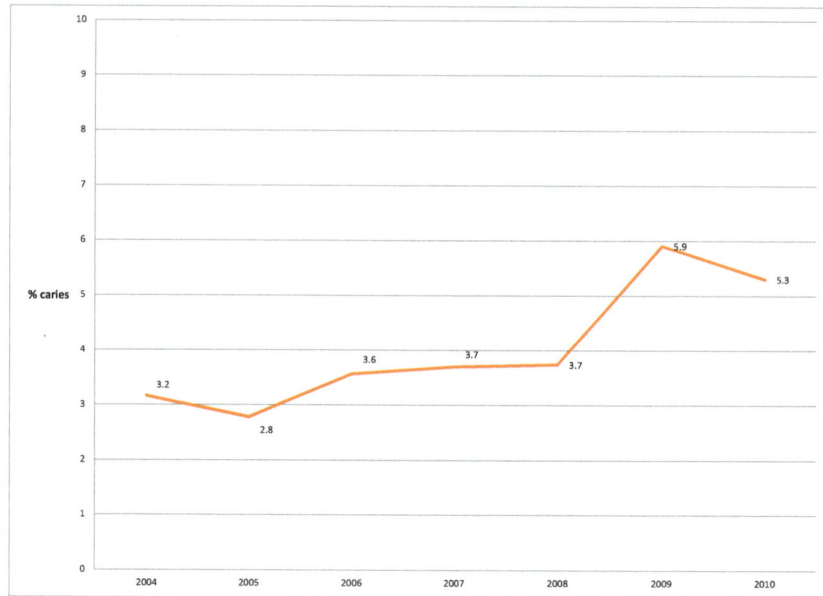

Figure 83. Percentage toddlers with carries, Aruba 2004–2010.

dental caries is being attributed largely to the increase in sugar consumption (amount and frequency) and the inadequate exposure to fluorides.

6.5.4 Nursing Bottle Syndrome by Year 2004–2010

Nursing Bottle Syndrome is a unique pattern of dental caries caused by allowing the child to feed from a nursing bottle containing milk or juice or from the breast, for extended periods of time. The upper front teeth are most commonly affected.

The prevalence of Nursing Bottle Syndrome has increased steadily from less than 2 percent in 2004 to 3.5 percent in 2010, see Figure 84.

The term "Nursing Bottle Syndrome" suggests that the primary cause of caries is the inappropriate bottle feeding. The current evidence suggests that although the use of a sugar—containing liquid in a baby bottle at night—time may cause dental caries.

6.5. P6ercentage Toddlers Who Have Used Fluoride by Year 2004–2010

The use of fluorides to reduce dental caries has been proven effective in numerous studies. Fluoride protects teeth in two 106 ways, systemically and topically. Systemic fluorides are those ingested into the body.

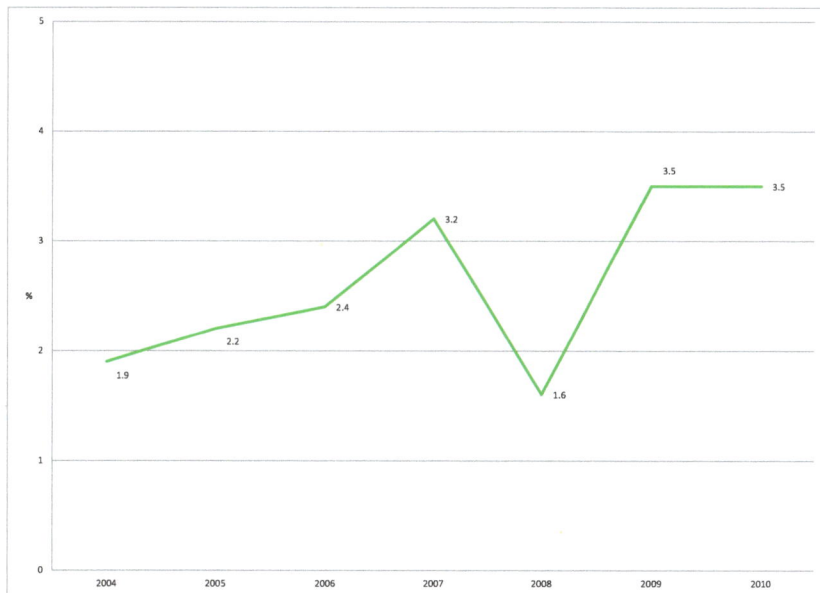

Figure 84. Nursing bottle syndrome by year, Aruba 2004–2010.

In the "Nutrition and Dental Care " clinic, the use of fluoride tablets was specifically measured. From 2004 to 2010 the percentage of toddlers who have used fluoride tablets decreased steadily from 36.2 to 11.9, Figure 85. The guidelines recommend brushing the infant's teeth as soon as they start to erupt, with fluoride toothpaste (with the appropriate concentration), early visits to the dentist (starting at two years of age) and the use of topical fluorides if necessary.

6.5.6 Toddlers with Teeth Demineralization, Percentage by Year 2004–2010

During the oral exam the presence of "white spots" or demineralization of the enamel is also recorded. The demineralization of the enamel is the earliest macroscopic 4 evidence of caries. The enamel surface overlying the lesion is intact. Demineralization occurs at the subsurface level.

Toddlers with white spots are referred immediately to their dentist for topical fluoride treatment. Parents are also 2 instructed to take extra preventive measures.

From 2004 to 2010 the percentage of toddlers with white spots increased steadily from 1.6 to 3.7, see Figure 86. The percentage increase of toddlers with white spots corresponds to the increase in prevalence of dental caries.

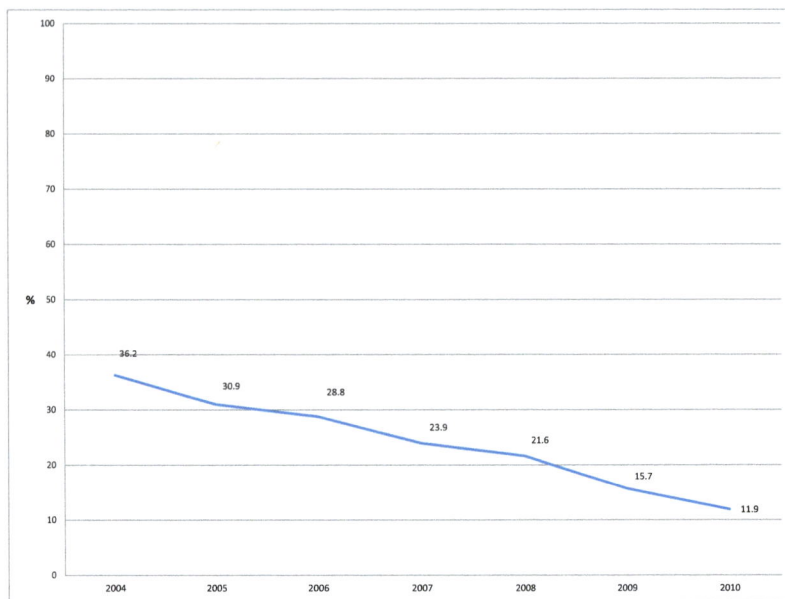

Figure 85. Percentage toddlers using fluoride per year, Aruba 2004–2010.

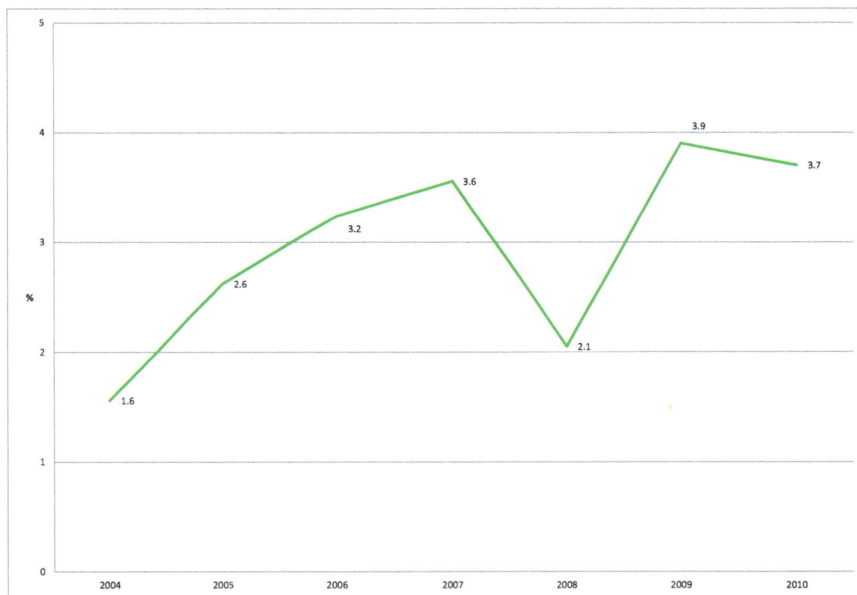

Figure 86. Percentage toddlers with teeth demineralization, Aruba 2004–2010.

6.5.7 Toddlers with Fractured Teeth, by Year 2004–2010

Facial traumas that result in fractured, displaced or lost teeth can have significant negative functional, esthetic and psychological effects on children. An estimated 30 percent of preschool children suffer injuries to the primary dentition. The greatest incidence of trauma to the primary teeth occurs at 2 to 3 years of age, when motor coordination is developing. In Aruba the percentage of toddlers with fractured teeth increased from 9.9 in 2004 to 11.4 in 2009. In 2010 the percentage of toddlers with fractured teeth doubled. The increase in percentage of toddlers with fractures from 11.4 in 2009 to 24 in 2010, see Figure 87.

6.6 Child/Youth Abuse

In 2008, a pilot study was conducted on the nature and the prevalence of child abuse on Aruba (Guda, 2008). This pilot survey focused on the number of cases of child abuse reported to schools and to other governmental and nongovernmental organizations in charge of providing care, support, guidance to children and families in general, and to victims of child abuse, in particular. This survey revealed that in 2008, 182 cases of child abuse were reported. The majority of these (25.3 percent) involved physical neglect of a child (see Figure 88).

Both girls and boys were victims of child abuse, girls representing a slightly higher percentage of reported cases (52.5 percent) when compared to boys (47.8 percent).

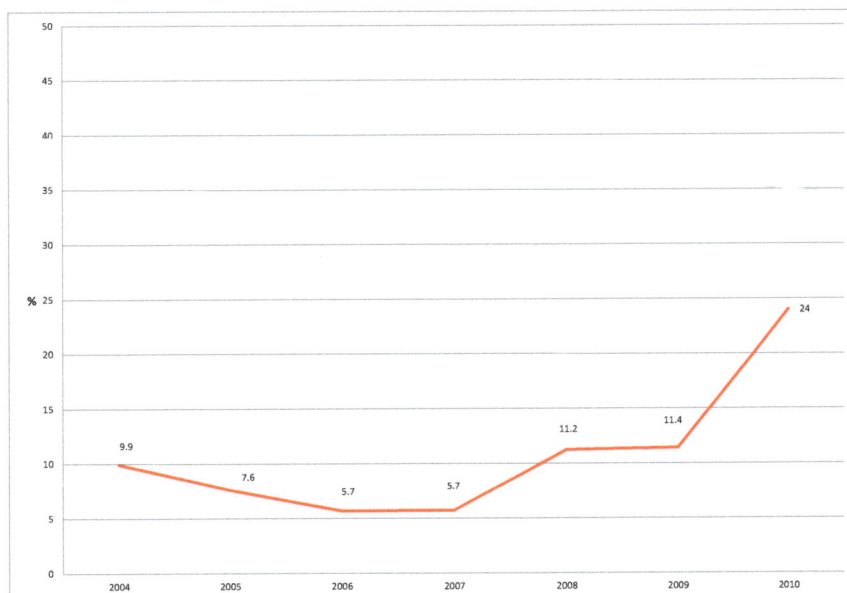

Figure 87. Percentage toddlers with fractured teeth, Aruba 2004–2010.

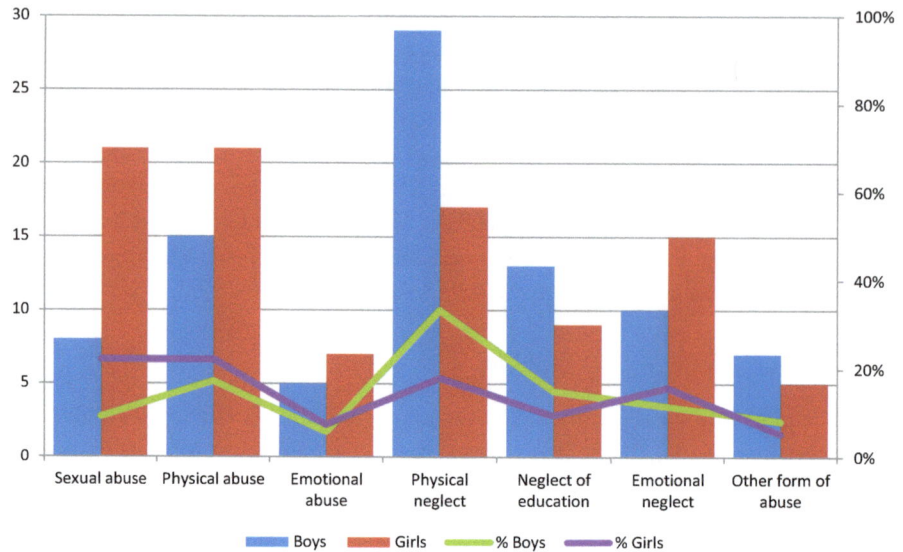

Figure 88. Prevalence and nature of child abuse by gender.

However, the nature of the abuse differed between boys and girls. Boys were more often subjected to physical neglect (33.3 percent), whereas girls were more often subjected to sexual abuse (22.1 percent) or physical abuse (22.1 percent; see Figure 84).

When considering the age of the children, the data obtained showed an increase in reported cases as age progressed up to the age of 16 years, where there was a visible drop in the number of reported cases (see Figure 89). As age progressed, there was also a shift in the nature of the abuse being reported. In children up to age 5 years, physical neglect was the most often reported type of abuse (41.7 percent), followed by emotional neglect (29.2 percent). In children between 6 and 11 years of age, physical neglect was still the most often reported type of abuse (34.2 percent), followed by physical abuse as the second most often reported type of abuse, representing 26.0 percent of the total number of reported cases. In adolescent children between 12 and 17 years of age, neglect of education took first place, followed by physical abuse and sexual abuse, representing both 17.6 percent of reported cases (see Figure 90).

Overall, when assessing the damaging effects of the abuse, the findings of the study indicated that in the majority of the reported cases of child abuse there was mention of moderate (33 percent of total) to serious (37 percent of total) consequences for the child. There were no reports of fatal consequences.

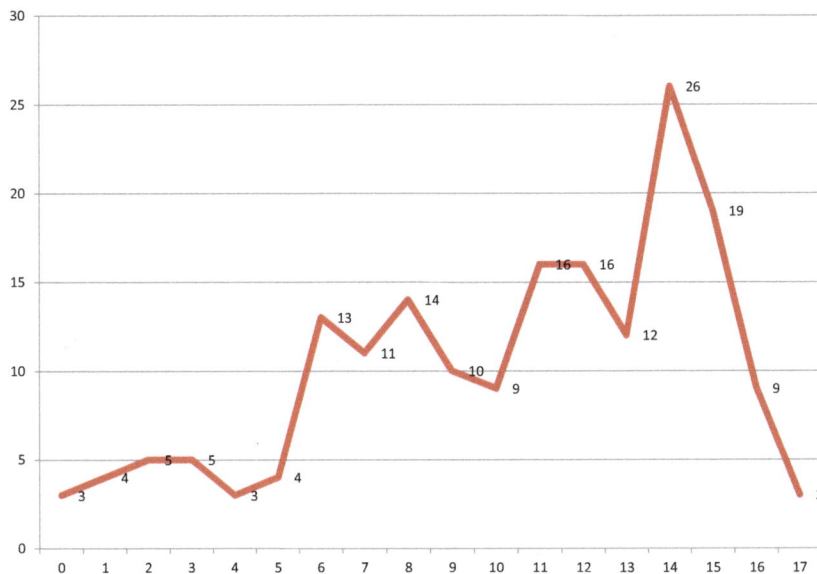

Figure 89. The number of reported cases of child abuse by age of the child.

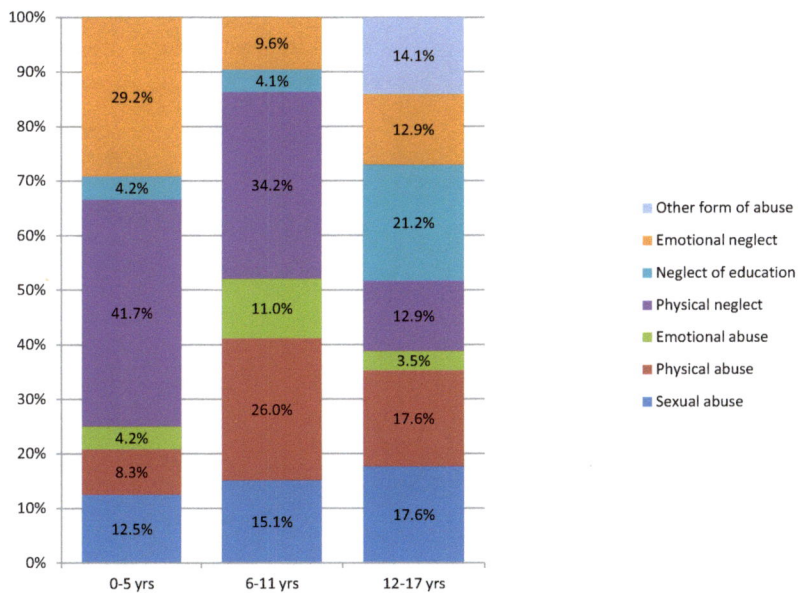

Figure 90. Type of child abuse by age category.

6.7 Teen Pregnancy

Teen pregnancy and childbearing bring substantial social and economic costs through immediate and long-term impacts on teen parents and their children. (CDC, 2012)

Teen pregnancy has its effects on the health costs, high school dropout rates among girls with the consequence of lower educational achievement, more health problems and probable unemployment as a young adult. (CDC, 2012)

These effects remain for the teen mother and her child even after adjusting those factors which increased the teenager's risk for pregnancy, such as growing up in poverty, having parents with low levels of education, growing up in a single-parent family, and having poor performance in school. (Singh et al., 2003)

Aruba is not different from other countries in the region and the world. The birth rate of teenage pregnancy for age category 15 to 19 years is about 40 live births per 1,000. This rate has been steady for the past 10 years.

As Figure 91 shows the regional birth rates teenage pregnancies of Aruba and the USA are about 4 times higher as compared to the birth rates of the Netherlands. The teenage birth rates for the USA have shown a steady decrease from 2008 up to 2011. In Aruba however there is a slight decrease only from 2010 to 2011. The teenage birth rate for the Netherlands has been steady for about the past 8 years. This birth rate is less than 10 live births per 1,000 girls between the ages of 15 and 19 years.

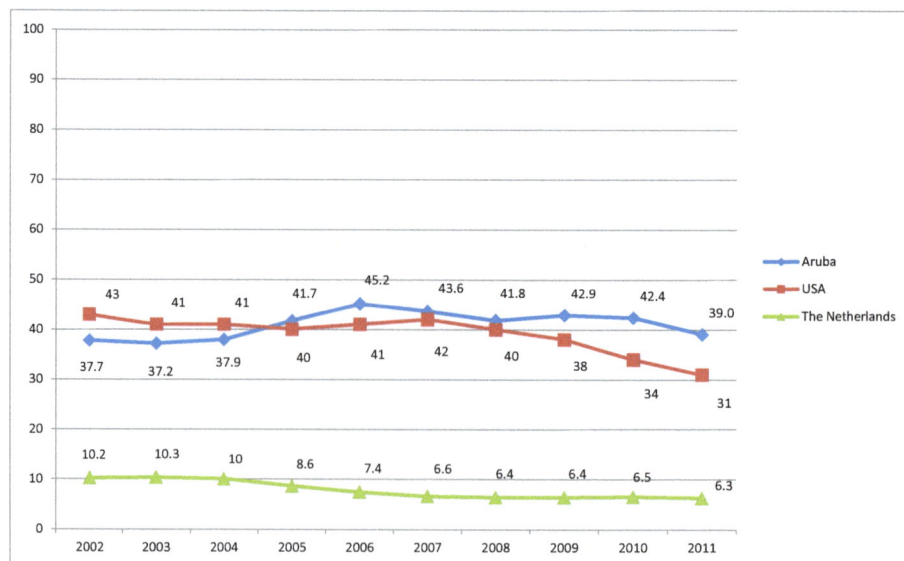

Figure 91. Birth rate teenage Pregnancies 15–19 years.

When comparing the birth rate of Aruba with other European countries, the difference is significant. Switzerland has the lowest rate between European countries, 4.3 per 1,000 with the United Kingdom having the highest, 23.6 per 1,000. The latter is half the birth rate of Aruba, see Figure 92.

However when comparing the teenage live birth rate of Aruba with countries in the American region, the Aruban rate is similar to the rates of North America, which is the second lowest birth rate worldwide, see Figure 93.

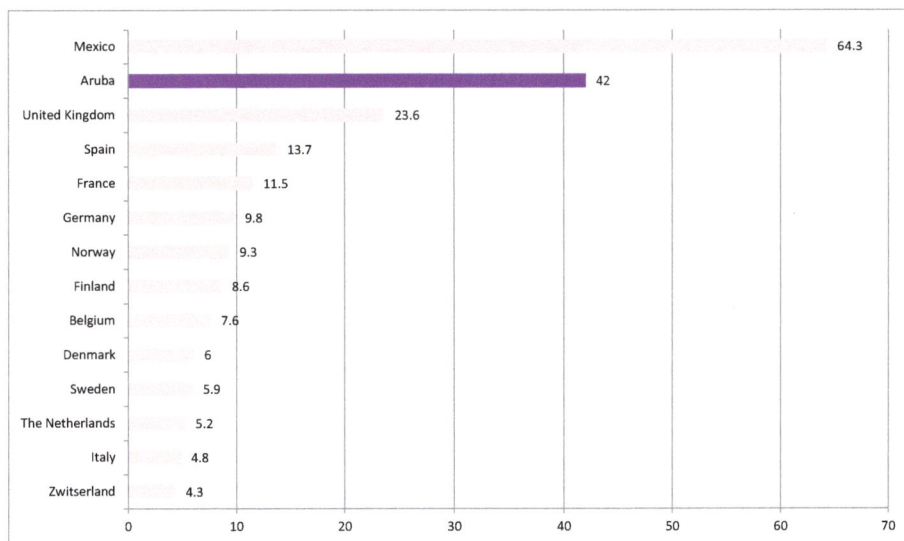

Figure 92. Live birth rates European countries.

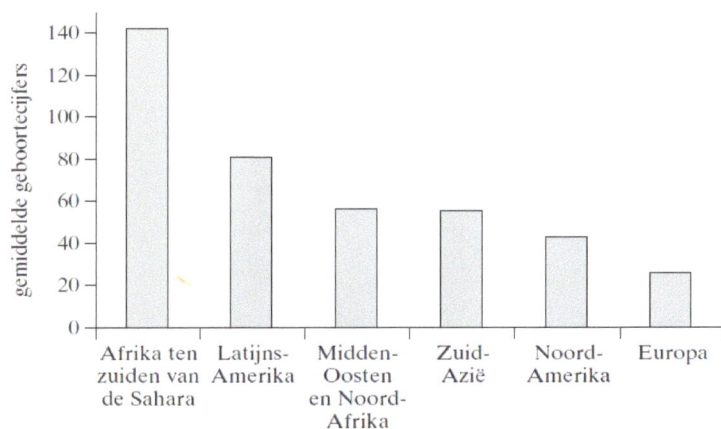

Figure 93. Live birth rates, 15–19 years for different regions worldwide, 2003.

6.7.1 Abortion

Teen pregnancies cannot be evaluated without taking into consideration the abortion numbers among teenagers. In the Treffers study it is stated that about 35–70 percent of the teenage pregnancies are interrupted. These data are from industrialized countries that have reliable data concerning abortions. The Netherlands have a low abortion percentage, which is 8.6 percent among teenagers between 15–19 years. In the document "Teenage pregnancies in Aruba" by the Social Economic Council (Sociaal Economische Raad) of Aruba, it is stated that the abortion data received from the hospital, is just the tip of the iceberg. As further stated in this document, it is known that abortion does occur in private practices of general practitioners and also at home, with the many negative consequences for the health of the mother. Figure 94 presents the absolute number of live births together with the absolute number of abortions.

Table 20. Abortions per year, Aruba 2002–2005.

Year	No. of abortions (15–19 yrs)	Nr. of abortion per 1000 (15–19 yrs)	% teen pregnancies (15–19 yrs)
2002	16	5	24
2003	34	11	24
2004	7	2	22
2005	23	7	23

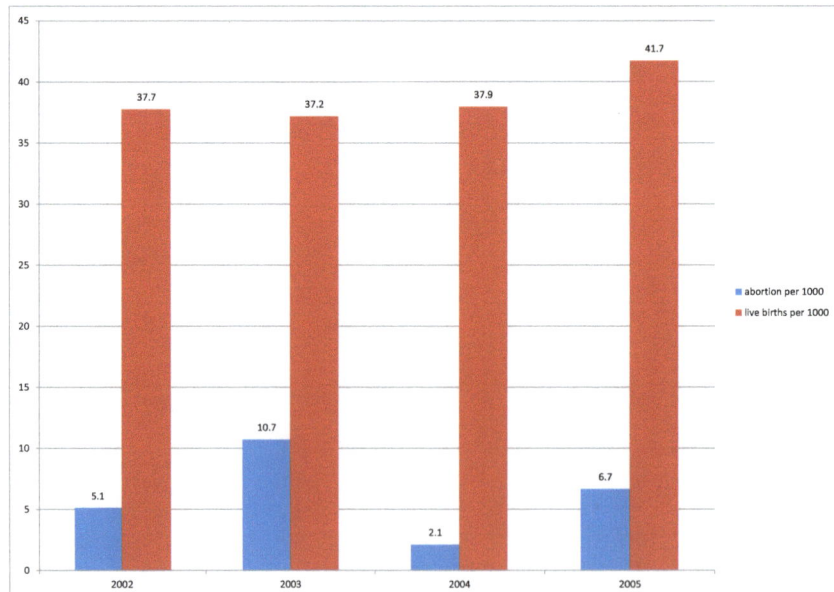

Figure 94. Number of total live births and abortions per year in Aruba, 2002–2005.

Health Monitor Aruba 2017

168

The abortion percentage for the USA which has a similar teen live birth rate as Aruba, is only 2.4 percent. For Aruba this percentage is around 24 percent, taking this into consideration, the abortion percentage in Aruba is high. But when comparing the Aruban abortion percentage with the Treffers' study, abortion percentage of Aruba is lower than 35 percent. Table 20 shows the absolute number of abortions per year, from 2002 to 2005. In this same table the abortion rate per 1,000 is showed together with the percentage of teen pregnancies per year in the age category of 15–19 years.

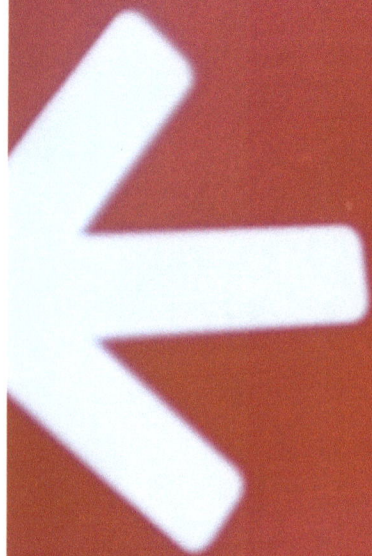 Accide

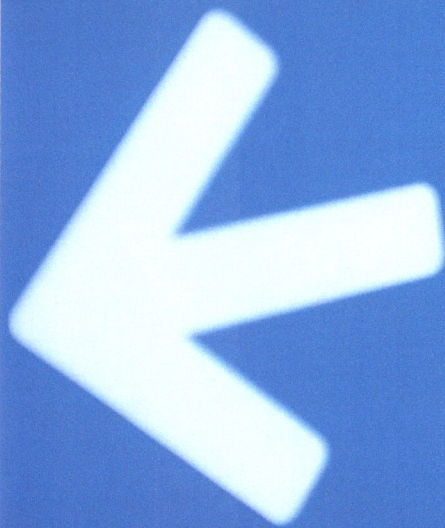 Main

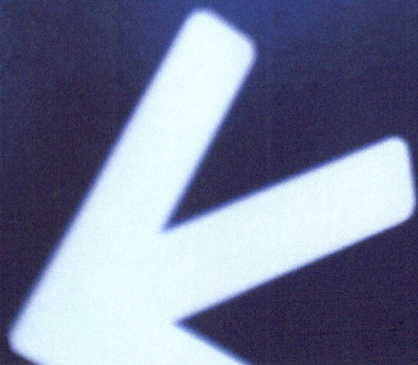 Outp

7. PROVISION, DEMAND AND SUPPLY OF HEALTH CARE TO THE ARUBAN POPULATION

In this section, attention is placed onto the provision of health care. After all, health and the provision of (health) care are 114 strongly correlated. This chapter provides insight into a number of aspects in terms of health care use, demand and supply of health care from the perspective of the General Health Insurance of Aruba (AZV).

7.1 Health Care Use

AZV uses a financial administrative registration system which makes it impossible to quantify information on the health care use of Aruba. This system only registers and administrates the finances of the different health services, e.g. the general practitioner care service is financed by means of a flat-fee. This means that the frequency of the use of health care by a patient cannot be extracted from this database. The financial information presented was taken out of the AZV the annual account for 2011 and from information available of health care professionals contracted by AZV.

7.2 Supply of Health Care

In the Aruban health care system a distinction is made in the accessibility of the client to the first and second line of care. Client can independently contact care providers in first line of care, without a referral. This applies to e.g. a general practitioner, the dentists, physical therapists and midwives. Highly specialized medical care, inpatient care (the second line of care) is offered by the Dr. H. Oduber Hospital and medical specialists in private practices. A client or patient is referred to the second line through the first line of care.

Specialized care, not available on the island, is referred to specialized care providers in the Netherlands, USA, Curaçao, Bonaire, Colombia and Venezuela.

7.2.1 General Practitioners

On December 31st, 2011 there were a total of 32 General practitioners' (GP) practices and a total of 39 general practitioners (GP's) providing general practice care to the population. Two third of the GP's were male (61.5 percent, $n = 24$) and about a third (38.5 percent, $n = 15$) were female. This percentage is similar to the Netherlands where 37 percent of the GP's are female and 63 percent are male.

The Aruban general practice sector is organized in 26 solo practices (81.3 percent), 5 dual practices (15.6 percent) and one group practice (3.1 percent). Steps were taken in 2010-2011 to improve the accessibility to the general practice services to the population. Six additional GP's were contracted by AZV and were placed in the most densely populated districts of the island. A total of 17.2 million florins were paid by the executive body of AZV for general practice services for the Aruban population.

Figure 95 illustrates the distribution of the GP practices over the island; it depicts the distribution of the general practice services amongst the population. A clear correlation between the population density and the size of the practice can be noted.

7.2.2 Physical Therapists

A total of 22 physical therapist private practices with a total of 28 physical therapists provide physical therapy services to the population. More than two third (64.3 percent, $n = 18$) of the physical therapists were female and 35.7 percent ($n = 10$) of the physical therapists were male. The percentage of female physical therapists is higher than the national Dutch percentage of 53. The Aruban physical therapy sector is organized into 81.82 percent (18) solo practices, 13.64 percent dual practices (3) and one group practice (4.55 percent). A total of 4.7 million florins were paid by AZV for physical therapy care in 2011. Figure 96 shows the distribution of the physical therapists practices over the island.

7.2.3 Midwives

There were 8 midwives in private practices on the island from which 2 of them were male and 6 female. The midwives are accessible from their own practices as well as from different locations on the island.

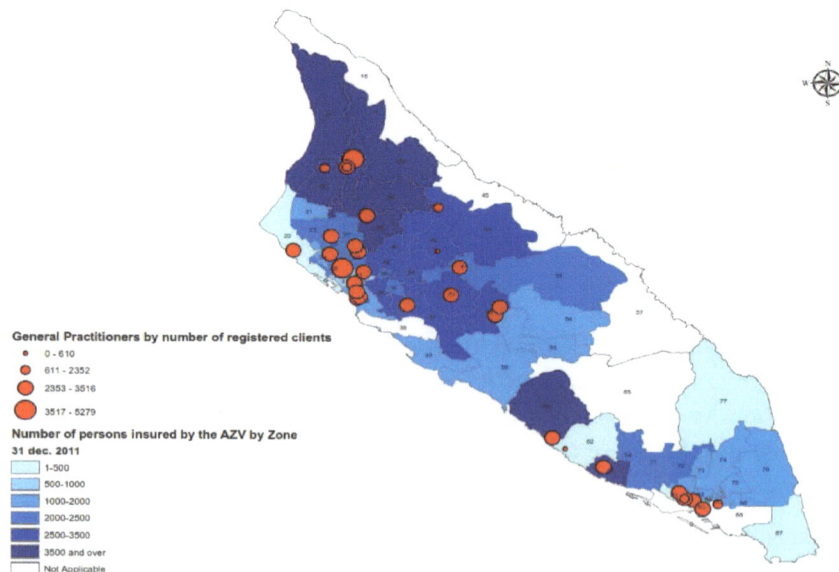

Figure 95. Distribution of the PG practices over the island, Aruba 2011.

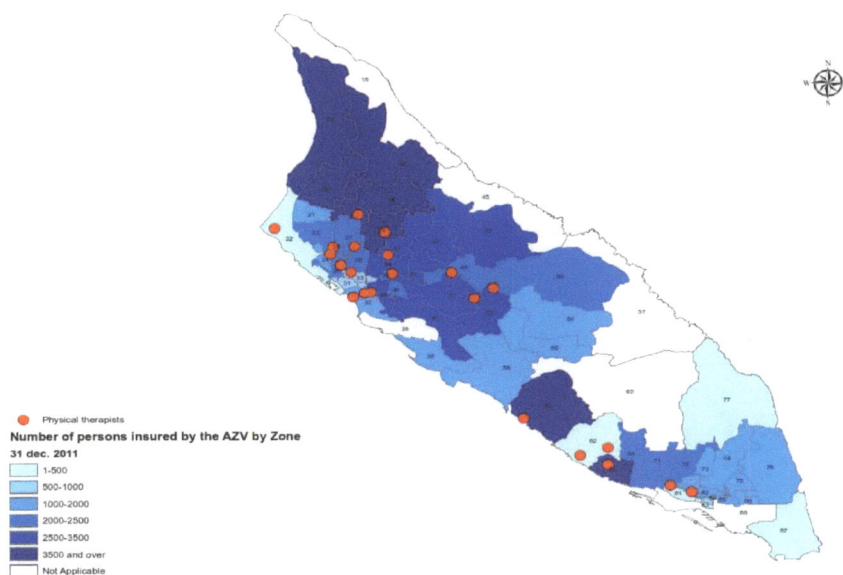

Figure 96. Distribution of the physical therapist in private practices over the island, Aruba 2011.

7.2.4 Dentists

On December 31st, 2011 there were a total of 19 dentist private practices distributed over the island. For the geographical distribution of the dentists on the island see Figure 97.

7.2.5 Second Line Health Care

In the second line of care, the more specialized and more expensive care is provided by our local hospital or by medical specialists in private practices. The specialized second line of health care provided by the hospital is excluded from the distribution of medical specialists observed in Figure 98. This figure refers to the medical specialist care in private practices.

The following medical specialties are provided in 2011 in private practice:

- Internal medicine (3ftes)
- Gynecology/ obstetrics (2 ftes)
- Orthopedic surgery (4 ftes)
- Ophthalmology (2 ftes)
- Plastic Surgery (1 fte)
- Dermatology (2 ftes)
- Psychiatry (2 ftes)

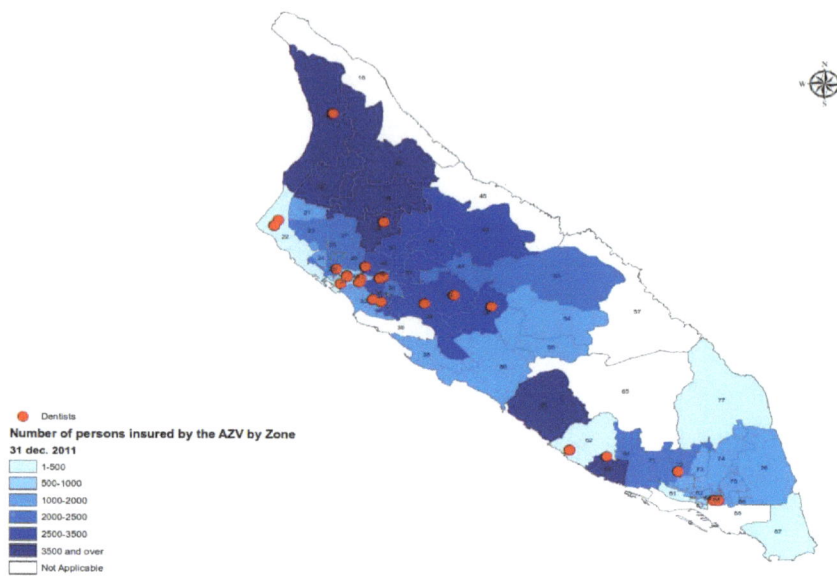

Figure 97. Distribution of dentists on the island by density of persons younger than 18 years old, Aruba 2011.

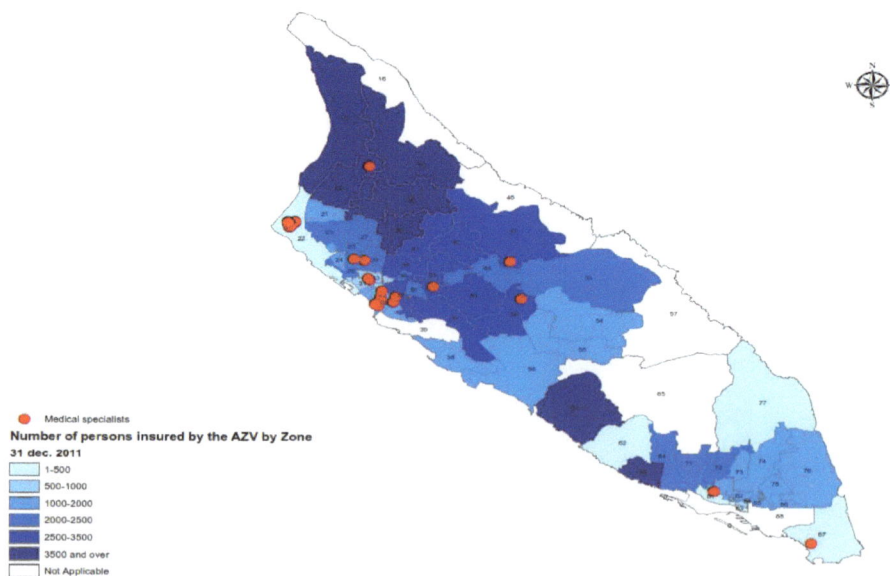

Figure 98. Distribution of second line health care services, Aruba 2011.

- Neurosurgery (1 fte)
- Ear-Throat-Nose (2 ftes)
- Neurology (1 fte)
- Gastroenterology (1 fte)
- Urology (1 fte)
- Cardiology (4 ftes)
- Pain clinic (1 fte)
- General Surgery (5 ftes)

The total amount paid by AZV for medical specialist care in private practice in 2011 was 24.6 million florins.

7.2.6 Supply of Pharmaceutical Care

On December 31st, 2011 Aruba had a total of 18 pharmacies. The pharmacies provide medication and medical related products to the population. In 2011, 2 out of the 18 pharmacies were owned by a pharmacist. The distribution of the pharmacies over the island can be observed in Figure 99. A direct correlation can be noted between the density of the population and the size of the pharmacy. A total of 72.8 million florins were paid by the AZV for the total pharmaceutical care of the population in 2011 of which 65 million were directed to medication and 6.5 million to medical related products.

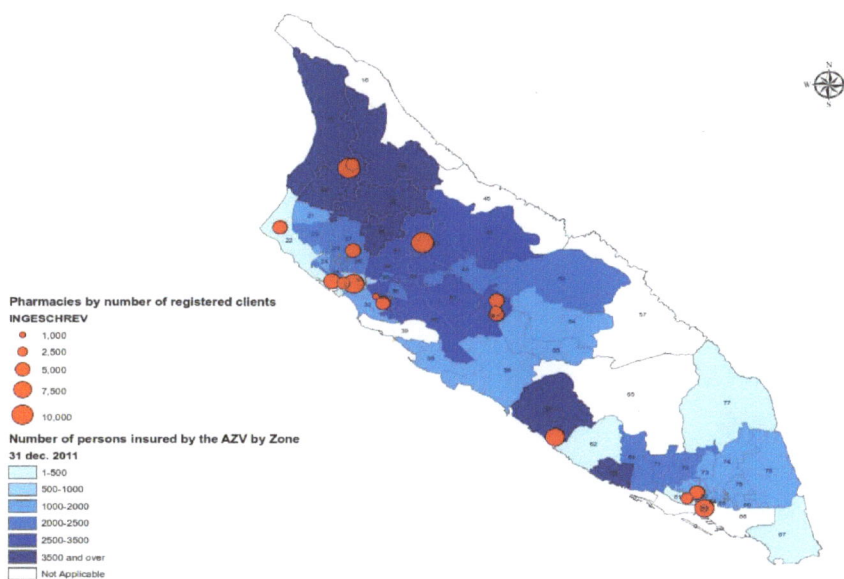

Figure 99. Distribution of the pharmacies over the island, Aruba 2011.

7.3 Hospital Admissions

Aruba has one hospital with about 300 beds. In Figure 100, the number of total clinical admissions per year is illustrated. This information is provided by the Dr. H. Oduber Hospital.

A decrease in the clinical admission is noted from 2006 to 2008; from 2007 to 2008 this decrease was of almost 10 percent (9.3 percent), see Figure 100. From 2008 to 2009 a small increase has been noticed (+1.3 percent). The admissions are further analyzed by age categories and are illustrated in Figure 101.

As Figure 101 shows, persons in the age category 15–44 years are the most admitted to the Dr. H. Oduber Hospital, followed by the age category 45–64 and the age category 0 years, see Figure 101.

As the Medisch benchmark Dr. H. Oduber Hospital showed, the age category 15–64 years occupies about 50 percent of all beds in the Dr. H. Oduber Hospital. The average hospitalization day of a patient is 8.1 days. Patients in the age category 65 years and up had a minimum of 11.1 hospitalization days to a maximum of 14.2 hospitalization days in 2009, whereas for the age category 15–44 this was 6.2 hospitalization days in this same year.

This means that although the age category 15–44 years has the highest number of clinical admissions, the age category 65 and up has the highest number of hospitalization days in the hospital, meaning that although the younger age category

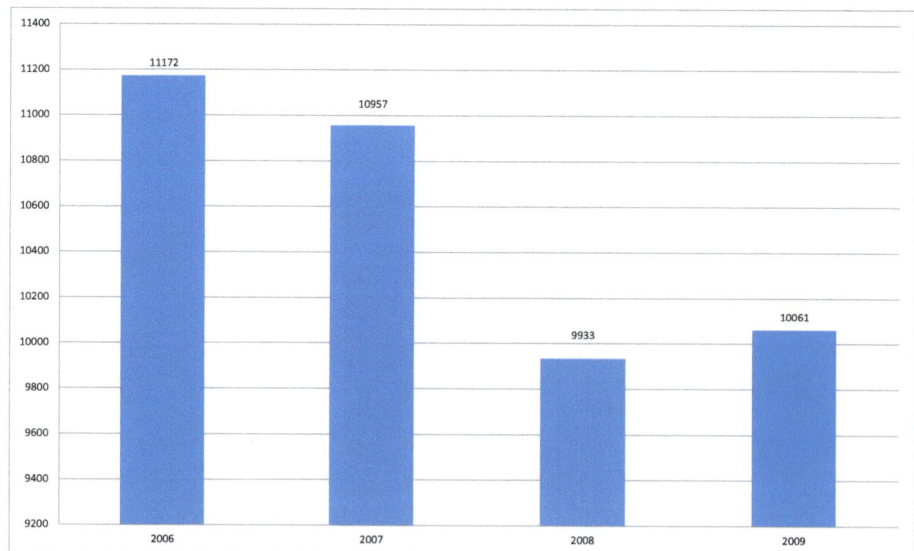

Figure 100. Total number of hospital admissions per year, Dr. H. Oduber Hospital, Aruba 2006–2009.

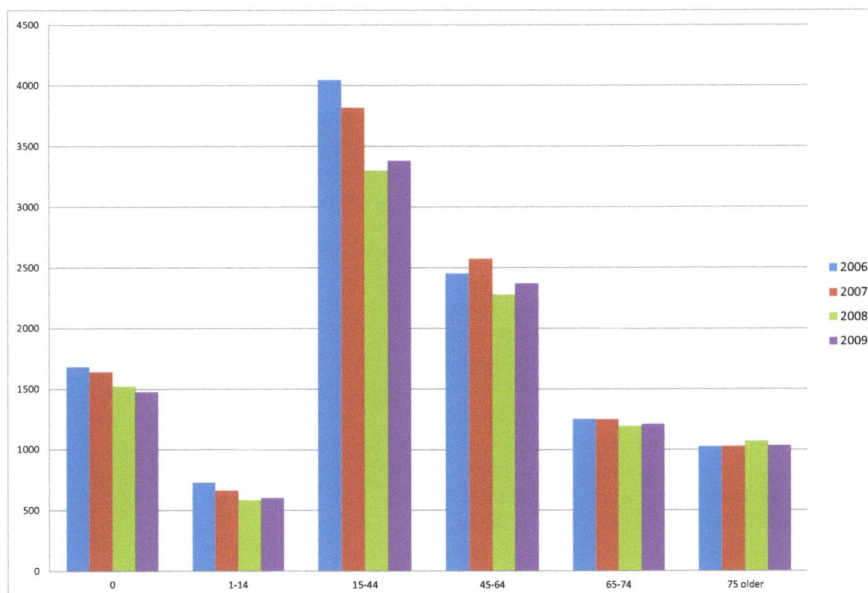

Figure 101. Total number of clinical admission per age category, Dr. H. Oduber Hospital, 2006–2009.

is admitted the most, their number of days admitted are less compared to the age category of 65 plus years (KIWA Prismant, 2012).

7.3.1 Admission by Diagnosis

Admissions are categorized between elective admission and emergency admission. An elective admission is where a patient has been booked in to be admitted to hospital rather than coming in as an emergency. The booking is usually made after the patient sees a hospital specialist. The patient will then be placed on a waiting list until it is their turn to be admitted (KIWA Prismant, 2012).

Emergency admission patients are admitted through the Emergency Department. These are seriously injured or ill patients who need immediate treatment (KIWA Prismant, 2012).

Elective Admissions

The following graph illustrates the elective admissions by diagnosis during the period 2006 to 2009; a selection has been made of the top 15 of the most common admissions.

As Figure 102 shows, eye disease is the most common cause of admission through the period 2006 to 2009, followed by arthropathies and dorsopathies and special aftercare.

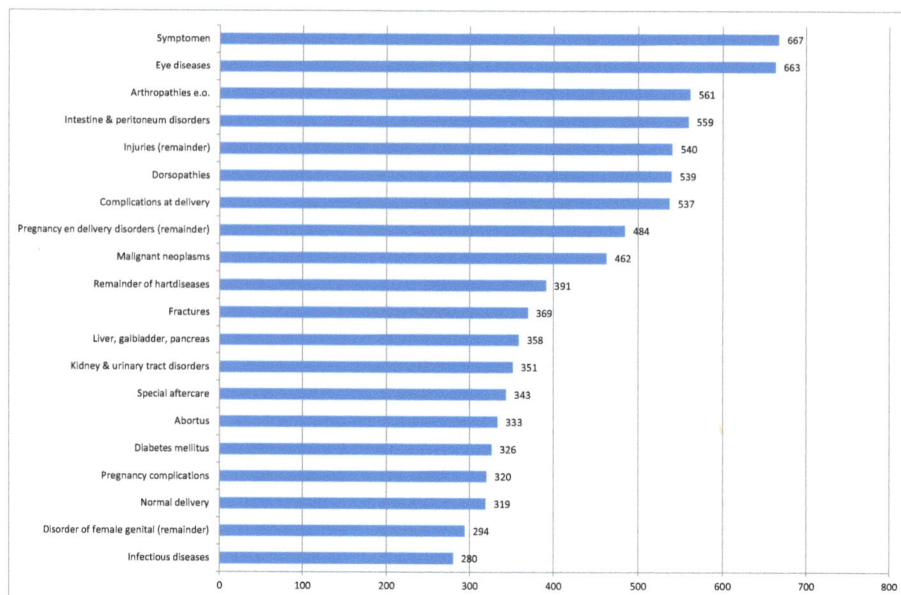

Figure 102. Elective admissions by disorder or disease at the Dr. H. Oduber Hospital, Aruba 2006–2009.

Emergency Admissions

The emergency admissions distributed are during the period 2006 to 2009 as follows, see Figure 103. In 2007 the emergency admissions have reached a peak, 9504 emergency admissions; from 2008 to 2009 the emergency admissions had a decrease of about 44 percent. This decrease was due to the fact that live births were registered under the correct administrative code during that year.

Diagnoses for emergency admission differ from the elective admission, since the patients need immediate care for their disease.

As Figure 104 shows, live births or deliveries are registered as emergency admissions, although this is not the correct admission registration for emergency admission. This is the most common type of emergency admission followed by complications at delivery and symptoms. Symptoms are subjective and in this case difficult to specify as a specific disease. Live births are more than 10 percent of the total emergency admissions from 2006 to 2009 (KIWA Prismant, 2012).

In the top 5 of the emergency admission are also intestine & peritoneum disorders, injuries and remainder of heart diseases. Overall complications at delivery, pregnancy complications and pregnancy and delivery disorders dominate the diagnoses for emergency admissions.

Other diagnoses that are of importance are e.g. abortions, which during this same period there were 1005 elective admissions for all age categories as well as through the emergency admission. Cerebrovascular disorder is also a diagnosis which had 122 about 1098 elective admissions including emergency admissions.

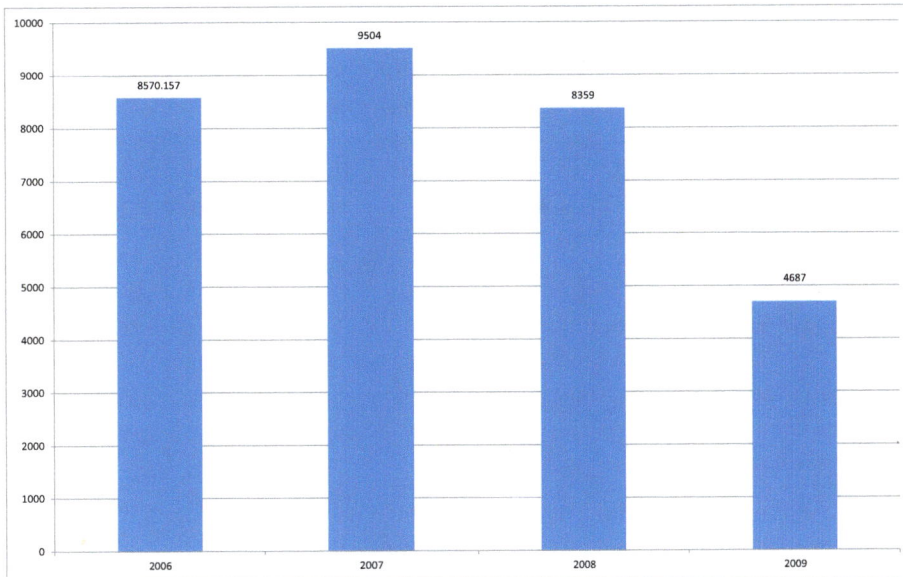

Figure 103. Emergency admission at the Dr. H. Oduber Hospital, Aruba 2006–2009.

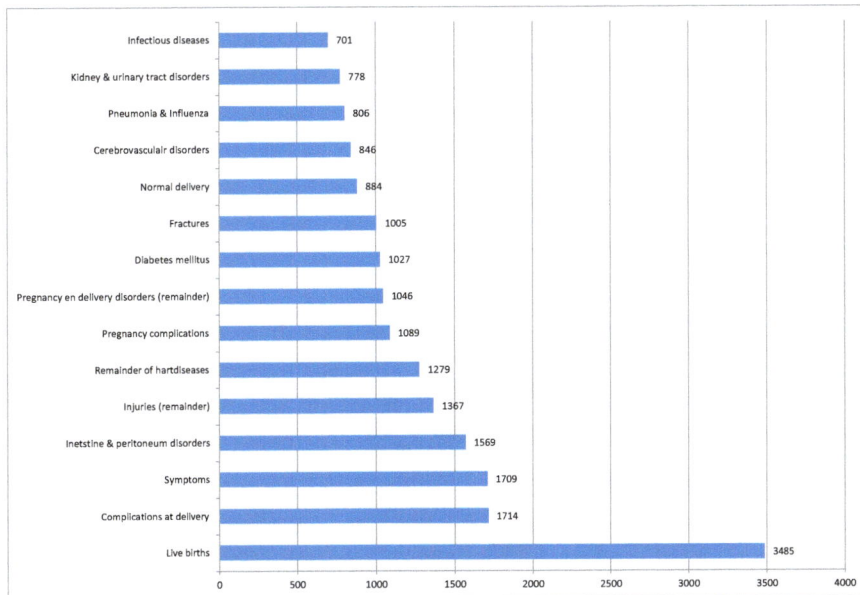

Figure 104. Total number of clinical admission per age category, Dr. H. Oduber Hospital, 2006–2009.

7.4 Healthy Baby Clinics

The Department of Public Health of Aruba is the only provider of the vaccinations of the National Vaccination Program. Through the White Yellow Cross (WYC) distribution is made possible using the different locations it has on the island. Vaccinations are administered by the youth health doctors of the Department of Public Health. The White Yellow Cross (WYC) organizes healthy baby clinics at six different locations on the island: Noord, Oranjestad, Dakota, Santa Cruz, Savaneta and San Nicolas. For a small yearly family-fee these clinics provide consultations by physicians and nurses (9-10 times in the first 15 months) and also provide vaccination during the first five years of life of the newborn.

Besides provision of vaccination and consultation nurses of the WYC also perform a hearing screening on the newborns. In 2010, 1277 babies underwent a hearing screening test. This neonatal hearing screening is performed at a small extra fee. Consultations during the first years of life provide early detection of congenital problems and nutritional and educational advice at an early age may help prevent health risks later in life.

In 2010 there were 1231 newborns registered at the baby clinics at the WYC which is higher than the official registered births at the Population Registry Office of Aruba. One of the reasons for this discrepancy might be that babies from undocumented mothers are registered at the WYC but not at the Population Registry Office, see Table 21.

Table 21. Live births White Yellow Cross and Population Registry office of Aruba.

Year	White Yellow Cross registered births	Registered births	%
2010	1231	1141	7.8
2009	1293	1213	6.2
2008	1389	1319	5.0
2007	1406	1339	4.8
2006	1477	1227	16.9

In this program, a child during their first 15 months of life receives 5 physician consultations and 5 nurse consultations. After this 15-month period, the child gets only 1 consult thereafter.

In 2010 there were 211 referrals to the family physician, where the following were detected, see Table 22.

Table 22. Health problems detected in newborns in 2011.

Health problems	Number of cases detected
Heart murmur	38
Strabismus (possible eyesight problems)	17
Atopic dermatitis	33
Hip dysplasia (probable)	35
Urological problemsproblems	16
Overweight	6

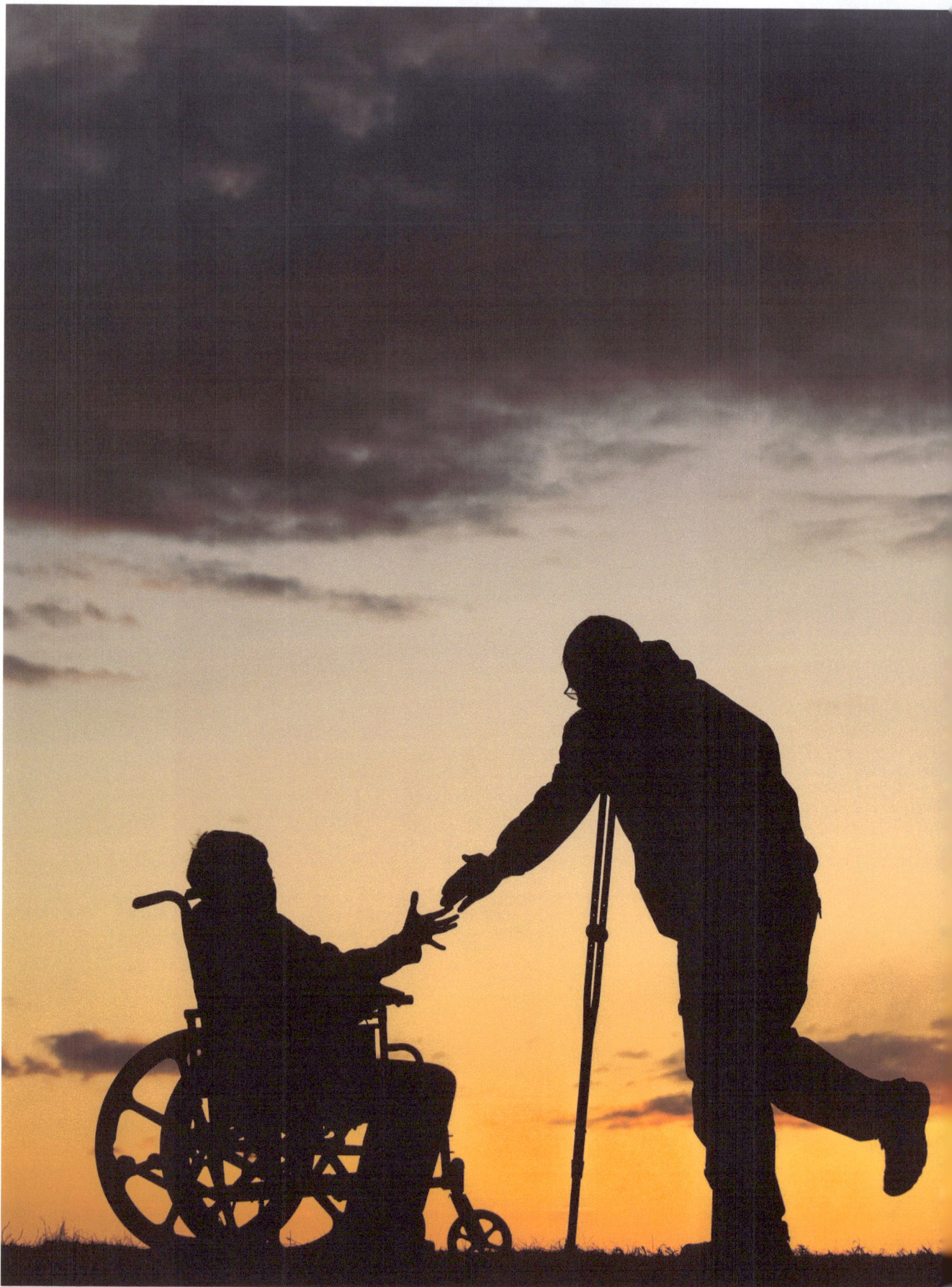

8.1 People with Mental and Physical Disabilities

Persons with disabilities often belong to the most vulnerable groups in society. Compared to the general population, they are at greater risk of experiencing limitations when performing daily activities and/or experiencing restrictions of participation in society. There are different types of disabilities in different domains, visual domain, hearing domain and mobility domain.

During the 2010 Aruba Census, a total of 6,955 individuals (2947 males and 4007 females) reported having a disability on at least one domain of functioning, representing 6.9 percent of the population of Aruba. The prevalence of disability increases almost exponentially with increasing age. Between ages 60 and 64, 11.1 percent reported having a disability, and in persons ten years older (between ages 70 and 74), the prevalence of disability doubled to 22.6 percent. Between ages 85 and 89, more than half of all persons 61.1 percent reported having a disability in at least one domain of functioning (see Figure 105A). Moreover, although persons 65 years and older represented 10.4 percent of the total population of Aruba, they accounted for

Where the role of sex in the prevalence of disability is concerned, worldwide, females are most affected by disability. However, in Aruba, the prevalence of disability in females has for decades been very similar to that in males. According to the 2010 Aruba Census, 7.6 percent of females and 6.1 percent of males were affected by disability.

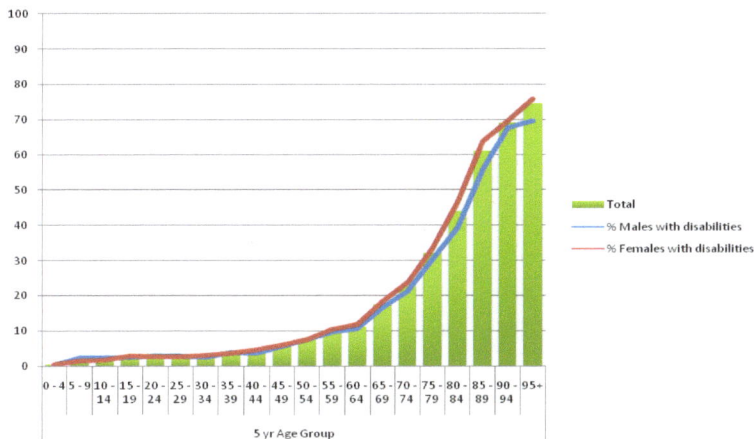

Figure 105A. The prevalence of disability by age category and sex.

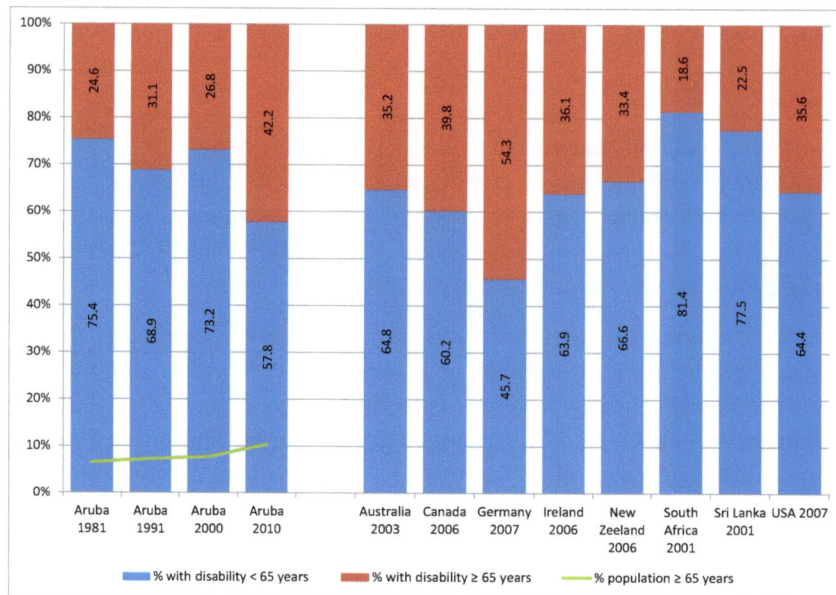

Figure 105B. Distribution of ages within disability populations (World report on disability, 2011).

Overall, disabilities were most often reported in the visual domain of functioning, followed by disabilities in mobility (see Table 23).

Table 23. Number of persons with disability by domain of functioning.

Domain of functioning	Number of persons with disability*		Prevalence of disability (%)*	
	Males	Females	Males	Females
Seeing	1242	1852	2.8	3.7
Hearing	660	635	1.5	1.3
Mobility	1061	1867	2.2	3.5
Cognition	638	809	1.3	1.5
Self-care	424	623	0.9	1.2
Communication	547	521	1.1	1.0

As age increases, a steep increase is observed in the prevalence of disabilities in mobility and self-care and in the number of functional domains for which persons reported having a disability (see Figure 106).

In total, 26.9 percent of persons with disability (on at least one domain of functioning) were in need of help with personal care and/or household chores.

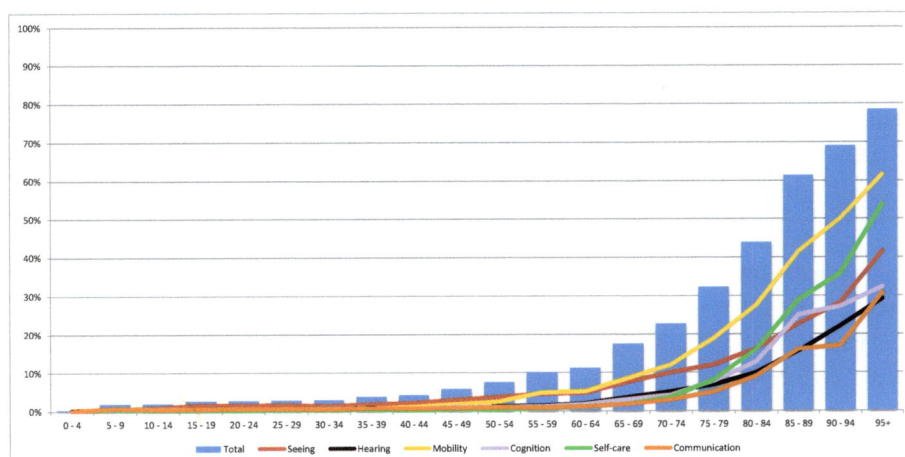

Figure 106. The Prevalence of disability by domain of functioning and age.

Those most in need of personal care were females, older persons and persons with disabilities on more than one domain of functioning. In addition, persons with a disability in self-care (94.1 percent), communication (70.6 percent) or cognitive functioning (55.6 percent) were more in need of help when compared to persons with a seeing (18.8 percent) or hearing (24.1 percent) disability.

Of persons with disability needing help, 6.7 percent reported not receiving the help and assistance they needed (5.5 percent of males, and 7.6 percent of females). These persons were on average younger than persons who did receive help and reported having a disability on a fewer number of domains of functioning compared to persons who received help.

Nearly a quarter of persons with disability not receiving help lived in a one-person household, whilst the majority of persons with disability receiving help lived in extended households, where help was more readily available. The help and assistance was mainly provided by family members who lived in the same household as the person with disability (71.0 percent).

In total, during the 2010 Aruba Census, 344 persons with a disability and in need of help were living in an institution. This group consisted of more females than males (210 and 134, respectively), who lived primarily in a home for the elderly (88.1 percent). Overall, the results of the 2010 Census revealed that as the age of persons with disability increases (and thus the number of domains on which they had a disability), the percentage receiving help from family members inside the 128 household decreases, accompanied by an increase in the percentage receiving help from others who were paid to provide the help needed and also by an increase in the percentage of persons with disability being admitted to an institution.

8.2 Female Commercial Sex Workers

As stated by the National Ordinance (LV BZ, 1994); "Person of the female sex, who commits adultery with persons of the opposite sex, profession or habit, are required to register in person at the Ministry of Justice or by an official to be designated." As the Ordinance further states, this person is required to register at the Department of Public Health who is in charge of the medical screening.

The Service of Infectious Diseases of the Department of Public Health is in charge of the screening of the female commercial sex workers (FCSW) that are employed by the San Nicolas Bar association. This association represents 30 bars in San Nicolas where these FCSW operate; each bar is allowed to have a maximum of 4 FCSW at one bar at a time. A working permission for 3 months is granted once they pass their medical screening.

The medical screening consists of a weekly medical screening for STI's conducted by a General Physician appointed by the Department of Public Health. At the arrival and registration of the FCSW the laboratory tests for Syphilis and HIV tests are conducted. Also the PPD (Mantoux) skin test to detect the presence of antibodies against Tuberculosis and a chest X-ray for detection of pulmonary tuberculosis are conducted. These tests are done by the Service of Infectious Diseases of the Department of Public Health.

From 2006 to 2010 the Service of Infectious Diseases received a total of 1913 work permission requests specific for FCSW. About 3 percent of the requests were denied,

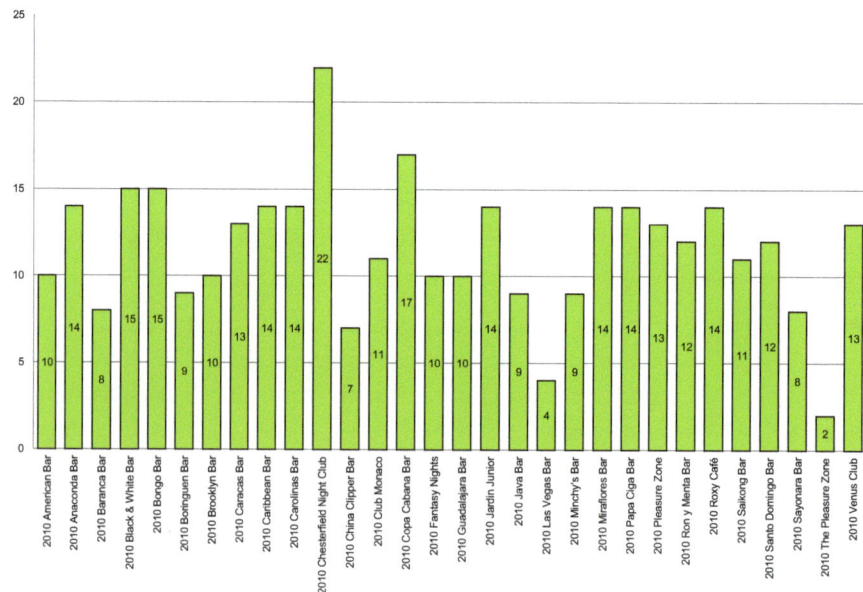

Figure 107. Total numbers of commercial female sex workers per bar, Aruba 2010.

from which 0.6 percent ($n = 11$) tested positive for syphilis, 0.5 percent ($n = 1$) tested positive for HIV and 0.3 percent ($n = 6$) had a positive PPD test.

In 2010 The San Nicolas Bas Association had 30 bars where the female FCSW operate. These bars are all located in San Nicolas. There is no bar association in the capital of the island for FCSW, there is no structure in place for the FCSW in the capital. These FCSW are considered as illegal FCSW. However these illegal FCSW are operational, exposing their health and their client's to risks. There are no registrations of the FCSW in the capital of Aruba. Most of the registered FCSW originate from Colombia, their age ranges between 18 and 50 years old, see Table 24 for the distribution of the age categories.

Table 24. Age distribution of FCSW, Aruba 2006-2009.

Age category	Number
18–24	457
25–44	1448
45–64	8
Total	1913

During their working period, the FCSWs as stated above undergo a medical checkup at the General Physician appointed by the Department of Public Health of Aruba. Refusal of this weekly check up will result in immediate deportation of the FCSW to the country of residence.

REFERENCES

Globocan, 2008. *Estimated cancer Incidence, Mortality, Prevalence and Disability-adjusted life years (DALYs) Worldwide in 2008.* Globocan website available online: http://globocan.iarc.fr/.

Pan American Health Organization, n.d. *Health Topics: Cancer.* PAHO website 2012, available online: http://new.paho.org/hq/index.php?option=com_content&view=article&id=292%3Acance r&catid=1866%3Ahsd0201a-cancer-home&Itemid=3855&lang=en.

Globocan, 2008. *The Data base.* Globocan website available online: http://www-dep.iarc.fr/ WHOdb/WHOdb.htm.

Martinez G, Copen CE, Abma JC. *Teenagers in the United States: Sexual activity, contraceptive use, and childbearing, 2006–2010. National Survey of Family Growth. National Center for Health Statistics. National Vital Health Stat.* 2011;23(31).

Singh S, Darroch JE. *Adolescent pregnancy and childbearing: levels and trends in developed countries.* Fam Plann Perspect. 2000;32(1):14–23.

National Campaign to Prevent Teen and Unplanned Pregnancy, *Counting It Up: The Public Costs of Teen Childbearing* 2011.

Perper K, Peterson K, Manlove J. *Diploma Attainment Among Teen Mothers.* Child Trends, Fact Sheet Publication #2010-01: Washington, DC: Child Trends; 2010.

Hoffman SD. *Kids Having Kids: Economic Costs and Social Consequences of Teen Pregnancy.* Washington, DC: The Urban Institute Press; 2008.

Kirby D, Laris BA, Rolleri L. *The Impact of Sex and HIV Education Programs in Schools and Communities on Sexual Behaviors Among Young Adults.* Scotts Valley, CA: ETR Associates; 2006.

Sociaal Economische Raad, 2007. Tienerzwangerschappen in Aruba.

Wilk van der, E. and Harbers, 2012. *Overgewicht: Zijn er verschillen tussen Nederland en andere landen?* Volksgezondheid Toekomst Verkenning, Nationaal Kompas Volksgezondheid. Available: http://www.nationaalkompas.nl

Algemene Ziektekosten Verzekering Aruba, Jaarrekening AZV 2011.

Kenens RJ, Hingstman L., 2009. *Cijfers uit de registratie van fysiotherapeuten.* Peiling 2008. Nivel.

Staring, J., "*An analysis of Mental Health in Aruba and the collaborating forces within the mental healthcare services.*" Dissertation, University of Aruba. 2010

National Institute of Mental Health, n.d. Schizophrenia. Available online: http://www. nimh.nih.gov/health/publications/the-numbers-count-mental-disorders-in-erica/index. shtml#Schizophrenia.

Gommer, A. & Poos M., 2010. *Prevalentie, incidentie en sterfte naar leeftijd en geslacht.* Volksgezondheid Toekomst Verkenning, Nationaal Kompas Volksgezondheid. Available: http://www.nationaalkompas.nl/gezondheid-en-ziekte/ ziekten-en-aandoeningen/psychischestoornissen/schizofrenie/cijfers-schizofrenie-prevalentie-incidentie-en-sterfte-uit-de-vtv-2010/

Public Health Agency Canada, 2002. *A report on mental illness in Canada.* Public Health Agency Canada website. Available: http://www.phac-aspc.gc.ca/publicat/miic-mmac/chap_2-eng.php.

National Institute of Mental Health, n.d. *The Numbers Count: Mental Disorders in America.* National Institute of Mental Health website, available: http://www.nimh. nih.gov/health/ publications/the-numbers-count-mental-disorders-in-america/ index.shtml

Schoemaker et al., 2012. *Hoe vaak komt depressie voor en hoeveel mensen sterven er aan?* Volksgezondheid Toekomst Verkenning, Nationaal Kompas Volksgezondheid.

Bilthoven: RIVM, Available: http://www.nationaalkompas.nl> Nationaal Kompas Volksgezondheid\Gezondheid en ziekte\Ziekten en aandoeningen\Psychische stoornissen.

World Health Organization, 2012. Suicide prevention (SUPRE). Programmes and projects: Mental Health. WHO website, available: http://www.who.int/mental_health/prevention/ suicide/suicideprevent/en/.

Bertolote, M., and Fleischmann, A., *A global perspective in the epidemiology of suicide.* Suicidologi 2002, arg.7, nr. 2.

Lanting, L. & Stam, C. *Hoe vaak komt zelftoegebrachte letsel voor en hoeveel mensen sterven eraan?* In: Volksgezondheid Toekomst Verkenning, Nationaal Kompas Volksgezondheid. Bilthoven: RIVM, Avaialble: http://www.nationaalkompas.nl> Nationaal Kompas Volksgezondheid\Gezondheid en ziekte\Ziekten en aandoeningen\Letsels en vergiftigingen\ Zelftoegebracht letsel.

Centraal Bureau voor de statistiek NL, 2012. Aantal zelfdoden stijgt naar 1647. CBS NL website, available: http://www.cbs.nl/nl-NL/menu/themas/bevolking/publicaties/artikelen/ archief/2012/2012-3668-wm.htm

Mc Main, S., 2012. *Hope for the Chronically Suicidal Patient, an interventional study.* Clinical trials website, available: http://clinicaltrials.gov/ct2/show/NCT00154154.

World Health Organization, 2001. Global Prevalence and incidence of selected curable sexually transmitted infections overview and estimates. WHO website, available: http://www.who.int/hiv/pub/sti/who_hiv_aids_2001.02.pdf

World Health Organization, 2012. Tobacco. Health Topics, WHO website, available: http://www.who.int/topics/tobacco/en/.

World Health Organization, 2012. Alcohol. Media Centre, WHO website, available: http://www.who.int/mediacentre/factsheets/fs349/en/index.html

Centraal Bureau voor de statistiek NL, 2012. Overleden 10–19 jarigen door zelfdoding per woonprovincie, 2000–2008. CBS NL website, available: http://www.cbs.nl/nl-NL/menu/themas/ gezondheid-welzijn/cijfers/incidenteel/maatwerk/2009-zelfdoding-jongeren-provincie-mw.htm.

The Department of Public Health Aruba, 2012. Department of Pathology of the National Laboratory Aruba.

KIWA Prismant, 2012. Medische benchmark Dr. Horacio E. Oduber Hospitaal, Aruba 2006–2009.

Chapter 3

HEALTHY AND ACTIVE LIFESTYLE:

WINDOWS ON A VISION IN MOTION — PREVENTION-FOCUSED COMMUNITY POLICY IN ARUBA FOR REDUCING DISEASE BURDEN AND MORTALITY RATES

WITH REFLECTIONS BY DR. RICHARD VISSER, MINISTER OF PUBLIC HEALTH AND SPORTS

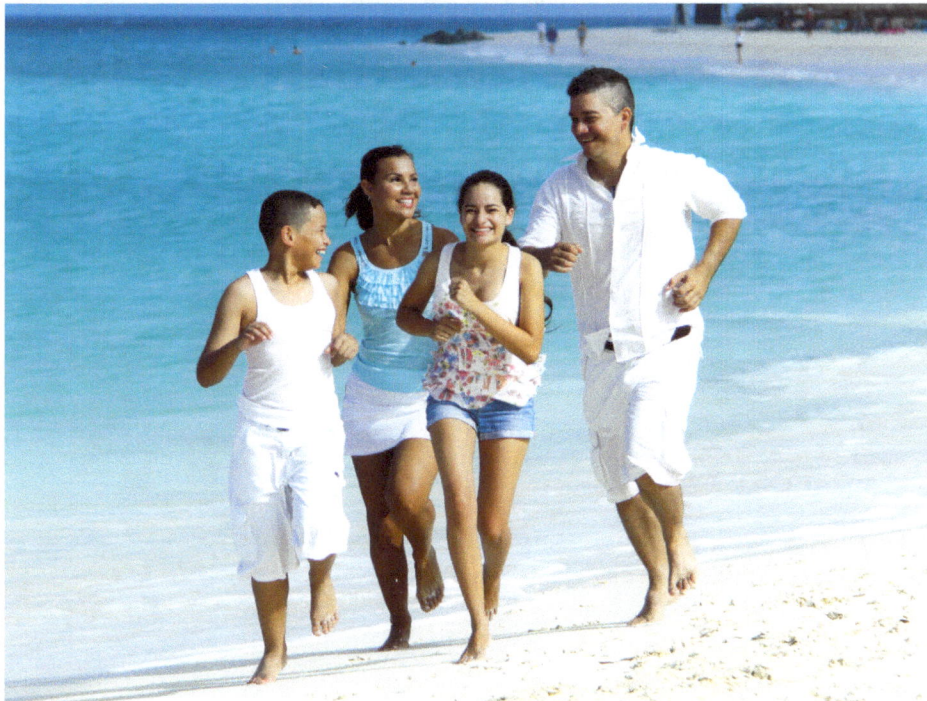

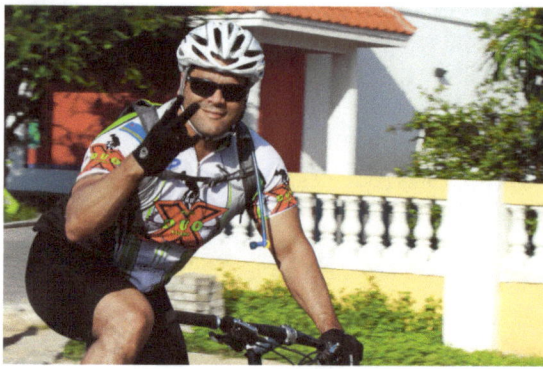

This publication—*Healthy and active lifestyle. Windows on a vision in motion*—gives a picture of the prevention-focused, community-based policy of the Minister of Public Health and Sports of the Government of Prime Minister Mike Eman, Dr. Richard Visser. The key objective of that policy is to prevent and/or reduce the disease burden and mortality rate in Aruba, caused by the obesity epidemic and other non-communicable diseases (NCDs), such as cardiovascular diseases, diabetes, cancer, pulmonary diseases, and depression. In the process, appropriate attention will still be paid to the fight against infectious diseases, such as dengue.

At the same time, it is being taken into consideration that health is more than just the absence of disease. Healthy people are absent less frequently, learn better, produce more, and are happier. In addition to disease prevention, including adequate treatment, the vision of a healthy and active lifestyle also entails health promotion. The health policy is characterized by the promotion of a whole-of-government and whole-of-society approach.

In his contribution, titled *Healthy and active lifestyle. Reflections,* Minister Visser outlines the national operational health vision. He also elucidates his personal and professional motivation in this respect. A crucial reference of the vision is the *National Plan Aruba 2009–2018: to fight overweight, obesity, and related health issues,* which was adopted unanimously by Aruban Parliament.

The text is followed by *Windows* on a vision in motion, pages with photographs illustrating the Aruban efforts and results in the area of public health and sports.

Under the heading *Literature consulted,* mainly the health effort of Aruba in the area of reporting, research, and policy development can be found. That effort offers a rich source to all those who wish to study the themes discussed in this publication more closely.

In *Literature consulted,* reference is also made to the website www.paco.aw on which *The Aruba Call for Action on Obesity* and all other contributions to the *Pan American Conference on Obesity,* with special attention to *childhood obesity* (PACO I and II) are published. The leading role of host Aruba in the creation of the international forum PACO laid the foundation for the admission in 2012 of Aruba, Curaçao, and Sint Maarten as Associate Members to the Pan American Health Organization (PAHO). The PAHO, well over 110 years old, is the oldest international public health organization. It also serves as the regional office for the Americas of the World Health Organization (WHO), the health organization of the United Nations.

Ministry of Public Health and Sports

Aruba, February 2013

HEALTHY AND ACTIVE LIFESTYLE

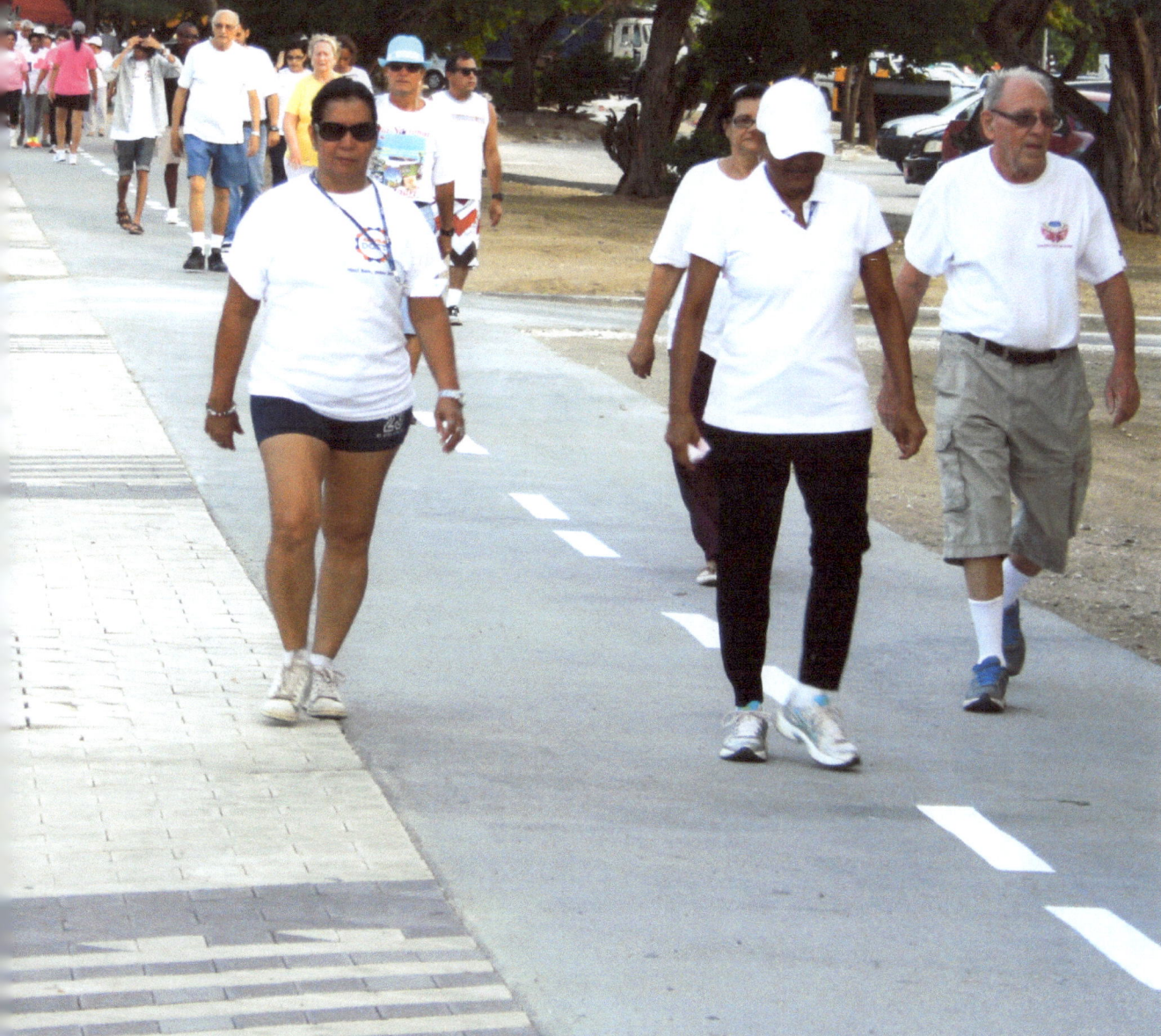

REFLECTIONS

I was eight years old when my father passed away. Obesity played a key role in his premature death. If he had lived a healthier life, I would probably have had a father for a longer time. Unfortunately, my personal story is the story of Aruba. Our island belongs to the world's 'best' insofar as the prevalence of obesity is concerned, as also evidenced by my doctoral research into overweight and obesity among schoolchildren in Aruba.

NATIONAL PLAN ARUBA 2009–2018 AND NCDS

Obesity is a non-communicable disease (NCD). Unlike an infectious disease, it is non-transmittable. It is also an important risk factor for other NCDs, such as cardiovascular diseases, diabetes, cancer, pulmonary diseases and depression. The NCDs are the biggest health challenge both worldwide and in our island. They form the most important disease burden, have the highest mortality rate, and generate the highest health care costs. The NCDs form an impeding factor to education and economic development. The rapid growth and extent of NCDs undermine the functioning and quality of life of families and communities.

Obesity and other NCDs are not a natural disaster; they can often be prevented and, in many cases, be treated as well. Smoking, alcohol abuse, unhealthy eating habits,

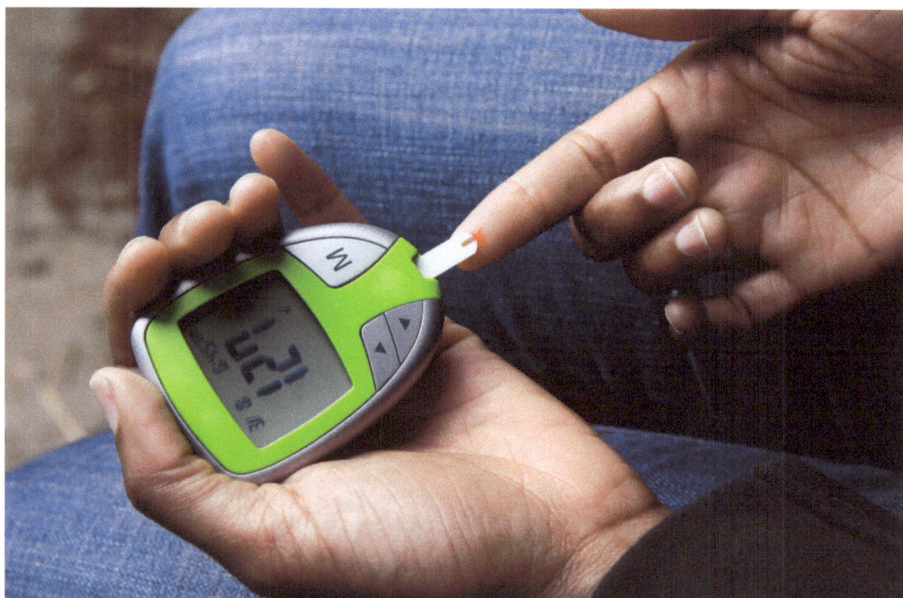

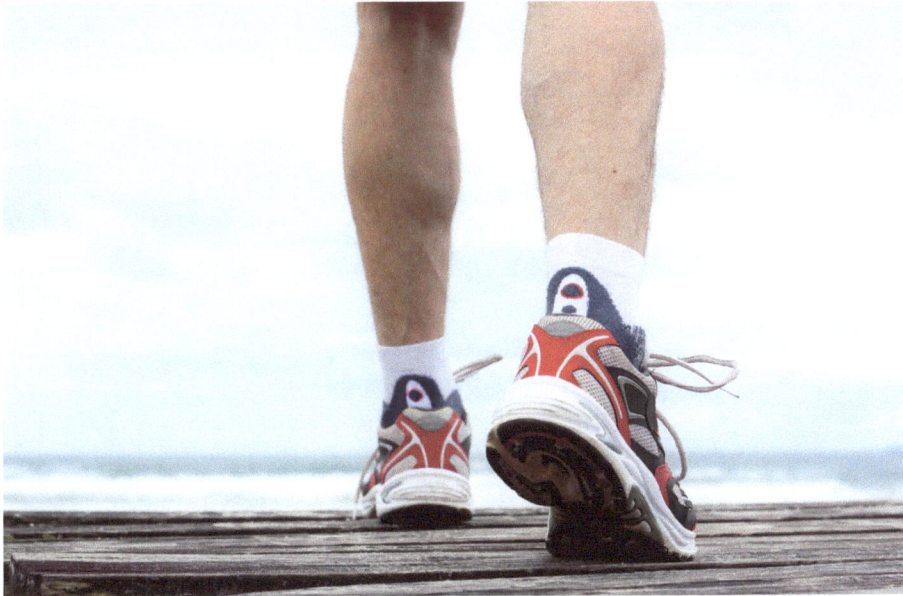

physical inactivity, lack of social commitment, and a weak socioeconomic status can be tackled. It is necessary to opt for prevention and social responsibility. Aruban Parliament unanimously approved the *National Plan Aruba 2009–2018: to fight overweight, obesity, and related health issues* (Special Obesity Committee, 2008). As a researcher and son of Aruba, I was honored to be able to draft the *National Plan Aruba 2009–2018*.

SUSTAINABILITY AND COMMUNITARIANISM

In 2009, I took office as the Minister of Public Health and Sports in the Government under the leadership of the innovative Prime Minister Mike Eman. New points of reference were also assigned to the public health and sports policy. Sustainability and communitarianism. Strategic partnership within the Kingdom of the Netherlands. The development of a European (Latin) American and regional liaison function.

As a result, Aruba was designated host for the meeting of epidemiologists and other experts in the area f the fight against infectious diseases of the four countries of the kingdom.

The accent on prevention and a life-course approach in the policy on public health and sports seamlessly integrated with the concept of sustainability, the main focus of which also lies on the generations to come.

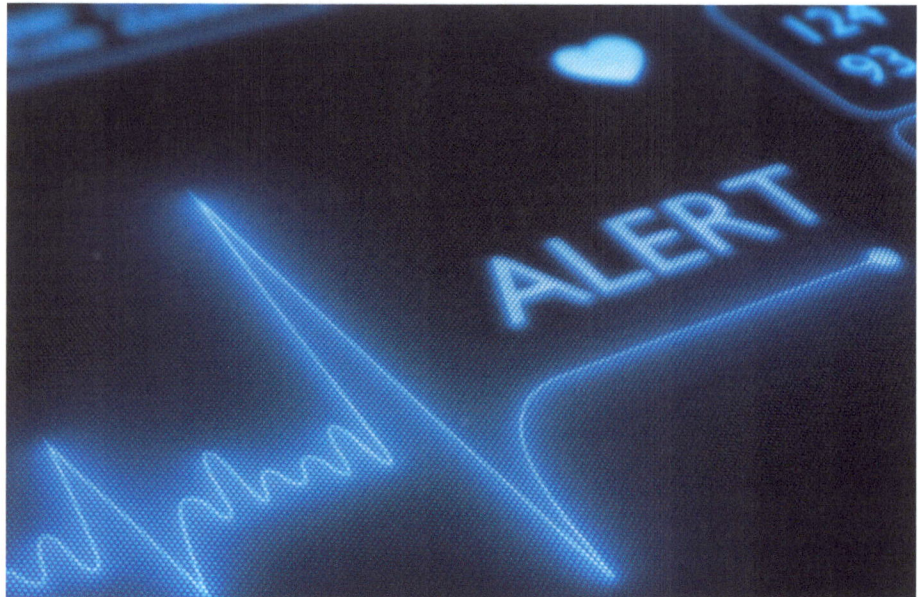

The community-based approach offered a stimulus for the concept of a new health officer: the Public Health Officer (PHO) in the district *(bario)*. He or she will work on a local intersectoral health policy together with officials of other government agencies in multifunctional accommodations. As a result of that approach, the idea that health is not only a matter of health care but of the *whole-of-government and the whole-of-society* as well was also incorporated into the policy. The Green Gateway, *Scol Saludabel* (Healthy School), the Linear Park, and the enforcement of traffic safety are examples of contributions to public health by sectors other than the (curative) care sector. Aruba is heading towards a comprehensive health policy and has opportunities to side with the best countries in this area. It could be one of the first islands/countries in the Americas to implement the Finish state-of-the-art model—'Health in All Policies'.

The concept of a strategic partnership in the area of public health care, notably disease prevention and health promotion, was implemented in the form of a productive cooperation between the Directorate of Public Health ('DVG') of Aruba and the Municipal Health Service ('GGD') of The Hague. Aruba took the initiative at a Kingdom level in the area of the (international) fight against infectious diseases. As a result, Aruba was designated host for the meeting of epidemiologists and other experts in the area of the fight against infectious diseases of the four countries of the Kingdom. Under the leadership of the National Institute of Public Health and Environmental Protection ('RIVM') and financially facilitated by the Dutch Ministry of Public Health, Welfare, and Sports ('VWS'), the experts from the Kingdom laid

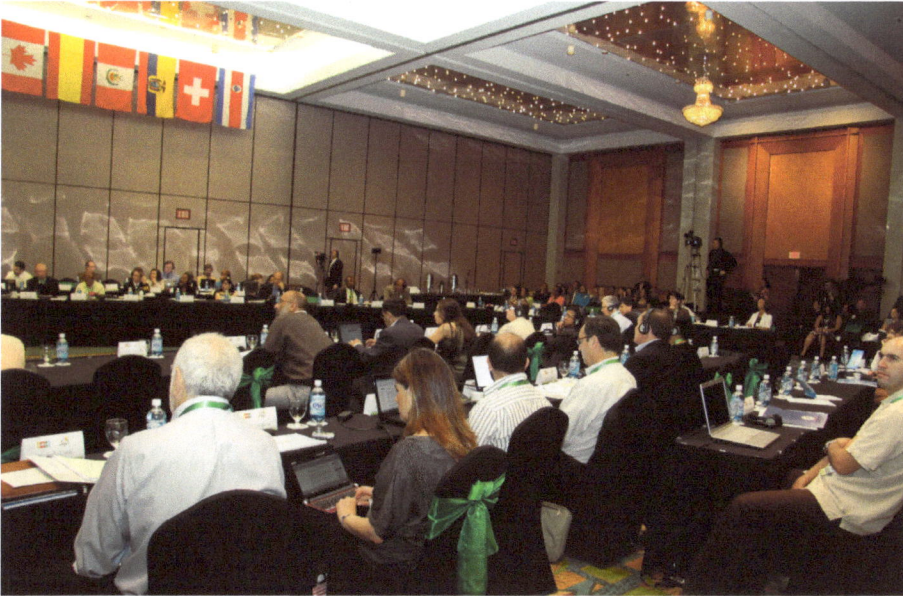

the foundation in Oranjestad for Kingdom policy on the implementation of the International Health Regulations (IRH) of the World Health Organization (WHO).

PAN AMERICAN CONFERENCE ON OBESITY (PACO)

Nos baranca tan stima [Papiamento name for Aruba] also played a leading role at a regional and international level. Aruba was the initiator and host of the first *Pan American Conference on Obesity, with special attention to childhood obesity* (PACO) in 2011, which was opened by Prime Minister Mike Eman. Experts, professionals, and public health ministers from dozens of countries in the Americas and Europe shared multidisciplinary knowledge, best practices, and networks. As a result of PACO I and II, the latter was held in 2012, Aruba received great regional appreciation in the area of the prevention of obesity and NCDs. Chilean Parliament praised Aruba for its contribution to public health in Latin America and the Caribbean.

The health-related effort of Aruba within the kingdom of the Netherlands and the Pan American Health Organization (PAHO) resulted in Aruba's associate membership of the PAHO in 2012.

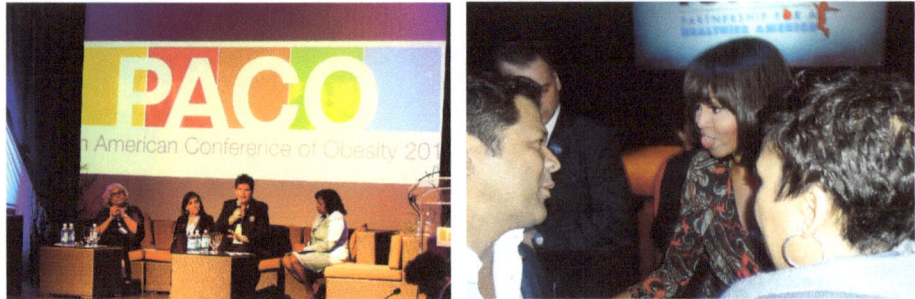

During the *United Nations High-Level Meeting on Non-Communicable Disease Prevention and Control NCD* in New York in September 2011, the Minister of Public Health and Sports of Aruba spoke on behalf of the Kingdom of the Netherlands. During this international top forum of heads of state and government leaders, I explained the contribution of PACO I. *The Aruba Call for Action on Obesity,* as adopted by PACO I, found its way in the *Political Declaration of the High-Level Meeting of the General Assembly of the United Nations on the Prevention and Control of Non-Communicable Diseases* (2011). Never before did an Aruban initiative acquire a place in a normative public health statement of the world community.

The health-related effort of Aruba within the Kingdom of the Netherlands and the Pan American Health Organization (PAHO) resulted in Aruba's Associate Membership of the PAHO in 2012. Until then, Aruba was indirectly represented by representatives of the Kingdom. Aruba obtained its own vote within the PAHO, an emancipatory event that marked an expansion of the Status Aparte within the health organization of the western hemisphere. Of course, Curaçao and Sint Maarten also obtained the PAHO Associate Membership, together with Aruba.

The PACOs also offered the local physicians, public health professionals, and other persons concerned a learning environment. Healthcare is a knowledge-intensive undertaking, in which knowledge development and knowledge sharing are cross-border activities. Sharing in evidence-based knowledge and best practices, as presented by top experts and renowned public health services during the PACOs, directly contributes to the health policy and the quality of the care offered in Aruba. The themes of the PACOs fit in with the *National Plan Aruba 2009–2018.*

'INSTITUTO BIBA SALUDABEL Y ACTIVIO (IBISA)'

The concept of a *healthy and active lifestyle* puts into words a health vision that does not only include the treatment of physical and mental diseases, but also the prevention of diseases and the promotion of health in the different stages of life as a social and professional assignment. This vision is in line with the modern requirements and standards. Dr. Carisse F. Etienne, the recently elected new PAHO Director, made the following statement in her confirmation speech on January 22, 2013:

> *Let me be clear: Providing universal health coverage means ensuring that the entire population has access to necessary health services—prevention, promotion , treatment, and care without fear of financial catastrophe or impoverishment.*

Professional, personal, and social responsibilities complement each other in the new Aruban health vision. A care policy should be supported by a health policy in which attention is paid to lifestyle-related socioeconomic and physical environmental factors. In addition to care providers, the *whole-of-government* and the *whole-of-society* should contribute to health and perform in the best possible way. Not only because the 'right to health' is one of the internationally recognized human rights, but also because health is more than just the absence of disease. Healthier and physically active citizens learn, study, and produce better and more. They are happier. It is with good reason that the United Nations consider the rapid growth of NCDs one of the most important threats to social, cultural, and economic development.

A healthy lifestyle requires more than just individual responsibility. It is influenced by *inter alia* knowledge (health literacy), socioeconomic status, and social cohesion. This thought led to the prioritization of a prevention institute in the *National Plan Aruba 2009–2018*. This institute has materialized in the form of the 'Instituto Biba Saludabel y Activo (IBiSA)', the National Institute for Healthy and Active Living. The IBiSA focuses on sports and education, nutrition, and public mental health (amplition). By means of the 'Bus di Salud' *[Health Bus]*, it has made personal prevention accessible to schools, companies, and districts. In addition, it analyzes risk factors and gives personal health advice based on biometry.

The convergence of public health and tourism in the area of Health and Wellness (H&W) is an innovative development. A new example of intersectoral cooperation, as a result of which, in this case, public health care contributes to another sector. The growing awareness of health—certainly in the United States, which, just like Aruba, is facing

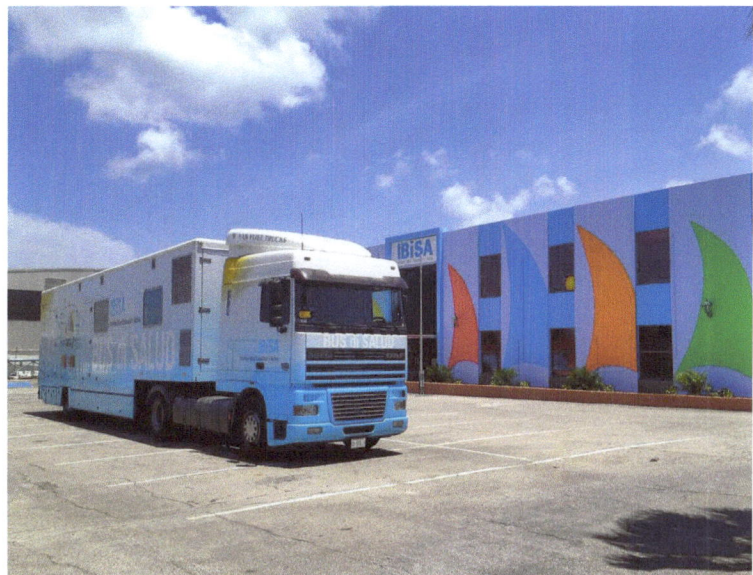

an enormous obesity problem—also becomes manifest in the tourism demand. A healthy vacation, in which healthy relaxation, sports and exercise, healthy nutrition, and a social gathering are provided by the tourism offerings, gives you more: returning home well rested and revitalized. Most progressive hotels aiming at sustainable tourism offer more H&W services. In this respect, the cooperation between the Ministry of Public Health and Sports and a large high-rise hotel is unique. The hotel has adopted the health promotion program of IBiSA, including the 'sailing boat'. Health information in the lobby, a healthy kitchen, more exercise programs, followed by marketing activities, consisting of approaching tourists who are interested in a healthy vacation.

The tourist population forms an important segment of the local market. A change in the tourism demand towards healthier products may also be helpful to making the local supply in supermarkets and restaurants healthier. The necessary change of the obese environment into a more health-promoting environment cannot be accomplished without paying attention to the tourism market. H&W tourism is a sustainable method that can contribute to that change. A renewed tourism identity of Aruba—in which not only *One Happy Island* but the *One Healthy Island* has a place as well—can contribute positively to the health of the Aruban population.

More emphasis was placed on the relationship between sports and health. The cycling event 'Cyclovia Educativo', during which sports activities are carried out in public space, has become incorporated in the Aruban workout landscape, after having overcome some growing pains. The 'Lotto pa Deporte', the subsidy

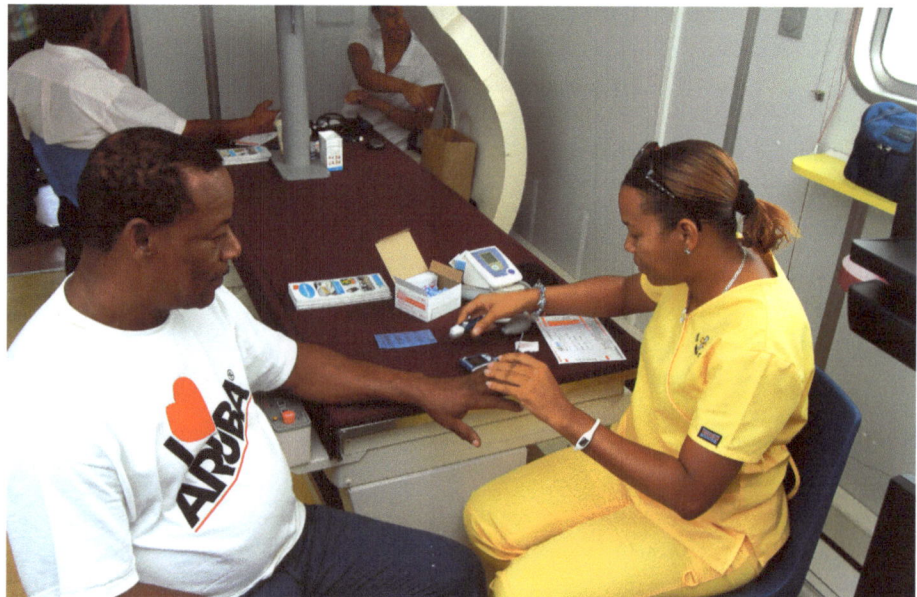

policy, and the organization of sport-loving Aruba were modernized. Conditions for semiprofessional top-class sports activities were established. The 'Centro Medico Deportivo Aruba' [*Medical Sports Center Aruba*] has materialized, so that sportsmen and sportswomen can be accompanied in healthy sports. Aruba organized different international sports events: the International Beach Tennis Tournament, the International Taekwondo Tournament, the International Beach Volleyball Tournament, the Pro-Windsurf Event, soccer clinics by Barcelona and AC Milan, Copa Andre Ooijer, and the Clinic of Demy de Zeeuw. Facilitated by the 'Comité Olympico Arubano (COA)' [*Olympic Committee Aruba*], Aruban athletes participated in the 2012 Olympics in London.

STRENGTHENING CURATIVE CARE

Primary health care, the level at which the general practitioner plays a key role, is of strategic importance to Aruban health care and the prevention and treatment of NCDs. In addition to being the gatekeeper for secondary health care (medical specialist and hospital care), it is the level at which the patient can be offered care (possibly) for life and within the psychosocial context of the patient. Primary health care has been strengthened by engaging more general practitioners and practice nurses. The electronic patient record has materialized in general practitioner care. With a view to developing care that is more responsive to the increasing lifestyle-related health problems, 'IBiSA' has initiated a pilot *Exercise is Medicine,* together with some general practitioners. In this pilot, exercising is used as a treatment method.

Secondary health care, the level at which specialist treatment, counseling, and rehabilitation take place, the Dr. Horacio E. Oduber Hospital (HOH), the only hospital in Aruba, plays a key role. It offers the local population consisting of 120,000 people care and service. Also, the 1.5 million tourists visiting the island each year are assured of qualitatively good medical specialist care. The make the hospital future-proof, the Government and parties concerned decided on *The 2037 HOH Master Plan.* The project file *Dr. Horacio E. Oduber Hospital Expansion & Renovation. Executive Summary: Master Plan & Schematic Design Report (2012)* contains the projection and calculations of an ambitious trajectory for the expansion and renovation of the hospital. This will take place in four phases until 2037.

The renovated hospital will accommodate inter alia the following: a cath lab/intervention surgery room, a new laboratory, improved admission capacity, expansion of outpatient clinics, a modernized emergency room, and a new psychiatric complex. Telemetry, completely digitalized imaging, new pharmacological technology, a wellness & rehabilitation center, and a healing garden will enable the new HOH campus to better respond to the changing demands for care. These new requirements are also caused by the aging population and the NCD challenge.

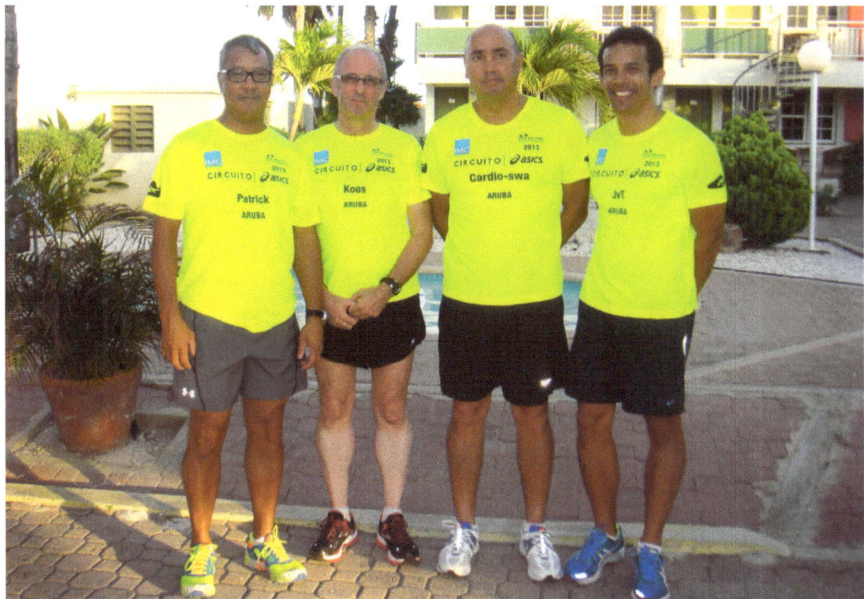

The Government has decided on the structural and professional improvement of the 'Instituto Medico San Nicolas (ImSan)' [*Medical Center San Nicolas*]. For that purpose, it decided to enter into a Strategic Partner Agreement with Baptist Health South Florida, the largest health care organization in South Florida. Based on a multiannual action plan, the parties are working on an oncology center for the treatment of cancer patients, so that they and their families no longer have to travel to foreign care institutes. By means of high-quality chemotherapeutical and radiotherapeutical care, ImSan should receive international accreditation, so that it can also be active in the area of medical tourism. ImSan will also become a center for NCDs with facilities for urgent care, a diabetes clinic, kidney dialysis, wound treatment, and ophthalmology. Cooperation with John Hopkins Medicine is also in store.

The Mental Health Care Committee (2013) denominated the lack of coherence and capacity in Aruban mental health care. Improvements are necessary. An important improvement is the restructuring of addict care. Prevention, shelter, counseling, treatment, and aftercare have been improved. Fragmentation has been replaced by a coherent organization structure, while the quality of care has been improved by hiring addict experts. An electronic patient record has been created. An important paradigm shift in a humanitarian sense was the complete transfer of addict care from Justice to Public Health.

When organizing the curative care facilities, the concept of public health to reduce health differences caused by socioeconomic circumstances should play an important role. The accessibility and reachability of care should be organized as much as possible with the patient in mind, also *pariba di brug,* the eastern part of the island that is less developed from a socioeconomic point of view than *pabou di brug,* the western part.

COST CONTROL, QUALITY, AND LIFE EXPECTANCY

Since 2001, a general health insurance ('AZV') has been effective in Aruba. This gives each resident of Aruba the right to (curative) health care. The annual reports of the AZV Executive Body show that the removal of the 'partitions' between all sorts of insurance arrangements, dating from the period before the introduction of the AZV, also contributed to cost control. The average cost increase during the years of my ministership amounted to 4%. Within the AZV system, the AZV Executive Body could make contractual agreements with care providers and care institutes with regard to quality and efficiency. It is remarkable that the alarming trend of a decreasing life expectancy that was established at the end of the previous century has been reversed in the past decade of the AZV, according to data of the Central Bureau of Statistics (CBS). Although the relationship between the re-increasing life expectancy and the AZV has not been examined, it is known that accessibility to medical care is an important, positive factor insofar as life expectancy and quality of life are concerned.

Just like other sectors of government policy, health care also faces budgetary challenges. The special, humanitarian nature of this sector deserves administrative attention, however. *Penny wise, pound foolish* could mean a high price here: unnecessary complications and death caused by insufficient capacity and quality. Increasing morbidity caused by failing prevention and health promotion. Financial policy in care and care institutes should be based on in-depth knowledge of care and humanitarian awareness, so that the household finances are in order, and the quality of the care is good. As we already saw before, health is not only a cost

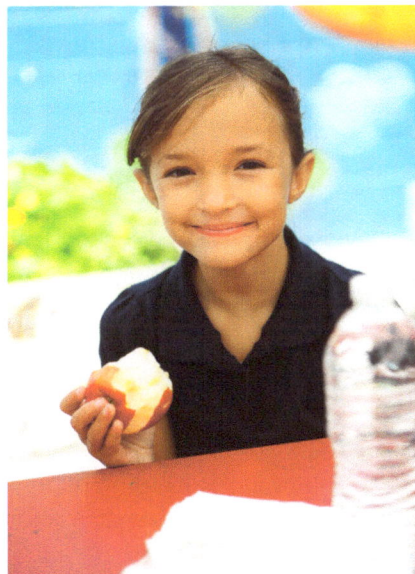

item, it mostly generates revenue. Efficiency forms part of quality and not the other way round.

To meet both the requirements of the quality of care and cost control, as well as to promote the harmonization of different types of care, the policy for all stakeholders has been worded unambiguously in the Public Health Care and Curative Care Framework Letters.

HEALTH MONITOR, INSPECTORATE, AND HEALTH LEGISLATION

The center for the development of policy in the area of public health care and the central organization of public health care (including youth health care, the prevention of infectious diseases, health promotion) is the Directorate of Public Health, 'DVG'. Since I took office, the DVG has vigorously tackled the challenges in the area of transparency, good governance, professionalization, and a positive working atmosphere and contributed significantly to public health care. A big success was the cooperation of different government agencies in the Food and Beverages Action Team, which took care of the hygienic control of many food establishments. Aruba received its *Health Monitor* for the first time, which provides an overview of the current health situation of the population. The *Health Monitor* makes it possible to develop and evaluate data-based health policy, also with regard to the prevention of infectious diseases, such as dengue.

> *Standards and laws without enforcement are toothless. An additional reason in this respect is the circumstance that, also because of the small scale, the self-regulating capacity of occupational groups in care is very limited insofar as quality assurance is concerned.*

The DVG also contributed to the conceptualization and draft legislation that should make an independent Health Care Inspectorate possible in Aruba. A strong Inspectorate is essential to a good quality of care. Standards and laws without enforcement are toothless. An additional reason in this respect is the circumstance that, also because of the small scale, the self-regulating capacity of occupational groups in care is very limited insofar as quality assurance is concerned. Also having regard to the broad knowledge domain of medicine and health care, the accomplishment of sufficient capacity for the Inspectorate is a big challenge. Therefore, the draft legislation provides for the possibility of structural cooperation within the Kingdom.

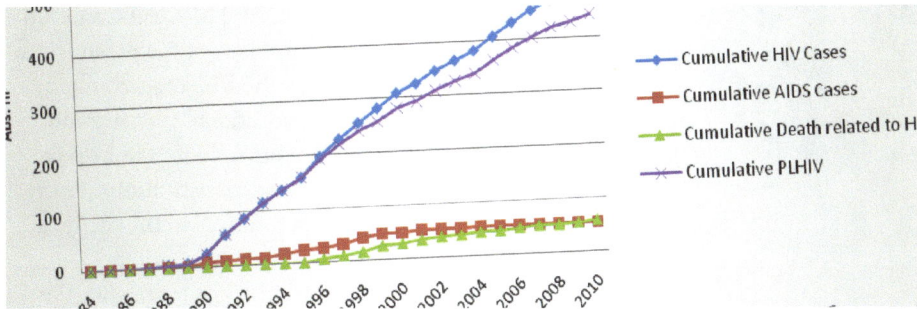

400		● Cumulative HIV Cases
300		■ Cumulative AIDS Cases
200		▲ Cumulative Death related to H
100		✕ Cumulative PLHIV
0		

To be able to face contemporary and future challenges, modernization is also necessary in the area of health legislation. Thus, the Government is obligated pursuant to the draft National Ordinance on Public Health to prepare a health policy in addition to the care policy. Draft national ordinances in the following areas are ready to be debated: ambulance care, medical appliances, communicable diseases (infectious diseases), quality of health care, care in psychiatric hospitals, and individual health care professions. With the cooperation of the Government and Parliament, I expect to be able to accomplish the modernization of health legislation in Aruba during this government period and thus to provide legal safeguards for the *whole-of-government* and *whole-of-society* approach.

LANDSKINDEREN

Dutch nationals born in Aruba [*the so-called 'landskinderen'*] and persons considered equivalent to them also study medicine in countries outside the Kingdom of the Netherlands. Consequently, they do not fulfill the requirement of registration in the 'BIG' [*Individual Healthcare Professions*] register in the Netherlands or in Aruba. In order to maintain quality assurance, on the one hand, and, on the other, to deal with the exceptional educational situation in Aruba, several problem-solving methods have been developed together with physicians involved, the Horacio Oduber Hospital, the 'Instituto Medico' [*Medical Institute*] San Nicolas, and the 'Vrije Universiteit'

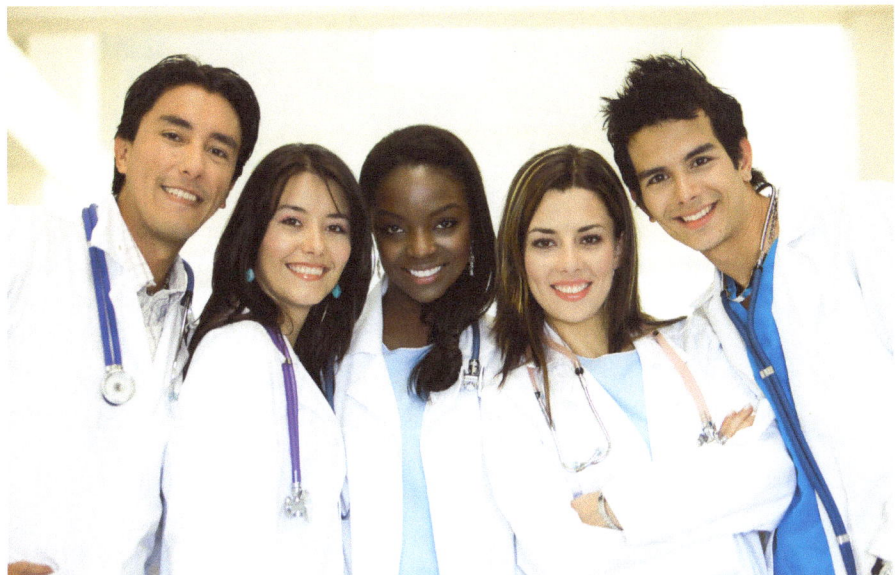

[*Free University*] Medical Center in Amsterdam. Part of the persons can still obtain the BIG registration by means of additional training and refresher courses with the help of aforementioned institutions. For others, alternatives in the medical professional practice will be developed in accordance with the statutory regulations.

NEW GUIDE FOR HEALTHY LIVING

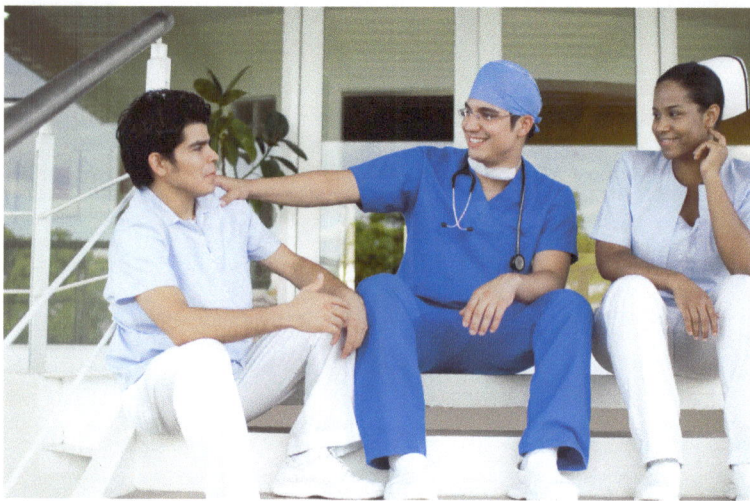

Guide for Healthy Living™

Air and Water
Breathe clean air and drink plenty of pure water.

Balance
Consume foods in the proper proportion, as the size of the sails indicate.

Variety
Eat foods from every group (sail) every day.

Safety
Healthy nutrition means a strong base of foods that don't harm the body in any way.

Sun
Avoid excessive exposure to direct sunlight and use proper protection (clothing and sunscreen).

Family Union
Share meals and physical activity with your family to maintain closeness and communication.

Physical Activity
As a family, enjoy moderate to intense exercise for 30–60 minutes every day.

Fats — Meats & Dairy — Water — Bread/Cereals, Rice — Fruits & Vegetables

BALANCED NUTRITION

PHYSICAL ACTIVITY: Exercise for 30–60 minutes

SVB AND ITS AMBITION

According to the law, the Social Insurance Bank, or the SVb, is charged with the implementation of five important programs within the framework of social security in Aruba. The main objective of the SVb is to implement legislation in an effective and efficient manner, while providing high-quality services to its customers.

The employees of the SVb are the most important resources in the performance of the duties assigned to the SVb by law. Based on this line of reasoning, the SVb

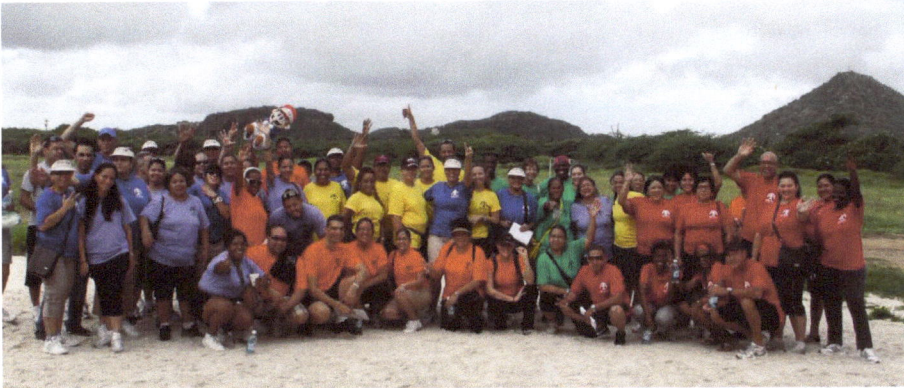

strives for ensuring that its employees dispose of the knowledge and skills necessary for their work, and that they have pleasure in performing their work. The SVb acknowledges that the health, well-being, and vitality of its employees also are of great importance to the organization.

For this reason, the human resource policy of the SVb is aimed at, on the one hand, maintaining the knowledge and skills of the employees at an adequate and up-to-date level and, on the other, at maintaining and promoting good physical and mental health of the employees. In its pursuit of achieving last-mentioned objective, the SVb applies the following strategies:

1. A human resource policy that emphatically appreciates the contribution of the employees to the organization in the achievement of its objectives by offering the employees the opportunity to continue developing their potential, by giving them acknowledgement when appropriate, and by taking into account the needs of the employee, depending on his or her stage of life.

2. The creation of a healthy and pleasant working environment by providing for workplaces that are as much as possible adapted to the employees, by giving the employees ergonomically adjusted furniture, by automating repetitive work as much as possible, by creating more space for work that requires knowledge (work enrichment), by stimulating a pleasant atmosphere between co-workers and, whenever necessary, supporting the engagement of professionals from outside.

3. The promotion and stimulation of a healthy lifestyle of the employees by creating opportunities to exercise and at the same time stimulating the employees to make use of other opportunities to exercise within our community. Furthermore, the SVb wants to be a source of information and guidance for its employees as to how to accomplish and maintain a healthy life.

The SVB strives for ensuring that its employees dispose of the knowledge and skills necessary for their work, and that they have pleasure in performing their work.

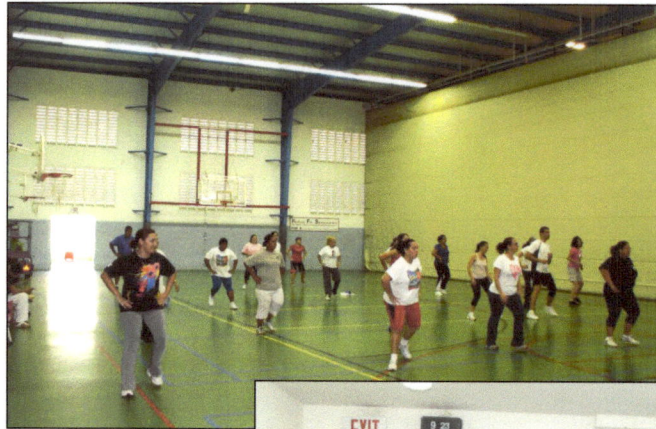

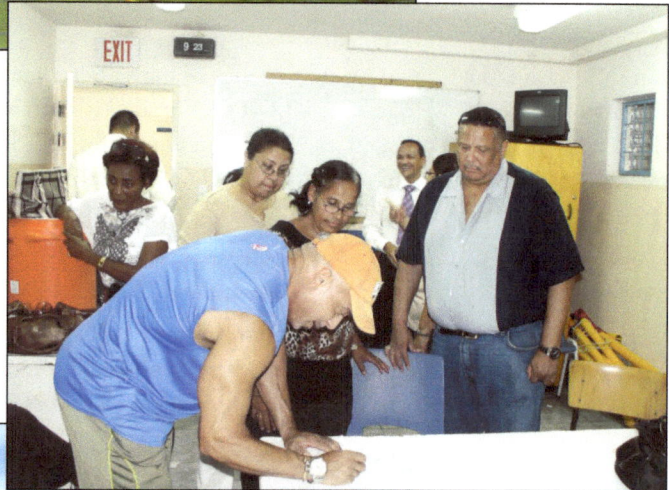

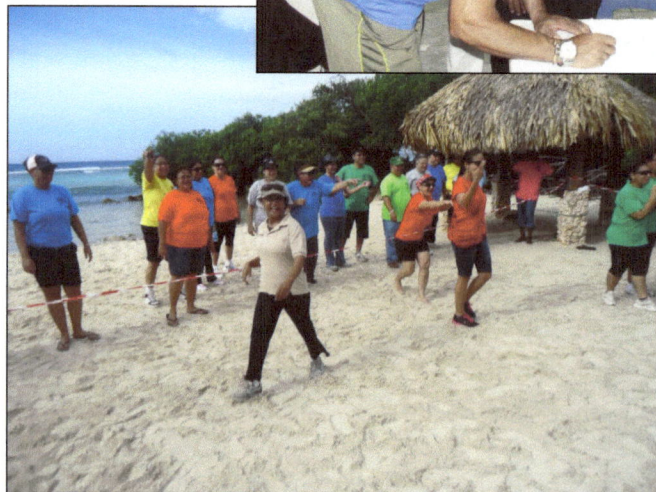

In the process of transforming into the type of organization the SVb wants to be, the SVb will use both conventional and modern and creative tools. In this mission, the SVb considers as its natural partners the Ministry of Public Health and Sports, IBISA, DESPA, Team Mission, Okido, and others that will be identified on the way towards reaching its goal. The SVb is confident that its experience will be useful in this process, and that, within the framework of the implementation of the sickness and accident insurance, this experience can be shared with other employers, in order to stimulate others to consider the health of employees a very important resource.

LEADING BY EXAMPLE

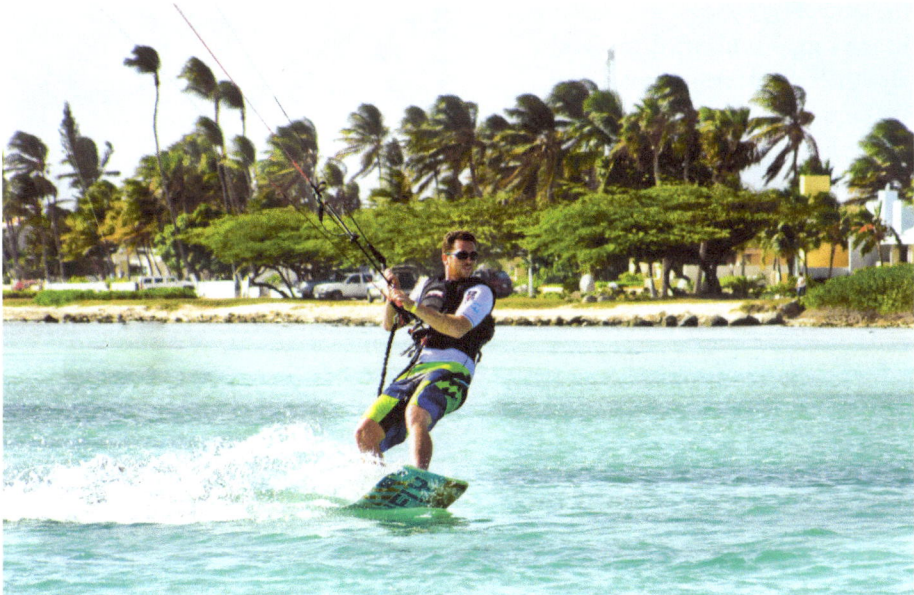

YOUR HEALTH STARTS TODAY.

Health care is a strongly differentiated and complex sector. Each specialty or each type of care has its own scientific and professional references and benchmarks. Therefore, it is unfeasible to give an exhaustive enumeration of care challenges. In these Reflections, a choice has been made to illustrate a vision in motion; any topic not mentioned here is also important in the land of care providers. Insofar as health care is concerned, the Aruba Health Team is formed not only by the curative care sector, but by the public health care sector, the domestic care sector, the occupational health care sector, the addict care sector, the numerous NGO health organizations, such as the White-Yellow Cross, the care insurers, and the health management as well. In addition, the fight against NCDs requires an Aruba Pro-Health Community, in which the Government, schools, sports organizations, the corporate sector, labor union movements, churches, charity associations, women's and youth organizations, the media, and, last but not least, the individual citizen take health initiatives.

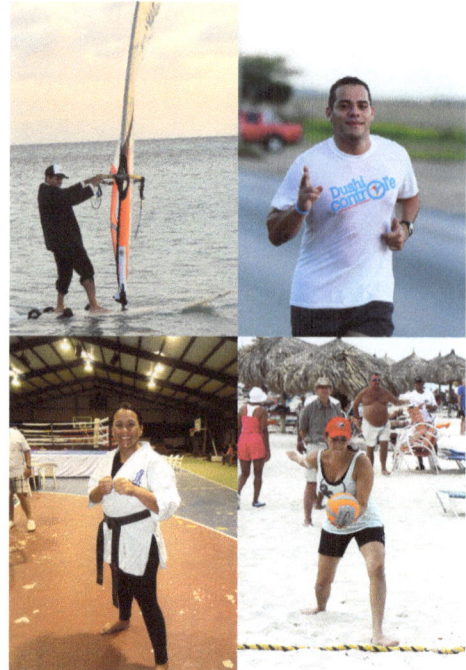

> *Insofar as health care is concerned, the Aruba Health Team is formed not only by the curative care sector, but by the public health care sector, the domestic care sector, the occupational health care sector, the addict care sector, the numerous NGO health organizations, such as the White-Yellow Cross, the care insurers, and the health management as well.*

Your health starts today. By making healthy choices. By going to bed on time. By eating and drinking healthier. By exercising 150 minutes or more a week. By investing in living together. By timely calling in medical assistance, whenever necessary. By looking up information about health. Health starts with a healthy example. Insofar as the vitally important aspect of health is concerned, let us also

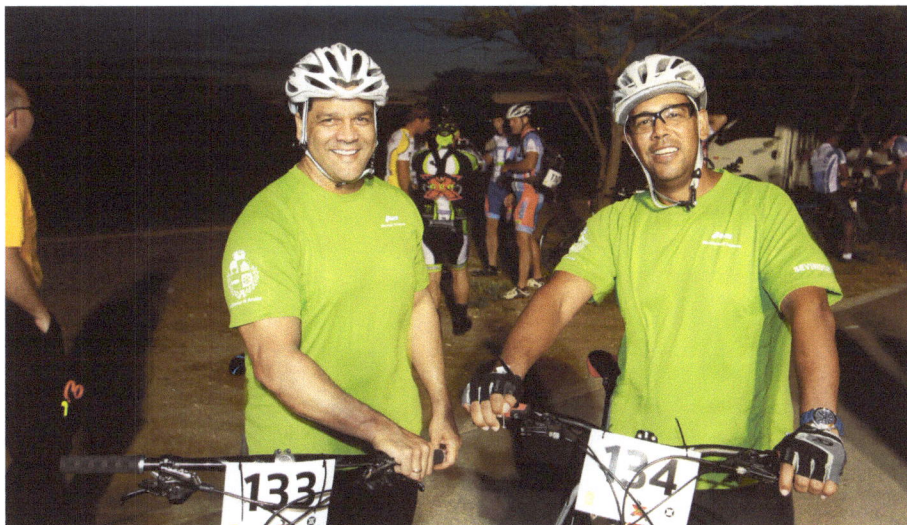

opt for the effective method at home, at work, in school, in the entire country: leading by example. Thus, we will create a health culture in Aruba.

Dr. Richard Visser

Minister of Public Health and Sports

WINDOWS ON A VISION IN MOTION
Three-Legged Stool

Comprehensive health care is symbolized by means of the *three-legged stool*. The seat represents the health system of Aruba. The three legs supporting the seat symbolize cure and care (curative care), public health care, and self-care, respectively. It is all kept together by *good governance*. In the health vision, with the *three-legged stool* as a metaphor, not only the idea of prevention, but the shared responsibility of the community, professionals, and the individual citizen/ patient can be recognized as well.

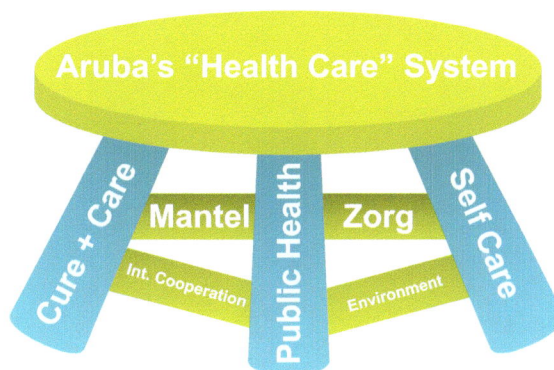

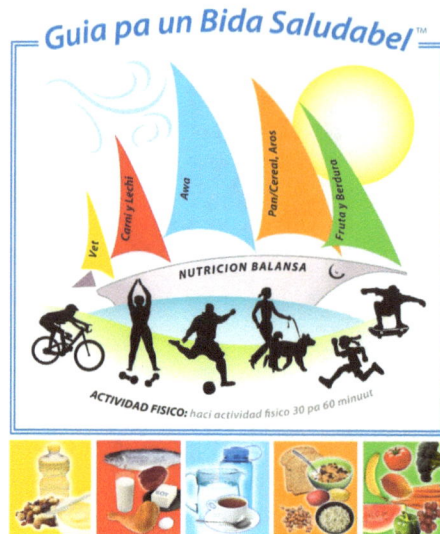

The 'Sailing Boat'

The 'sailing boat' with the colored sails is the symbol of health promotion in Aruba. Drinking water, much emphasis on vegetables and fruit, and sufficient exercise are important elements of the message. However, psychosocial factors, such as an active family life, are also reflected in the 'sailing boat'. The building of 'IBiSA' and the 'Bus di Salud' can be recognized in the 'sailing boat'.

Health Monitor

The Health Monitor provides an insight into the health situation and health determinants. It makes a data-based health policy possible. The first *Health Monitor* of Aruba has materialized.

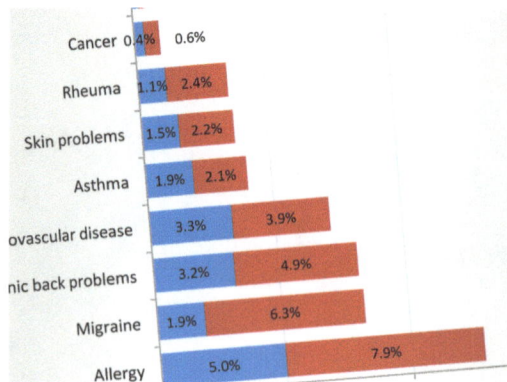

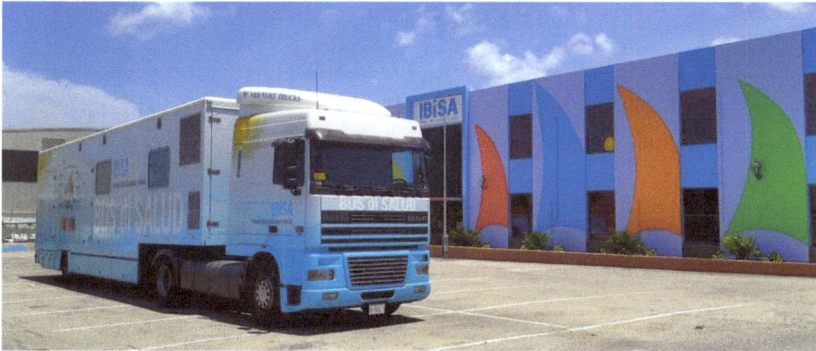

'Bus di Salud' and 'Ibisa'

More than 3000 people had free access to Personal Prevention (PP) through the 'Bus di Salud'. After an examination, they received an explanation of individual health risk factors and received personal lifestyle and health advice. By making Personal Prevention widely accessible, Aruba plays a leading role in the Kingdom. The Netherlands also endeavor to make Personal Prevention accessible to each citizen (www. preventweb.nl). The 'Bus di Salud' is a project of the newly established institute for healthy and active living, 'Instituto Biba Saludabel y Activo, IBiSA'.

Strengthening Directorate of Public Health (DVG)

The fight against dengue is a big challenge for DVG, the public health authority of Aruba. The DVG also is a trendsetter in policy development. Two important policy memoranda on health promotion and healthy nutrition (see Literature consulted) were drawn up. The DVG has worked on the strengthening of the organization and the composition of an Organization Book, clearly describing the duties and powers of all officials.

Pan American Conference on Obesity

Experts, professionals, and ministers of public health from dozens of countries of the Americas and Europe shared multidisciplinary knowledge, best practices, and networks. In 2013, PACO III will also be held in Aruba (www.paco.aw).

Recognition in the United Nations

On behalf of the Kingdom of the Netherlands, Minister Visser addressed the General Assembly of the United Nations about the fight against obesity and NCDs.

Aruba Associate Member of PAHO

Aruba obtained its own vote within the Pan American Health Organization (PAHO), an emancipatory event that marked an expansion of the Status Aparte within the health organization of the western hemisphere.

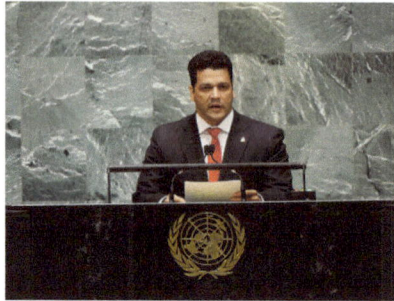

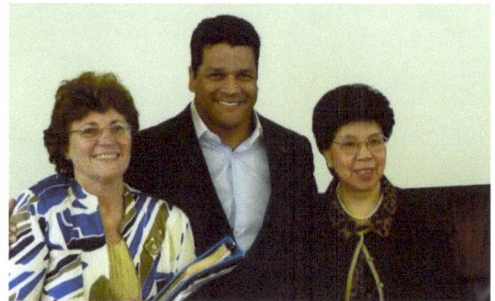

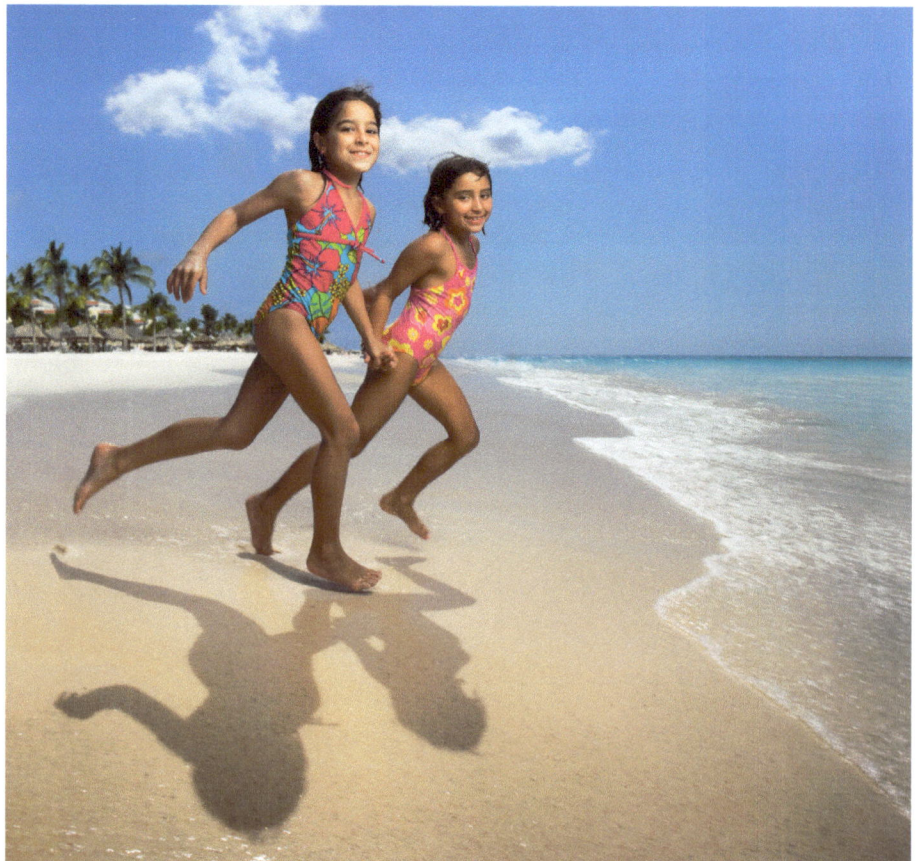

The Hospital Is Expanded and Renovated

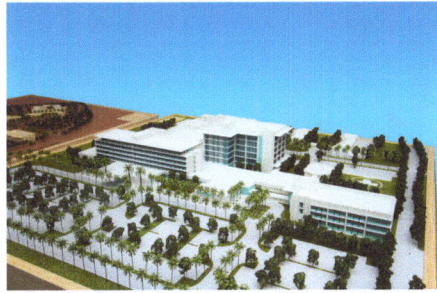

'To make the hospital future-proof, the Government and parties concerned decided on The 2037 HOH Master Plan.'

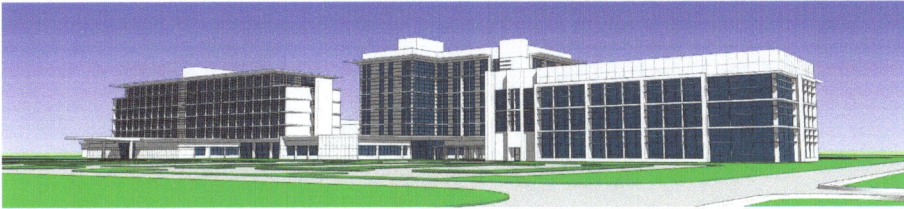

A state of the art, our renovated and expanded hospital of Aruba. An investment of 250 million florins in health and top of the line technology.

Care Renewal in San Nicolas

An oncology center where chemotherapy and radiotherapy for cancer patients will become possible will be accommodated in the 'Instituto Medico San Nicolas (ImSan)'.

ImSan Center of Excellence in Oncology, Diabetes and Urgent Care. In collaboration with Baptist Health International. Transforming Aruba in to a destination for world class Health Care.

Addict Care Has Been Restructured and Modernized

The new 'Centro di Motivacion' [*Motivation Center*] for drug addicts placed under conservatorship. The improvement of both preventive and therapeutic addict care marks a strengthening of mental health care in Aruba.

More Attention Is Paid to Sports and Exercise

Dr. Joel Rajnherc, Director of 'ImSan': "People practice sports and exercise more. I now see people studying the food labels in the supermarket. A change towards healthier living is gradually taking place." A relationship is established between sports, exercise, and health in the new health vision. Therefore, the government organization for the promotion of sports and exercise, 'Idefre', has been incorporated in 'IBiSA'.

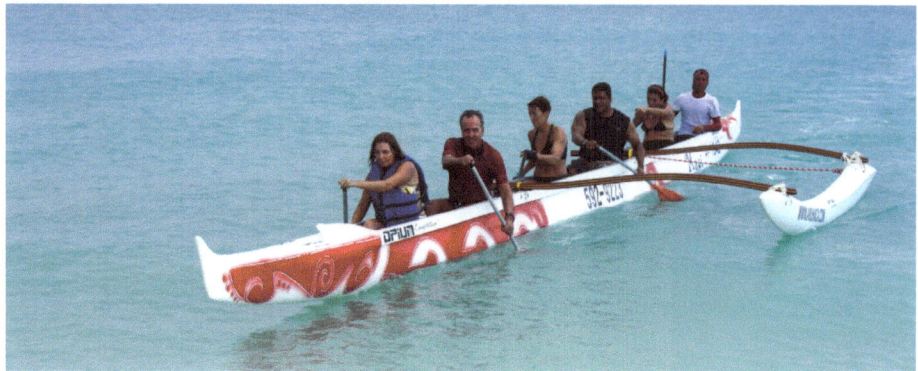

Leading by Example

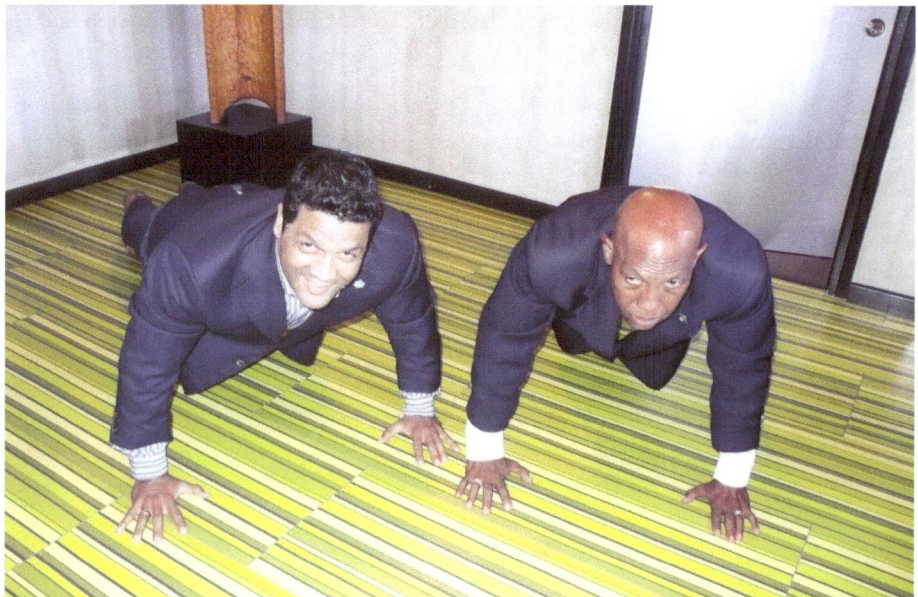

LITERATURE CONSULTED

Food and Beverages Action Group, Actions 2010.

Medical Assistance and Coordination Alert Schedule, Management Team DVG, Directorate of Public Health 2012.

Disaster Alert System, DVG.

Aruba, Situation Analysis of HIV/STIs (1985–2010) and Strategic plan for HIV/STIs (2012–2016), developed in collaboration with the PAHO HIV Caribbean Office (PAHO) and with financial support of the European Commission, Pan American Health Organization, PAHO, December 2010.

Asbestos sheets/asbestos-containing materials, 'Dienst Technische Inspecties' [Department of Technical Inspections], November 20, 2009.

Baseline Assessment: the Drug Problem in Aruba. Survey Secondary Schools, 'EPB' [Junior Secondary Vocational Education] & 'EPI' [Senior Secondary Vocational Education], Results School Survey 2011–2012, University of Aruba.

Baseline Assessment: the Drug Problem in Aruba, Registration Care Institutes & Outpatient Drug Users, Final Report Part l, Center for Research & Development, University of Aruba, November 2012.

Baseline Assessment: the Drug Problem in Aruba, School Survey 2011–2012, Final Report Part II, Center for Research & Development, University of Aruba, June 2012.

Policy Document on Health Promotion 2011–2015. From Facts to Action. 'Departamento di Salubridad Publico Aruba, DESPA' [Department of Public Health Aruba], 2011 Policy Intentions Directorate of Public Health 2013, Directorate of Public Health/Department of Public Health Aruba, DESPA, 2013.

Decision of the Ministerial Council of November 1, 2011 (BE-68/11) concerning approval of the establishment of the 'Instituto Biba Saludabel y Activo (IBiSA)'.

'Bus di Salud', Health Profile of the Attended Population, September 2012, Report submitted to the Minister of Public Health and Sports, Dr. Richard Visser, L. Arango, Aruba, 2012.

Future Parents Course, White-Yellow Cross Aruba, August 2011.

Outlines of the Coordination of Health Care Training Programs, A.N.A. Kool, August 24, 2012.

Dr. Horacio E. Oduber Hospital Expansion & Renovation. Executive summary: Master Plan & Schematic Design Report, Bermello Ajamil & Partners, Inc., May 31, 2012.

Dr. Horacio E. Oduber Hospital, Maintenance Plan, October 13, 2009.

Shelter & Care Contingency Plan, Process 14, Organizational Part, draft, Land Aruba Disaster Response, adopted by the Minister of General Affairs, July 2010.

Combined Financial Report 2009, General Medical Expenses Fund, including the AZV Executive Body, Aruba, June 9, 2009.

Combined Financial Statements and Annual Report 2010, AZV Executive Body, March 31, 2011.

Coordinated Disaster & Incidents Response Procedure ('GRIP'), Aruba, Version April 12, 2011.

'ImSan', A Business Plan with a Shared Vision, Atlas Accountancy Tax Legal & Advisory Services, December 7, 2007.

Annual Planning 2011, DESPA, Directorate of Public Health.

Annual Planning 2012, DESPA, Directorate of Public Health.

Annual Planning 2013, DESPA, Directorate of Public Health.

Financial Statements 2010, Report of the Board of Directors of the 'Stichting Ziekenverpleging Aruba' [Nursing Foundation Aruba], Board of Directors.

Financial Statements 'Stichting Bloedbank' [Blood Bank Foundation] 2010, March 16, 2012.

Annual Report 2010, Communicable Diseases Service.

Annual Report 2011, Communicable Diseases Service.

Annual Report 2010, Hygienic Service Directorate of Public Health, March 2011.

Annual Report Veterinary Service 2010, for DVG.

Annual Report 2010, Yellow Fever and Mosquito Prevention, compiled by Roque Dirksz, April 2011.

Annual Report 2010, Youth Health Care Department Directorate of Public Health, Public Health Department Aruba (DESPA).

Annual Report 2011, Youth Health Care Department Directorate of Public Health, Public Health Department Aruba (DESPA).

Annual Report 2010, Policy & Information Department Directorate of Public Health Aruba.

Annual Report 2011, Policy & Information Department Directorate of Public Health Aruba.

Annual Report 2010, Epidemiology and Research Department Directorate of Public Health Aruba, March 2011.

Annual Work Plan 2011 of the Yellow Fever and Mosquito Prevention Department, compiled by Roque Dirksz, Head Yellow Fever and Mosquito Prevention, January 2011.

Curative Care Framework Letter 2011–2013, Minister of Public Health and Sports, November 2010.

Public Health Care Framework Letter 2011–2013, Minister of Public Health and Sports, 2010.

Land Aruba -Sports Facilities Inventory 1 (A modern outlook on the current situation and administration), Ministry of Public Health and Sports, Michael Paesch, 2012.

National Decree of September 28, 2011 No. 26 on the recommendation of the Minister of Public Health and Sports (concerns the establishment of the National Drug Council).

National Decree of June 11, 2012 on the recommendation of the Minister of Public Health and Sports (concerns the establishment of the prevention institute 'Instituto Biba Saludabel y Activo (IBiSA)').

National Laboratory Aruba, Annual Report 2010.

National Ordinance on Ambulance Care, final draft, September 15, 2011.

National Ordinance on Communicable Diseases, final draft, September 15, 2011.

National Ordinance on Quality in Health Care, draft, January 15, 2013.

National Ordinance on Medical Appliances, final draft, September 15, 2011.

National Ordinance on Public Health, final draft, September 15, 2011.

National Ordinance on Care in Psychiatric Hospitals, final draft, September 15, 2011.

Lung specialist HOH: 'Increased risk of mesothelioma after exposure to asbestos', 'Amigoe' October 8, 2011.

Memorandum of Understanding Mexico convention 1974, HAVA (dr. J. van Veen, Chairman), VMSA (dr. N. Lampe), AVSD (dr. A. Schwengle), ImSan (dr. J. Rajnherc), SZA (dr. J. Falconi), Minister of Sports and Public Health dr. R.W.M. Visser, Minister of General Affairs mr. M. Eman, L. Rafael-Croes, pediatrician, D. Alders, anesthesiologist, C.J. Lesire, physician educated in Costa Rica, B.L. Berkeley, physician educated in Costa Rica.

Disaster Response Environmental Consultations, Meeting October 12, 2011.

Motion of Aruban Parliament of June 18, 2010.

National Plan Aruba 2009–2018: to fight overweight, obesity, and related health issues, Special Obesity Committee, October 2008.

New Structure, New Organization Chart, Dr. Horacio E. Oduber Hospital.

Policy Document on General Nutrition and Exercise Guidelines for Aruba, Directorate of Public Health, IDEFRE, Advice 'ANDA' ('Asociacion di Nutricionista y Dietista Arubano' [Aruban Association of Nutritionists and Dieticians]).

Draft National Ordinance for the Adoption of the Budgets of the Ministries of the Land for the Year of Service 2012, Chapter E Policy Intentions Public Health and Sports, the Minister of General Affairs.

Overweight and Obesity: Prevalence, Characteristics, and Collective Prevention among Elementary School Students in Aruba 2004–2006, R.W.M. Visser.

Political Declaration of the High-Level Meeting of the General Assembly of the United Nations on the Prevention and Control of Non-Communicable Diseases, 2011.

Paying attention to what is missing in the lives of disabled persons. A research report on a needs assessment among disabled persons in Aruba, Drs. Carol Kock, Directorate of Social Affairs, November 2012.

Promotion Campaign 'Without breeding places there will be no mosquitos, without mosquitos there will be no dengue', Directorate of Public Health, October 2012 - January 2013.

Disaster Telephone List 2010.

Report of the Committee for the Restructuring of Mental Health Care, January 2013.

Social Psychiatric Service Annual Report 2010, Rafael S. Lopez, Head of the Social Psychiatric Service, March 2011.

Strategic Policy Plan 'Scol Saludabel' 2011–2016, Steering Group 'Scol Saludabel', November 2011.

Terms of Reference, Activity Train-the-Trainers—Addict Care "Project Drugs Master Plan", within the framework of Social (Neighborhood and Personal) Security. Part of the National Security Plan 2008–2012, Ministry of Public Health and Sports, August 10, 2011.

Terms of Reference, Prevention Sector—Addict Care "Project Drugs Master Plan", within the framework of Social (Neighborhood and Personal) Security. Part of the National Security Plan 2008–2012, Ministry of Public Health and Sports.

Terms of Reference, Restart Training Program Addict Education Aruba "Project Drugs Master Plan", within the framework of Social (Neighborhood and Personal) Security. Part of the National Security Plan 2008–2012, Ministry of Public Health and Sports.

Terms of Reference, ICT—Addict Care "Project Drugs Master Plan", within the framework of Social (Neighborhood and Personal) Security. Part of the National Security Plan 2008–2012, Ministry of Public Health and Sports, October 2011.

Terms of Reference, Activity 'HBO'[University of Applied Sciences] Training Program—Addict Care "Project Drugs Master Plan", within the framework of Social (Neighborhood and Personal) Security. Part of the National Security Plan 2008–2012, Ministry of Public Health and Sports.

Terms of Reference, Establishment Centro Colorado "Project Drugs Master Plan", within the framework of Social (Neighborhood and Personal) Security. Part of the National Security Plan 2008–2012, Ministry of Public Health and Sports.

Terms of Reference, Modernization Health Legislation, Directorate of Public Health (DVG), (2008-FDA-PA-076).

The Aruba Call for Action on Obesity, 2011, www.paco.aw.

The association between behavioral risk factors and the seroprevalence of HIV, hepatitis B and syphilis in the Aruban Prison: An epidemiological study, Dissertation, Ms. Maribelle M. Tromp, BAS, October 2012.

Nutrition and Exercise Task Force, Annual Report 2010, Directorate of Public Health, Idefre, February 2010.

Health Care Inspectorate Task Force, 2010.

www.gobierno.aw

www.overheid.aw

www.paco.aw

www.salud.aw

Department of Public Health.

www.despa.gov.aw

directie@despa.gov.aw / dbz@despa.gov.aw

vetservice@despa.gov.aw

spd@despa.gov.aw

jgz@aruba.gov.aw

IGZ@despa.gov.aw

Algemene Zorg Verzekeraar AZV, www.azv.aw.

Dr Horacio Oduber Hospitaal, www.arubahospital.com.

NGO's

www.witgelekruisaruba.org

www.alzheimeraruba.org

arubaheartfoundation@setarnet.aw

www.cvaaryba.com

www.maryjoanfoundation.aw

www.saba.org

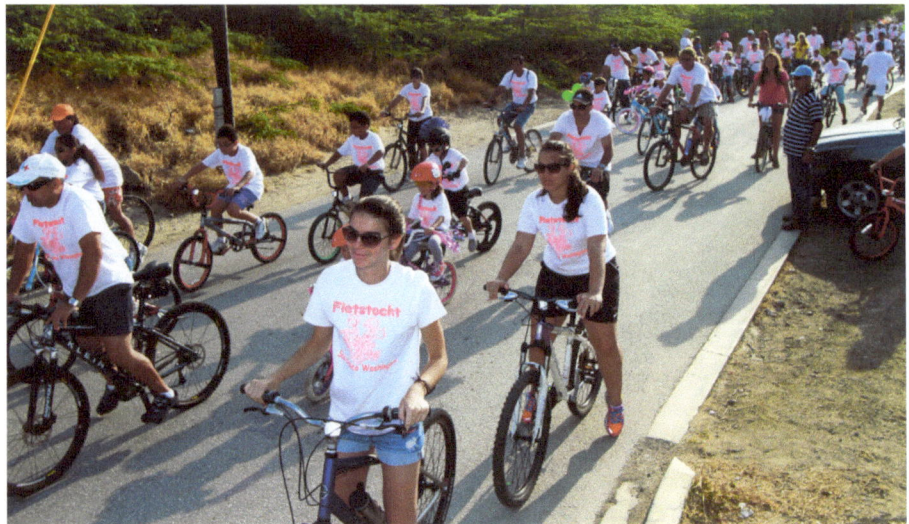

YOUR HEALTH STARTS TODAY.

By making healthy choices.

By going to bed on time.

By eating and drinking healthier.

By exercising 150 minutes or more a week.

By investing in living together.

By timely calling in medical assistance, whenever necessary.

By looking up information about health.

Health starts with a healthy example. Insofar as the vitally important aspect of health is concerned, let us also opt for the effective method at home, at work, in school, in the entire country: leading by example. Thus, we will create a health culture in Aruba.

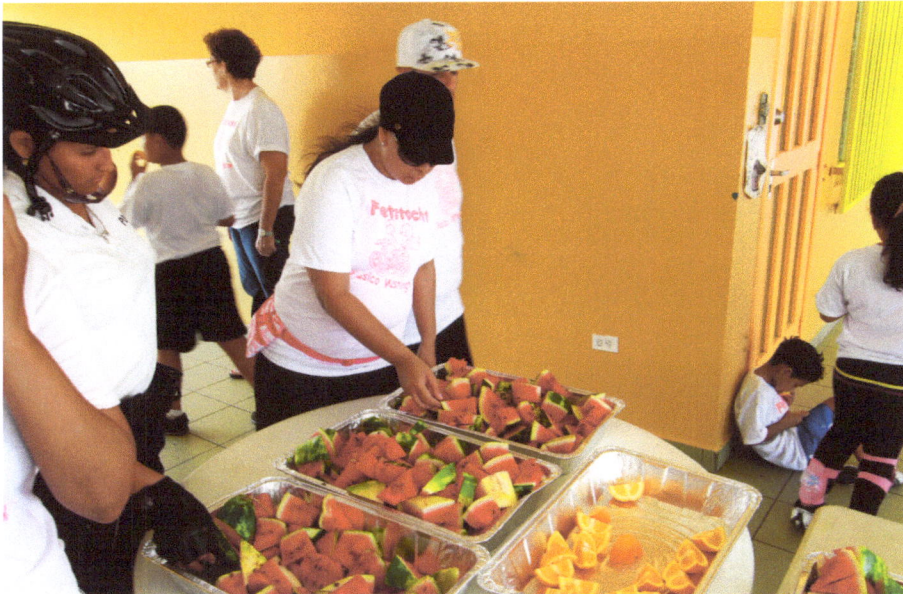

Chapter 4

A PROPOSAL OF GUIDE, SPECIFIC PLATFORM AND PHILOSOPHICAL FOUNDATIONS FOR HEALTHY LIVING: TOOLS FOR THE PREVENTION OF CHILDHOOD OBESITY

Richard Visser

Minister of Health and Sport of Aruba
drangelcaballerotorres@gmail.com

Abstract—This paper proposes three tools for the prevention of childhood obesity: a guide for healthy living, specific platform and philosophical foundations. A guide for healthy living explains the principal characteristics of balanced food and physical activity to prevent childhood obesity. The specific platform for childhood obesity prevention shows how it is possible to inform and motivate the population and stakeholders to act against the obesity. Philosophical foundations present the basis for obesity prevention. The holistic approach of these tools facilitates comprehension of the ways to prevent the childhood obesity.

Keywords—Prevention of Childhood Obesity; Guide; Specific Platform; Philosophical Foundations; Healthy Living

I. INTRODUCTION

Scientific publications clearly indicate that the alarming increase of childhood obesity constitutes a big problem for health and development. However, some parents, teachers and health providers, among others, do not recognize it as a serious issue[1, 2].

Obesity affects the rich and the poor, both genders and ethnicities, but its effect is not homogeneous in these population groups. Place of residence, educational level, as well as socio-cultural aspects, among others, influence the presence and development of obesity [3–5].

An urbanization rate of 80% or more in a high number of countries without access to active transportation, among other conditions, is conducive to physical inactivity as part of daily life. High demand and supply of food with a high content of fat and refined sugars coincide frequently with this sedentary lifestyle [6–8].

It is a known fact that today's children do not spend energy with the same frequency, intensity and duration when engaged in games and recreational activities as today's adults did 40 years ago. Today, in a majority of countries more than 50% of adults are overweight. Therefore, it is easy to see how this problem will increase if we do not act urgently and appropriately, against this epidemic.

Decreasing a sedentary lifestyle, at the individual level and the population level, is a complex issue and the procedures to make it sustainable and stable are not clear [9, 10].

Educating the population and creating healthy environments are the best solutions to facilitate a healthy lifestyle, but not all tools are known to achieve it. In the search for a solution to these problems, it is proposed that the population must be educated and an environment allowing the realization of healthy lifestyle must be made available, but the tools for its appropriate application are not in place [11–14].

To contribute to the solution of these limitations we propose a guide (see image below), a specific platform and a philosophy for healthy living.

II. A GUIDE FOR HEALTHY LIVING

People are living systems. As such, we have a remarkable ability to spontaneously adapt to changes that occur in our environment by modifying or altering our biological functions.

Metabolism is a critical biological function, consisting of a combination of chemical reactions that take place within the cells of every living organism over a period of time. It is the most important biological function because it releases the energy required for other types of biological functions to operate.

The process of metabolism cannot take place in the absence of two critical types of fuel. The first type of fuel is *oxygen*, which we take in from the external environment through our respiratory system. The second equally important fuel is the *nutrients* contained in the various food groups we eat as part of our diet. The process of metabolism can only function well if we consume the right type and amount of food, (i.e., nutrients) required to produce the level of energy our cells need to perform the functions we demand of them.

It is, therefore, important to know the actual amount of energy expended by each person. These energy requirements, in turn, determine the type and amount of energy needed and this, in turn, dictates the type and amount of food necessary to satisfy these requirements.

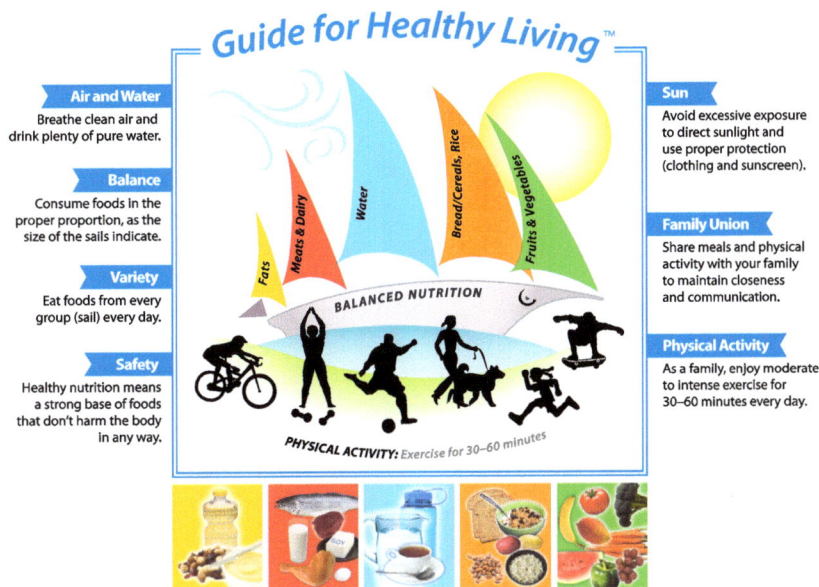

Guide for Healthy Living™

Air and Water — Breathe clean air and drink plenty of pure water.

Balance — Consume foods in the proper proportion, as the size of the sails indicate.

Variety — Eat foods from every group (sail) every day.

Safety — Healthy nutrition means a strong base of foods that don't harm the body in any way.

Fats

Meats & Dairy

Water

Bread/Cereals, Rice

Fruits & Vegetables

BALANCED NUTRITION

Sun — Avoid excessive exposure to direct sunlight and use proper protection (clothing and sunscreen).

Family Union — Share meals and physical activity with your family to maintain closeness and communication.

Physical Activity — As a family, enjoy moderate to intense exercise for 30–60 minutes every day.

PHYSICAL ACTIVITY: Exercise for 30–60 minutes

Exercise, which consumes energy and has a direct effect on metabolism is another important ingredient in our search for an optimum physical balance. This is an important condition for a perfect equilibrium between the nutrients obtained from and the amount of energy expended through exercise. Healthy nutrition, which involves the regular intake of various foods in recommended proportions, should therefore be based upon the need to provide sufficient fuel to support the energy one expends. It also requires increased water consumption and the consumption of large quantities of fruits and vegetables, which are critical elements in the five basic food groups comprising the food pyramid.

The "Sailing to Health," with its five sails, reflects this concept as it moves through a sea of plenty filled with sunshine, clean air, healthy food and physical activity on its journey toward a longer and healthier life.

Each of the sails propelling the ship forward represents a distinct food group. The three large sails represent the consumption of water, fruits and vegetables, and carbohydrates; the medium sail represents proteins; and the small sail represents fat. The size of each sail is correlated with the amount of food that should be consumed from the food group that it represents. And the anchor is the symbol for breastfeeding the healthiest start you can give your child. Some nutrients, including water are explained below about their properties:

A. Water (represented by a large blue sail)

Water is the principal component and most important element of every living organism, representing 50% or more of our total body weight. The importance of water as a nutrient is only exceeded by the importance of oxygen. Water is therefore represented by a large sail, reflecting the need to drink as much water as possible.

The physical and chemical characteristics of water make it an ideal medium for the distribution of chemical substances, found in the body-substances which are important to the metabolic process. Given its role as a general transport medium, water plays a direct part in enabling various biological functions to operate effectively.

The total amount of water found in the body changes with age. In the newborn, it comprises up to 75% of total body weight. The percentage of water decreases as one grows older, down to 55–65% of body content in adult men and 50–55% in adult women. This difference between men and women is due to the fact that women have less muscle and more fat tissue. In a physiologically ideal situation, a male individual of 20 years old and 1.83 m tall, with a body weight of 70 kg who is in good health should have a body water content of about 40 liters.

Total body water content remains relatively constant due to the action of two powerful reflex mechanisms: the sensation of thirst and a reduction in the volume of urine eliminated when total body water volume begins to diminish. Should the total body water content increase for any reason, the sensation of thirst tends to wane and the volume of water eliminated through the kidneys increases as well, producing the desired balance of body water content.

There are three principal sources of body water: water ingested as such; water found in food; and water generated by one's cells as a by-product of the metabolism of carbohydrates, fats and proteins.

The total amount of water ingested by an individual, either as water or as water contained in his diet, can vary widely, depending upon factors such as climate and type of food consumed.

For example, oranges, watermelons, cantaloupe and similar fruits have high water content per unit of weight, while the water content per unit mass of other foods, such as grains, legumes and tubers, is much lower. The need for water also increases in hot, dry climates and in situations involving increased respiration or what is known as "alveolar ventilation".

Urine is the principal channel through which water is lost from the body. The amount of water lost through the skin is extremely variable and may occur as sweat, which is noticeable, or "insensible perspiration", which is unnoticeable. It can also occur through fecal matter, the lungs and exhaled air.

It has been suggested that at least 1.5 liters of water should be consumed each day, but it is practically impossible to determine one's true water needs in a given situation with any degree of precision.

B. Fruits and Vegetables (represented by a large green sail)

Fresh fruits and vegetables must be part of a varied and nutritious diet. These foods provide significant amounts of vitamins, minerals, trace elements, dietary fiber and antioxidant nutrients that protect an individual's health and are active in the prevention of disease. A diet consisting of large quantities of fruits and vegetables is one that is high in both taste and nutrition. Fruits and vegetables are, therefore, represented by a large sail, indicating the need to consume large portions of these types of foods in your diet.

Consumption of fruits and vegetables increases the antioxidant content of one's diet which is currently thought to be a basic dietary requirement. Nutrition experts now recognize the contribution of fresh fruits and vegetables in helping to destroy or neutralize the oxygen-based free radicals generated as part of the human metabolic process, supporting the defense systems that reduce the adverse effects of these free radicals. The damage caused by free radicals, if extensive enough can harm the body's cells and make it difficult for them to adapt to change. It can even lead to cell death. The consequences of these changes can be severe, and have been linked to the development of arteriosclerosis, cancer, inflammatory bowel disease, neurodegenerative diseases, autoimmune problems such as rheumatoid arthritis, and the complications of diabetes.

Fruits should be eaten in their natural and fresh state, and salads should be eaten in their raw state due to the loss of vitamins and minerals that occurs during the cooking process.

Preference should be given to dark-green and yellow or orange vegetables, and to fresh vegetable juices with no salt or sugar added.

Fruits and vegetables also play a significant role in providing the required amount of dietary fiber. Not long ago, dietary fiber was thought to be an inert substance consisting largely of cellulose and having an insignificant influence on human health. However, it is currently suggested that insufficient fiber in the diet may contribute to the development of many diseases including colon and rectal cancer, diverticulitis, appendicitis, constipation, hemorrhoids, diabetes, and obesity.

Much research has been done on the relative importance of dietary fiber, and some controversy exists as to which foods should or should not be defined as dietary fiber. However, there is general agreement on the value of a number of properties characteristic of this element.

One important property of dietary fiber is its ability to retain water. This property makes a major contribution toward a well functioning digestive system. Dietary fiber also has the ability to form gels in the gastrointestinal tract, leading to increased glucose tolerance and lessening the absorption of cholesterol and salt. Another important property attributed to dietary fiber is its ability to absorb calcium, magnesium, zinc and iron. The fermentation of dietary fiber in the colon also produces two elements, gas and energy, that are necessary for proper colon function.

The consumption of a sufficient amount of dietary fiber therefore has a positive effect on the digestive system through increased fecal mass, increased stool fluidity, shortened intestinal passage time, dilution of solids found in the large intestine, excretion of nitrogen, fatty acids, cholesterol and salt through the feces, and the stimulated growth of beneficial bacteria. It also helps to reduce the absorption of carbohydrates, which increases glucose tolerance, reduces insulin requirements after meals, and increases the efficiency of glucose metabolism.

Currently, there is no definite agreement among researchers on the amount of dietary fiber that should be consumed daily, and there is even less agreement as to the type and variety of fiber that should be eaten.

It has been suggested that consumption of 15–30 grams daily is sufficient for a healthy adult, and 3–4 grams a day is recommended for children of two years old. No recommendations have been made for younger children. Diets providing 6 grams of fiber or more are considered to be rich in this nutrient, which should form a regular part of every person's diet.

Vegetables that should be eaten include chard, cabbage, lettuce, carrots, squash, beets, beans, peppers, onions, pumpkin, cucumbers, radishes, tomatoes, celery, eggplant, broccoli and okra, among others. Fruits that should be eaten include oranges, lemons, limes, grapefruit, mangos, papaya, bananas, guava, apples, pineapple, pears, grapes, apricots, peaches, coconut, cherries, mandarin, mango, anon, soursop, pineapple pear, coco, prunes, red currants, medlar, strawberries, cantaloupe and watermelon, among others.

The importance of consuming large amounts of fruits and vegetables is reflected in the large size of the green sail representing this food group. Remember, it is always better to eat the fruit (fiber) than drinking the juice because of less fiber and a low satiety rate.

C. Carbohydrates (represented by a large orange sail)

Foods containing carbohydrates are critical in that they provide the energy we need to function well and to lead an active life style. Of all the dietary elements, carbohydrates, represented by a large orange sail, has to be consumed most frequently in order to meet the body's energy needs. Sixty percent or more of an individual's total energy needs must be satisfied through this food group.

There are two basic types of carbohydrates: complex carbohydrates such as starch, and simple or refined carbohydrates such as sucrose, maltose, or lactose. Carbohydrates should preferably be eaten in the form of starch, which is absorbed into the bloodstream more slowly than simple carbohydrates. This slower absorption, as compared with the rapid absorption of simple carbohydrates, is beneficial because it does not produce the concentrated peaks of large glucose production that simple carbohydrates does and therefore it does not require the production of large quantities of insulin by the pancreas. When combined with adequate amounts of soluble dietary fiber, carbohydrates will be digested more slowly, thereby improving glucose tolerance so critical to the prevention and control of diabetes.

No less than 85% of carbohydrates eaten must come from starch, with the remaining 15% consumed through simple or refined carbohydrates. Foods containing high levels of starch include rice, wheat, corn, barley and rye. It is important that these foods should be designated as "whole grain," that is, grains that have not had their shell completely removed or depleted through industrial processing. Pasta is also an excellent source of carbohydrates, and pastas too should be "whole grain." Other sources of carbohydrates include potatoes, yucca, and bananas, among others. Foods containing high concentrations of simple or refined carbohydrates, which should be consumed in limited quantities, include jam, candy, donuts, cakes, cookies, sugary beverages and other foods containing large quantities of sucrose, maltose or lactose.

D. Proteins (represented by a medium red sail)

Food containing large amounts of protein is represented by a medium red sail, suggesting that this type of food should be consumed in smaller amounts. Foods containing protein should satisfy 10–15% of an individual's total energy needs. However, the fundamental nutritional purpose for consuming proteins is not their use as an energy source but rather their role in the process of cell multiplication and the repair of body tissues. Proteins are made up of simpler structural units known as amino acids. There are currently 22 different types of amino acids.

Amino acids too are classified as essential and non-essential. Non-essential amino acids can be synthesized from carbohydrate and nitrogen residues, whereas essential amino acids cannot be produced in this way and must be obtained through one's diet.

Proteins must be digested before their constituent amino acids can be released and subsequently absorbed. The digestion of protein begins in the stomach and is completed in the small intestine, with help from the pancreas. The nutritional quality of the proteins found in food depends, among other things, upon their digestibility and upon their biological use and importance once they have been digested and their constituent amino acids absorbed. A protein is considered complete from a nutritional perspective if it contains all essential amino acids in the correct proportions, as is true for milk and egg proteins.

Dietary proteins can also be of animal or plant origin. Animal proteins tend to have a higher amino acid score and a higher level of digestibility, adding to their nutritional value. Many experts believe that 50% of the total amount of protein consumed should be of animal origin and the remaining 50% of plant origin, although this may vary depending on the individual's life style, functional capacity and health.

Excellent sources of animal protein include low fat milk, free-range poultry, fish and eggs. Plant-based foods, such as grains and legumes or beans, make the greatest quantitative contribution in meeting an individual's protein needs, especially in developing countries. When grains and legumes are combined in appropriate proportions, amino acid mixtures that significantly reduce the actual need for animal-based proteins can be achieved. Vegetables, tubers and other starchy foods provide very little protein, and any protein obtained from these foods is of poor nutritional quality. It decreases the consumption of red meat and focuses more on eating healthier white meats.

E. Fats (represented by a small yellow sail)

Fats are represented by a small yellow sail, based on portion size and indicating that 25–30% of an individual's total energy needs should be met through this type of food.

The most common fats in the human diet are triglycerides and cholesterol esters. Triglycerides may be saturated or unsaturated, depending on the presence or absence of what are called "double bonds." If a fatty acid contains only one double bond between two carbon atoms, the fat is considered to be mono-unsaturated. Fat containing two or more double bonds are considered to be poly-unsaturated. Of the total energy received through the ingestion of fat, 5–10% should be in the form of saturated fats; another 10% in the form of mono-saturated fats; and the remaining 10% as poly-saturated fats.

Fats may have an animal or plant origin. Animal fats are generally saturated fats. Food containing this type of fat is also generally rich in cholesterol. With the exception of coconut and palm oil, fats originating in plants, known as oils, contain a greater amount of unsaturated fat.

The fats we consume may be visible or invisible. Visible fats include fats used for cooking, such as oils, lard or bacon, or those served at the table, such as butter, cream cheese or margarine. Because this type of fat is visible, it can be easily avoided. Non-visible fat, on the other hand, cannot be seen, even though it is present in many foods we eat. These fats can be found in meat, fish, eggs, milk, and nuts, among others. Fats are also classified as being non-essential or essential, depending upon the body's capacity to synthesize its own fatty acids. The non-essential group consists of fat produced by one's own body, and essential fatty acids must be supplied through one's diet in quantities equivalent to 3–5% of an individual's total energy needs.

Excessive fat consumption is associated with many medium and long-term health implications. This is especially true of foods rich in saturated fat and fatty acids. Limited consumption of pork, beef, lamb, bacon, lard, butter, chicken skin, cream cheese, whole milk and fatty cheeses is therefore recommended. Coconut, palm and avocado oils also have high saturated fat content. Fats that are liquid at room temperature, in contrast, (good fats) are rich in polyunsaturated fats and can be found in vegetable oils such as olive, soy, corn, sunflower, sesame and peanut oils. Cold water fish such as salmon contain Omega 3 DHA fatty acids beneficial for brain development.

When preparing food rich in fat, especially fried foods, it is important to avoid overheating the fat or reusing it to the point where its essential qualities are altered. This can produce toxic substances in the fat leading to various illnesses, including cancer.

F. Physical Activity

The principal messages to promote physical activity must include the following: exercise around 30 to 60 minutes at day. Also, it is necessary to use the opportunity to involve the whole family, starting by breastfeeding and physical activity at school that are essential building block and have to be part of their development and curriculum. Exercise at any age has also shown to be the best medicine against obesity and other Non Communicable Diseases (NCD's) and even at higher ages focusing on resistance exercise can decrease one's chances of getting certain cancers. It, improves one's metabolism and organ functions all is a must at any age. Exercise is even prescribed by a growing number of physicians.

III. SPECIFIC PLATFORM FOR THE PREVENTION OF CHILDHOOD OBESITY

The specific platform for the prevention of childhood obesity is a set of plans and programs designed to inform, motivate, promote and implement effective measures against this disease. This platform should be directed at all possible stakeholders in the health and the wellness of children. The recognition of obesity determinants indicates that solutions to this problem require a multi-sectorial and multi-level participation in order to create and develop healthy environments and to decrease obesogenic conditions.

In this multi-level and multi-sectorial work, the coordination of all strategies and actions to stop this epidemic is important and the responsibility to offer safe information that allows the identification of the behavior of the disease and its determinants belong to the health sector. The multi-level work to prevent obesity implies international, national and local efforts; for it is impossible to confront this epidemic without considering its determinants at these levels. The consideration of the national and local conditions is critical when aspiring to the success of prevention.

Local and national plans as well as the Pan American Conference on Obesity with Special Attention to Childhood Obesity series facilitate the execution of effective interventions to promote physical activity and healthy food, both of which contribute to the prevention of childhood obesity. Obesity prevention must be addressed based on the life course approach at all stages with special attention to the pre-conception period, first stages of life, school years, and also workplaces and communities.

In order to prevent the increase of morbidity and mortality due to obesity, there is a need to initiate community interventions programs on a grand scale, directed at increasing physical activity and sustainable options to consume healthy food, especially for children. Obesity prevention is a task involving everyone, individuals, families, communities, and governments, among others. It is not enough to create healthy environments if individuals do not know how to use them, and without healthy environments they cannot be physically active and eat healthy food.

Childhood care must be a catalyst in the prevention of obesity but it requires better demonstration of the negative effects of childhood obesity on health and development. Also, details of the cause-effect relationship of this epidemic and a more effective procedure for its prevention are required.

Parents, teachers, health providers, leaders of public opinion, policymakers and all stakeholders of wellness and people's health require more and better information on the associations of the determinants with the direct causes of obesity. On many occasions parents and teachers interpret that childhood obesity is an expression of wellbeing and beauty. They also believe that this condition will be lost in adulthood.

Changing these interpretations into accepting that childhood obesity is one of the principal health and development problems is the basis for the prevention of this problem. Stakeholder's participation in the childhood obesity prevention work in different sectors as education, culture, economy, policy, government, law, health, infrastructure, citizen safety, trade, agriculture, industry, among others, depends on whether or not they are sufficiently informed and motivated about their role in the presentations and development of overweight and obesity. The specific platform to prevent childhood obesity allows for properly educating parents, teachers, health providers and the entire population, as well as for informing and motivating in the different sectors of society those who are interested in topics that facilitate maintaining healthy lifestyles.

The specific platform for the prevention of childhood obesity creates a superior opportunity compared to attempting to revert this problem in adulthood. Prioritizing this in addition to presently protecting children, helps their future health and also contributes to halting the epidemic in the overall population.

It is necessary to observe that the characteristics and conditions that are considered in the strategies to prevent noncommunicable diseases have a high generalization level that comes short of clearly demonstrating the association between causes and effect of childhood obesity. These observations indicate that within the frame to control and prevent noncommunicable diseases, one must address the prevention of the presentation and development of childhood through a specific platform.

IV. PHILOSOPHICAL FOUNDATIONS FOR HEALTHY LIVING

Philosophy is the study of general and fundamental problems, such as those connected with reality, existence, knowledge, values, reason, mind, and language. Philosophy is distinguished from other ways of addressing such problems by its critical, generally systematic approach and its reliance on rational argument. The philosophy for healthy living allows us to understand why specific ways of living must be preferred. It also provides enough motivation for developing and maintaining lifestyle that prevents diseases such as childhood obesity.

Protecting children by developing habits and behavior that incite them to choose for the pleasure of being active and for healthy food means a different lifestyle from that prevailing in most countries where the philosophical foundations lead to a sedentary lifestyle and an unbalanced diet. These philosophical foundations are the result of associating excessive body weight with economic wealth and health, in addition to linking the underweight with malnutrition and poverty.

In these philosophical foundations one can find in one way or another, the causes that lead individuals to behaviors which science has demonstrated to be conducive to the presence and development of overweight and obesity, from denying obesity is a disease and limits societal development to ceasing to take care of the most valued treasure of any country – its infant population. The prevention of obesity implies changes in lifestyle, a philosophy that includes the search for wellbeing, better quality of life and an increase in longevity by enjoying moderate and intense physical activity and for healthy food; in others words, "the philosophy for healthy living".

This philosophy has a physiological basis that is observed in individuals in the first stage of life, when they naturally seek to exercise their muscles and receive the breastfeeding as the better food. The basis for the philosophy for healthy living lies in the equilibrium between energy intake and energy expenditure. It indicates precisely what we should eat and which physical activity we must perform.

Food intake must be in accordance with nutritional requirements and being active makes it easier for muscle and joints to keep their physiological capacity as part of the normal functioning of the individual. As is well known, in the feeding concept it is necessary to consider the type and the quantity of food, the manner in which it is prepared, the frequency of consumption, the location and the companies during meals, in addition to the way and how quickly the foods are consumed.

As to physical activity, we need to keep in consideration the types, way, frequency, and duration of the activity, as well as where and with whom we exercise. Eating healthily and be active require knowledge, perceptions, and objective and subjective decisions. They are part of the philosophy for healthy living. The philosophy for healthy living indicates how to find the solutions to the obesity problem, because it includes holistically and integrally, all its causes and determinants.

This philosophy also suggests in accordance with these integrated and interrelated causes, how to find a way to prevent or reverse these causes upon recognizing the skills needed to achieve this goal and the need to search for greater and better scientific knowledge about efficacious actions against obesity. This philosophy must be able to have an influence on politics, science, and all factors affecting society, including the concept of beauty and wellbeing, in addition to promoting the following principles "the most important thing once there is life, is health" and "to preserve health it is necessary to avoid being overweight or obese: obesity is not compatible with health."

The philosophy for healthy living leads to a deep conviction that all types of sedentary behavior or unhealthy food adversely affect health. At an individual level, the philosophy for healthy living suggests avoiding foods that can cause more harm than good and enjoying the effects of moderate and intense physical activity. Refusing unhealthy food should be the results of information, education and motivation that facilitate preference and taste by the healthy food.

Similarly preferring an active lifestyle must satisfy the individual's real interest. Motivation should be sufficient to act in a sustained manner and in correspondence with the decision to lead a healthy life. Practical examples of how to apply the philosophy for healthy living could be, at social and family activities, speaking while walking or running (substituting conversation with people sitting); swimming instead of lying on the beach; offering foods without reinforcing the intention of expressing good will along with the abundance of what is being offered; educating children and youth with good personal behaviors as opposed to rhetorical messages; also stimulating people to voluntarily decide to keep a good body weight.

In order to attain that the population acquire this life philosophy it becomes necessary to inform, educate, investigate, empower and increase the cooperation among all through specific projects at local, national and regional level. Among types of projects worth mentioning are those of a diagnostic nature and interventions against obesity; research on healthy food and physical activity; legislation that supports the prevention of obesity; creating human resources and education of the population, such as decreasing obesogenic environments and increasing healthy environments.

The evolution of the human species towards self-destruction and for attempting against its own health and development due to philosophical foundations incompatible with intelligence but with intelligence humanity is capable of overcoming these issues. These philosophical foundations that lead to a loss of life, sedentariness and the intake of unhealthy foods can and must be eliminated through everyone's committed participation, for the problem belongs to all, and for the well-being of all, everyone must be the solution by using the philosophy for healthy living.

V. CONCLUSIONS

The guide for healthy living, the specific platform and the philosophical foundations proposed in this paper are tools that help to prevent childhood obesity. They are the scientific basis to apply an integral approach to promote a healthy lifestyle with special attention to increased physical activity and healthy eating habits.

REFERENCES

[1] CL Ogden, MD Carroll, BK Kit and KM Flegal. Prevalence of obesity and trends in body mass index among US children and adolescents, 1999–2010. JAMA vol. 307, No. 5, 2012, pp. 483–90.

[2] Y. Wang, M. A. Beydoun, L. Liang, B. Caballero and S. K. Kumanyika, "Will All Americans Become Overweight or Obese? Estimating the Progression and Cost of the US Obesity Epidemic," Obesity (Silver Spring), Vol. 16, No. 10, 2008, pp. 2323–2330. doi:10.1038/oby.2008.351

[3] R. Kelishadi, "Childhood Overweight, Obesity, and the Metabolic Syndrome in Developing Countries," *Epidemiological Reviews,* Vol. 29, 2007, pp. 62–76. doi:10.1093/epirev/mxm003

[4] E. A. Finkelstein, J. G. Trogdon, J. W. Cohen and W. Dietz, "Annual Medical Spending Attributable to Obesity: Payer-and Service-Specific Estimates," *Health Affairs (Millwood),* Vol. 28, No. 5, 2009, pp. w822-w831. doi:10.1377/hlthaff.28.5.w822

[5] J. Bhattacharya and N. Sood, "Who Pays for Obesity?" *The Journal of Economic Perspectives,* Vol. 25, No. 1, 2011, pp. 139–158. doi:10.1257/jep.25.1.139

[6] G. Nyberg, E. Sundblom, A. Norman and L. S. Elinder, "A Healthy School Start-Parental Support to Promote Healthy Dietary Habits and Physical Activity in Children: Design and Evaluation of a Cluster-Randomised Inter-vention," *BMC Public Health,* Vol. 11, 2011, p. 185. doi:10.1186/1471-2458-11-185

[7] JJ Reilly. Assessment of obesity in children and adolescents: synthesis of recent systematic reviews and clinical guidelines. *J Hum Nutr Diet.* Vol. 23, No, 3, 2010, pp.205-11. doi: 10.1111/j.1365-277X.2010.01054.x

[8] T. Psaltopoulou, I. Ilias and M. Alevizaki, "The Role of Diet and Lifestyle in Primary, Secondary, and Tertiary Diabetes Prevention: A Review of Meta-Analyses," *The Review Diabetic Studies,* Vol. 7, No. 1, 2010, pp. 26–35. doi:10.1900/RDS.2010.7.26

[9] R. Kones, "Is Prevention a Fantasy, or the Future of Medicine? A Panoramic View of Recent Data, Status, and Direction in Cardiovascular Prevention," *Therapeutic Advances in Cardiovascular Disease,* Vol. 5, No. 1, 2011, pp. 61–81. doi:10.1177/1753944710391350

[10] H. Kitzman-Ulrich, D. K. Wilson, S. M. St. George, H. Lawman, M. Segal and A. Fairchild, "The Integration of a Family Systems Approach for Understanding Youth Obesity, Physical Activity, and Dietary Programs," *Clinical Child and Family Psychology Review,* Vol. 13, No. 3, 2010, pp. 231–253. doi:10.1007/s10567-010-0073-0

[11] M. Moodie, M. M. Haby, B. Swinburn and R. Carter, "Assessing Cost-Effectiveness in Obesity: Active Trans-port Program for Primary School Children-TravelSmart Schools Curriculum Program," *Journal of Physical Activity & Health,* Vol. 8, No. 4, 2011, pp. 503–515.

[12] J. M. Spahn, R. S. Reeves, K. S. Keim, I. Laquatra, M. Kellogg, B. Jortberg and N. A. Clark, "State of the Evidence Regarding Behavior Change Theories and Strategies in Nutrition Counseling to Facilitate Health and Food Behavior Change," *Journal of the American Dietetic Association,* Vol. 110, No. 6, 2010, pp. 879–891. doi:10.1016/j.jada.2010.03.021

[13] AM Hendriks, JS Gubbels, NK De Vries, JC.Seidell, SPJ Kremers and MWJ Jansen. Interventions to Promote an Integrated Approach to Public Health Problems: An Application to Childhood Obesity. J Environ Public Health, 2012: 913236. doi: 10.1155/2012/913236. PMCID: PMC3390054

[14] V Verbestel,S De Henauw, L Maes, L Haerens, S Mårild, G Eiben, L Lissner, LA Moreno, NL Frauca, G Barba, É Kovács, K Konstabel, M Tornaritis, K Gallois, H Hassel, and I De Bourdeaudhuij. Using the intervention mapping protocol to develop a community-based intervention for the prevention of childhood obesity in a multi-centre European project: the IDEFICS intervention. Int J Behav Nutr Phys Act, Vol. 8, 2011, pp. 82. doi: 10.1186/1479-5868-8-82. PMCID: PMC3169445

Chapter 5

LOOKING AHEAD— TECHNOLOGY AND BEYOND

https://vimeo.com/30170531

Where we need to be looking right now: *Gamification* or game-based learning combined with gameplay, which focuses on treating topics and ideas, as rules, action, decisions, and consequences instead of just feeding content to be assimilated.

If we look at the gaming world, we see that our kids are growing up with this technology and format as a natural extension of life, which is starting to merge into the entertainment industry, movies, radio, the medical field, military, and so on, to name a few areas affected.

Here are a couple of things to think about: When our kids get a new game, do they ask us for instructions? Do they need classes to learn how to play the game? The answer is no.

Learning, adapting, and improving are intrinsic to gamification. Gameplay starts them off simply and enables them to go through building blocks. Their social interaction with fellow players gets the gamers to the highest level of play. So how does it work? Well there are a few key elements at *play:*

1. Rewards that are immediate in nature

2. Curiosity—both sensory and cognitive

3. Challenge constantly motivates the player to take on a higher level of difficulty and understanding.

Games live all around us. Games went from the gaming hall (arcade) to the computer, to TV, to portable game players, and to our cellphones. Everyone has access to cellphones—

everyone! Young, elderly, poor, rich, sick . . . All over our planet, cellphones have taken over, so gamification would seem like a natural fit for educating the masses.

Our example is the *Guide to Healthy Living* that we created for Aruba, which is based on a sail boat that comes to life and teaches generations of kids about hygiene, healthy eating, exercise, and the environment. They play the Pirate game in which they get to conquer each island/level; in turn, they learn how to choose healthier options at the grocery store.

They start making healthier choices and know why!

Starting with the design of our *Food Guide,* through all of our public health educational and informative materials, and all the way through how we communicate, care, manage disease, and interface with our health data, has led us in turn to a new era in healthcare communication, analysis, and care.

For example, there are virtual hospitals, clinics, ICU's, urgent care facilities, home care resources, and the list goes on—cloud computing, cellular technology, and Mhealth devices are making it possible to do the impossible.

We live in times of great innovation, with exponential technological development and never before seen global connectivity. This revolution is redefining every aspect of our lives, no matter our socioeconomic background and geographical location. We are converging these technologies to change the face of healthcare.

Cloud-based medical platforms make it possible for patients, healthcare professionals, and plan administrators to collaborate seamlessly and securely collect and share clinical data from patient medical records, lab results, and in-home biometric devices for real-time risk assessments, diagnosis, and treatment.

With a device the size of a kernel of rice or a bio stamp/tattoo, we can monitor a person's vitals 24/7 from any location. Activity trackers, scales, blood pressure cuffs, glucometers, oximeters, virtual medical visits, and medication management systems are engaging patients in a new relationship with their health, healthcare providers, and their environment.

We are rapidly solving accessibility to quality care issues. Language and cultural barriers will be a thing of the past. This is current technology that any country can take advantage of.

For example, lifestyle coaching and tele-psychology are two areas that are taking advantage of these advances in the personal mobile technology arena. These advances, integrated with social media, can revolutionize how we create awareness, educate, deliver care, and impact our population.

This glimpse of things we are doing today is only the beginning.

Technology, biotech, nanotechnology, information tech, and medical sciences are merging to solve global health and wellness challenges.

Appendix 1

THE PANAMERICAN CONFERENCES ON OBESITY— IDENTIFYING STRATEGIES TO PREVENT OBESITY IN THE AMERICAS— PACO 1

INTRODUCTION

The Pan American Conference on Obesity with special attention to Childhood Obesity was held in Aruba from June 8th to 11th, 2011 with the participation of national, provincial and municipal government representatives; ministers, senators; minister's representatives, scientists, experts, journalists, and athletes from 22 countries of all the Americas.

The participants of the Conference were from Anguilla, Argentina, Aruba, Barbados, Belize, Chile, Costa Rica, Colombia, Cuba, Curacao, Dominica, Ecuador, El Salvador, Grenada, Guatemala, Mexico, Montserrat, Nicaragua, Surinam, St Kitts & Nevis, United States of America and Uruguay.

Experts from scientific associations such as the International Association for the Study of Obesity (IASO) with its representatives of Latin America and the Caribbean (FLASO) and North American (TOS), the Latin American Pediatrics Association (ALAPE), LATINFOOD, universities and international organizations including WHO, PAHO/ WHO, FAO and IOC, in addition to the multilevel representation (national, provincial, and municipal) and multi-sector such as health, sports, education, agriculture, and infrastructure participated in the preparation and the work session of the Conference.

During the Conference, strategies that can be applied to prevent obesity in the Americas were identified and the principal document was signed by the majority of the participants. The signed document is **THE ARUBA CALL FOR ACTION ON OBESITY** "Throughout Life . . . at All Ages" in order to help stop this epidemic in the Region.

THE ARUBA CALL FOR ACTION ON OBESITY "Throughout Life . . . at All Ages" is presented in this report with two addendum:

1. BREAKOUT GROUP SESSIONS DURING THE CONFERENCE

2. PREVENTING OBESITY IN THE AMERICAS: A CALL FOR CONCERTED ACTION prepared by The January Preparatory Group.

THE ARUBA CALL FOR ACTION ON OBESITY "THROUGHOUT LIFE . . . AT ALL AGES"

We, the participants of the Pan American Conference on Obesity with special attention to childhood obesity held in Aruba from June 8–10, 2011,

– Recognizing that data shows that obesity prevalence in the Americas has increased and in some cases doubled, affecting all ages, cultures, genders and especially children;

– Recognizing that the growing obesity epidemic needs to urgently be addressed;

– Recognizing that being overweight or obese during childhood has both immediate and long-term health outcomes. Increasingly, obese children are being diagnosed with a range of health conditions previously seen almost exclusively among adults, including high cholesterol, high blood pressure, type 2 diabetes, sleep apnea and joint problems. Moreover, being overweight or obese in childhood significantly increases the risk of overweight or obesity in adolescence and adulthood, which is very hard to reverse;

- Recognizing that under nutrition or obesity during pregnancy and during early infancy are risk for subsequent obesity and other non-communicable diseases;

- Recognizing that early prevention and priority to address childhood obesity is of critical importance;

- Recognizing that obesity has multiple causes such as unhealthy diet and physical inactivity, which are closely linked to an increasing "obesogenic environment" and associated to social determinants such as poverty, low education, food insecurity, cultural norms and lifestyle influences;

- Noting that obesity prevention requires multisectoral, multistakeholder and multi-level actions;

- Noting that obesity-associated NCDs have negative effects on the quality of life and direct economic impacts, including rising health care costs and reduced labor productivity, thereby impede economic development of all affected countries;

- Taking due account of the critical role of children for the development of countries, hence investments in health promotion and obesity prevention throughout life at all ages are essential for the social and economic development.

- Considering that a coherent, consistent message should be given globally emphasizing a comprehensive approach based on three principles: a) that primordial and primary prevention with a life course approach should be the central component of national programs to stem the obesity epidemic, b) that the multi-level focus should be working across all sectors to modify the 'obesogenic' environment that facilitates a positive energy balance and excess weight gain, and c) that developing self care skills, meaning actions taken by the individual to protect and promote their health and the health of their children, is imperative.

- Acknowledging that the 'obesogenic' environment shows wide variability across countries, and therefore any concerted regional action plan must allow for flexibility and adaptation to each local situation.

- Considering that, under the auspices of the Ministry of Health and Sports of Aruba, and the co-auspices of the Pan American Health Organization, a group consisting in members of Governments, non-governmental organizations, Academia, scientific experts and international organizations working on the fight against obesity, and the promotion of healthy weight, met in Oranjestad, Aruba from January 26–29, 2011 with the goal to discuss the current situation regarding the global obesity epidemic, and to propose a plan for concerted action;

– Noting that in recognition of the urgent need to address the obesity pandemic, the Minister of Health of Aruba initiated the Pan American Conference on Obesity with special attention to childhood obesity, held from June 8–10, 2011, in Oranjestad, Aruba, providing an opportunity to discuss the challenges of promoting healthy lifestyles, reducing childhood obesity and the related health issues, and to exchange effective strategies in the fight against obesity, especially in childhood;

Therefore, the participants of the Pan American Conference on Obesity with special attention to Childhood Obesity agree that it is necessary:

– To commit to the fight against childhood obesity and promote healthy weight by sharing strategies and actions contained with our respective governments, institutions and communities; and then promoting those strategies that are consistent with national circumstances.

– To support effective public policies and multi-level, comprehensive strategies to address obesity, based on three principles: a) that primordial and primary prevention with a life course approach should be the central component of national programs to stop the obesity epidemic, b) that the multi-level focus should be working across all sectors to modify the 'obesogenic' environment that facilitates a positive energy balance and excess weight gain, and c) that developing self care skills, meaning actions taken by the individual to protect and promote their health and the health of their children is imperative. At the same time, it is acknowledged that the 'obesogenic' environment shows wide variability across countries, and therefore any concerted regional action plan must allow for flexibility and adaptation to each local situation.

– To create, promote and sustain supportive environments that facilitate access to education, physical activity, healthy foods, and empower the individual to make decisions toward improving their quality of life.

– To implement the necessary policies that insure access to physical activity opportunities, and availability of healthy foods, breastfeeding promotion, utilizing strategies such as menu labeling and restricting the marketing of unhealthy foods and beverages to children via all media, including children's programs and sports.

– To promote access to healthy and affordable food options that are consistent with cultural and environmental factors, providing people with the opportunity to make healthy choices by, inter alia, working with manufacturers and retailers to produce and serve healthy food options, and by implementing programmatic nutrition standards and organizational policies to limit access to unhealthy foods, such as food procurement policies in schools, early learning centers, worksites and hospitals.

– To incorporate the collection of obesity data into chronic disease surveillance systems in member countries and monitor, measure and evaluate the progress made to reduce the prevalence of obesity and its associated risk factors.

– To foster collaboration and knowledge sharing on health promotion and obesity prevention among governments, non-governmental organizations, educational institutions and the private sector.

– To facilitate accumulation and exchange of knowledge on which projects and strategies have proved effective and in which settings. Such facilitation to be done through an alliance of collaborators that provide mutual assistance within and among the countries.

– To raise awareness on all levels in the community about the determinants of obesity across the lifespan, using consistent and actionable messages.

– To raise awareness that obesity has a significant impact on labor productivity, and therefore on the social and economic development of countries, and that investment in health promotion to prevent and reduce obesity supports personal and national economic growth.

– To implement a system to monitor and evaluate the effectiveness and impact of the strategies implemented, and assess the progress made in reducing obesity and increasing the labor productivity.

– To submit and present this call for concerted action to the United Nations High-level meeting on Non-Communicable Diseases, to be held in New York in September 2011.

BREAKOUT GROUP SESSION DURING THE CONFERENCE

In the Pan American Conference on Obesity with Special Attention to Childhood Obesity, breakout group sessions provided the following contributions:

Civil Society:

- Healthy Diet, Physical Activity, and Growth:
  - Monitoring actions of food industries and contribute to independent evaluations;
  - Use power of the media (e.g., blogs) to get the word out, identify offenders and counteract viral marketing of harmful foods and beverages to consumers;
  - Take a role in setting cost controls on physical activity apparel and equipment.
- Multisectoral/multilevel focus:
  - Educating existing consumer groups focused on other issues to foster alliances about win-win scenarios;
  - Form alliances across levels-local, regional, national, and multinational, in the same way the multinational corporations are organized, for parallel efforts.
- Life course approach-start early-at all ages:
  - Promotions including working together with different organizations dedicated to raising public awareness towards the protection of people and future generations.
- Context of the Americas:
  - Examine role of schools run by religious organizations in different countries, on issues as to whether they are required to follow government policies;
  - Link use of traditional foods and healthy eating to religious teaching;
  - Joint use agreements for church grounds and church spaces to the community.
- Engage decision makers and politicians:
  - Organize consumer groups/coalitions to influence policy makers;
  - Educate the community about the issues to get support;
  - Raise consumer voice to demand and protect rights;
  - Approach varies by country and also on whether laws and regulations are already in place or need to be put into place.

Academia:

- To facilitate accumulation and exchange of knowledge on which strategies have proved effective and in which settings through sustained, multisectoral collaboration, and in particular, to promote:

  • Linkages between academia and policy-makers;

- Compared to other chronic diseases, obesity has had less fundamental research into the causes, the reasons for its complications, and into treatments. More basic research is needed to be able to develop more effective prevention and treatment strategies:

  • Teaching tools, in particular distance education, to develop capacity and improve implementation.

Food Industry:

- Truthful and transparent nutrition labeling;

- Advertising must not be misleading or confusing;

- Development of healthy foods including food reformulation;

- Initiate and be involved in programs for healthy lifestyle.

Media and Communications Recommendations:

- Mass media should be regarded as "partners", not "antagonists" in the effort to combat obesity:

- There should be an examination of the current "conversation" and language about obesity with the intention of creating a sense of immediacy about the crisis.

- Each nation should make an effort to identify "champions, opinion leaders, and spokespersons" from various societal sectors to help promote the fight against obesity.

- With particular consideration of children, messages and information about obesity should be framed within the context of the World Health Organization "Declaration of Children's Rights" and should provide positive focus on healthy living (diet, etc.) and avoid focus on body image.

- Massages on obesity should be culturally appropriate, relevant, and should consider the characteristics (age, income levels, and education) of the targeted groups.

– Concerted effort should be made to educate the producers of popular and entertainment media about the misinformation and misapprehension that exist with regard to obesity, i.e., "obesity is caused by laziness". Effort should also be made to get media producers to incorporate positive and informative messages about diet, health care, exercise, etc. in their products.

– News media should be educated, informed, sensitized, and trained on the subject of obesity and its impact on public health, the economy, security, etc.

PREVENTING OBESITY IN THE AMERICAS: A CALL FOR CONCERTED ACTION

Preparations for the Conference included the making of the technical document (white paper) under the name "Preventing Obesity in the Americas: a Call for Concerted Action" to support the main document and to help in the obesity prevention. The document is as follows:

Under the auspices of the Ministry of Health of Aruba, a group of representatives of international organizations and scientific experts working on obesity met in Oranjestad, Aruba, from January 26-29, 2011. The goals of the meeting were to discuss the current situation in the countries of the Americas region regarding the global obesity epidemic and to propose a concerted action plan to confront this problem.

The group expects that this initiative will also be an important contribution from the region to the Global Summit on Non-Communicable Diseases of the General Assembly of Heads of State and Government, to be held in New York in September 2011.

Introduction

Obesity: A global problem for all countries

The old idea that obesity is a problem of abundance, affecting only rich countries, has been replaced by the hard reality that even the poorest countries in the world are facing problems of obesity and its consequences. Recent global obesity data show that the obesity prevalence in the Americas has increased over the past 20 years, and in some countries has doubled.

Obesity in the Americas and throughout the world is closely associated with economic and health disparities. Those who are poor may not have access to affordable, healthy foods, but often do have access to calories of low nutritious value, such as high-fat and high-sugar foods, resulting in excessive energy consumption. Likewise, opportunities for recreational physical activity and access to preventive health care may be limited. Excessive caloric intake and reduced physical activity will almost inevitably lead to excess weight gain and obesity, resulting in poor health for the population.

Many developing countries today face a 'double burden' of malnutrition in which obesity coexists, sometimes in the same family, with under nutrition, usually in the younger members of the family. This situation threatens the economic development of nations, because it dramatically raises health care costs and at the same time reduces productivity in the adult population.

Obesity in children is of special concern, as it conveys a high risk of continuing obesity in adulthood. Established obesity is extremely hard to reverse, demonstrating the critical importance of early prevention and early establishment of health seeking behaviors.

Because obesity involves multiple complex human functions and actions, such as eating habits, daily activities, food production, marketing, and cultural and lifestyle influences, it is not surprising that there is no simple direct solution to this problem.

Traditional research on the determinants of obesity focuses more on individual behaviors with less attention to the social and environmental contexts that facilitate and sustain certain behaviors, or detracts from others. Hence, it is clear that only multi-sectoral, multi-level programs will be able to stop and reverse the obesity epidemic.

Our approach centers on three principles: a) that primordial and primary prevention with a life course approach should be the central component of national programs to stem the obesity epidemic, b) that the multi-level focus should be working across all sectors to modify the 'obesogenic' environment that facilitates a positive energy balance and excess weight gain, and c) that developing self care skills, meaning actions taken by the individual to protect and promote their health and the health of their children, is imperative.

Background

The information on overweight/obesity trends in the region is still incomplete, since not all countries have nationally-representative, longitudinal surveys that would allow the tracking of changes in prevalence over time. However, there are numerous sub-national studies that can be used to estimate overall country prevalence. It is clear that overweight/obesity has increased dramatically since 1990.

Insufficient physical activity is the fourth leading risk factor for mortality with approximately 3.2 million deaths and 32.1 million disability adjusted life years (DALYs) (representing about 2.1% of global DALYs) each year being attributable to insufficient physical activity. Globally, 31% of adults aged 15 years or older were insufficiently active (men 28% and women 34%) in 2008. Among WHO regions, prevalence of insufficient physical activity was highest in the Americas where almost 50% of women and 40% of men were insufficiently active. The prevalence of insufficient physical activity rises according to the level of a country's income, with high-income countries having more than doubled the prevalence compared to low-income countries.

Worldwide, 2.8 million people die each year as a result of being overweight and an estimated 35.8 million (2.3%) of global DALYs are caused by overweight or obesity. In 2008, 35% of adults aged 20 years and older were overweight (BMI = 25 Kg/m2) (34% men and 35% of women). The worldwide prevalence of obesity has nearly doubled between 1980 and 2008. In 2008, 10% of men and 14% of women in the world were obese (BMI = 30 kg/m2), compared with 5% for men and 8% for women in 1980. An estimated 205 million men and 297 million women over the age of 20 were obese in 2008—a total of more than half a billion adults worldwide. The prevalence of overweight and obesity globally were highest in the WHO Region of the Americas (62% for overweight in both sexes, and 26% for obesity), with over 50% of women being overweight and half of these being obese.

In 2010, the estimated prevalence of overweight and obesity (above 2SD from weight for height median in children aged 0–5 years of age) was 40 million preschool children (about 6%) globally. Overweight and obesity prevalence in Latin American and the Caribbean countries is higher than the global average, at 6.9% or approximately 3.7 million children. Globally, the highest prevalence of overweight among infants and young children was found in the upper-middle income group, while the fastest rise in overweight was in the lower-middle income group. Low-income countries had the lowest rate, but overweight rose over time among all country income groups. The rising rates of overweight among infants and young children are associated with rising incomes.

Overall, it is clear that the entire region is in advanced stages of the nutritional transition, with a high degree of urbanization, wide penetration of commercial food markets, and globalized dietary sources. Over 80% of the population lives in an urban environment characterized by predominantly sedentary employment, mechanized transportation, and low levels of recreational physical activity.

A fully commercialized food chain results in a higher proportion of dietary energy consumed outside of the home, with less personal control over its content, increased dependency on food prices in consumption decisions, and influences of promotion and advertisement. This in turn has led to higher consumption of low-cost, energy-dense foods. Taken together, this situation of higher energy intake and reduced energy expenditure greatly favors excess weight gain in almost the entire population.

Determinants

A fundamental starting point to explore the multiple causes of obesity is the principle that in order to gain body weight, an imbalance must exist between the amount of calories consumed and the amount expended in metabolic and physical activity. A healthy non-pregnant adult must keep a zero balance in order to avoid weight gain. Thus, from this starting point, it follows that a person can gain excess weight by either consuming excessive dietary energy, or by expending too few calories.

The apparently straightforward phenomenon of energy imbalance is expressed in a complex fashion. Some of the key elements are summarized below.

Urbanization and Sedentary Lifestyle

Over 80% of the populations in the Americas reside in urbanized areas. This fact has important consequences for energy balance. The characteristics of urban lifestyle are powerful influences on individual and social behaviors related to food intake and physical activity. The urban environment also affects food availability and food purchasing patterns. All these factors favor a positive energy balance.

In terms of lifestyle, the energy demands of urban life are reduced relative to rural life. Labor is heavily mechanized and sedentary. Typical survival activities of rural living, such as walking long distances to obtain and then carry drinking water or firewood, or intensive physical work in the field, are nonexistent in the urban environment.

Typical leisure activities in the urban environment also have of low energy demands, such as watching television, surfing the internet, and playing video games. In addition, opportunities for recreational play for children may be limited by lack of public facilities, street violence, and poor physical activity education at school.

Dietary energy intake

The **food type and quantity** in the urban environment tend to depend on the commercial, cash market which typically is influenced by economic rather than health considerations. The penetration of supermarkets in the Region of the Americas continues to advance dramatically, and even in low-to-mid-income countries may account for one-third to one-half of all calories consumed. Given the high percentage of household budgets spent on food (typically over 50% of income), food choices are heavily influenced by promotions, discounts and subsidies, which may be used by food corporations to promote products that are often far from healthy for the population.

The **energy density** of low-cost foods tends to be high, providing more energy per unit of weight consumed. This is due to a number of factors, one being the dramatic and continuing decline in the price of vegetable oils worldwide, particularly relative to other sources of calories such as grains or rice.

The percent of **calories consumed away from home** is also increasing in many low income countries. This is an important phenomenon because consumers lose control of food quality and quantity when they eat foods prepared by others. In those circumstances, consumers tend to be influenced by price, appearance, and portion size, and not by nutrient quality, which may not be apparent at all.

Availability and cost of healthy foods

In contrast with the higher availability of energy-dense, nutrient-poor foods, in poor urban areas there may often be a limited availability of healthy foods. This problem also exists in poor urban areas of developed countries and is called "food deserts," areas where there are either no food stores or those that exist have limited or no selection of healthy foods. In addition, prices of healthier choices, such as fresh fruits and vegetables, may be prohibitive for a family already spending over half their income in food, as noted above.

All of these factors taken together result, on the one hand, in ample opportunity for overconsumption of calories, and on the other hand, reduced opportunities to spend those calories, either at work or leisure. Under these conditions excess weight gain is very difficult to avoid.

The school environment

In most countries children spend a substantial portion of the day at school, and often consume one or two meals there. They constitute, therefore, an ideal 'captive audience' for nutrition education and healthy eating. Unfortunately, the same is valid for those seeking to sell unhealthy foods. Some food companies have targeted schools for promoting and selling their products, and compete by offering cash compensation in exchange for exclusive access to schools. Several countries have begun to act against this practice, but it is still prevalent in many countries in the region. A particularly troublesome case is that of caloric beverages (soft drinks, fruitades, and sweetened beverages). Data from several countries indicate that almost half of the increase in energy intake over the past decade came from calorie-enhanced drinks. These have displaced milk and other more nutritive calorie sources, particularly in children and adolescents. Furthermore, penetration of vending machines for caloric beverages at schools has also greatly increased, providing opportunities and inducements to millions of children to consume nutrient-poor, 'empty' calories on a daily basis.

Options for preventive initiatives

Preconditions:

A basic condition in order to put into place an obesity prevention strategy for the Americas, and thus, to achieve the new health objectives require the involvement of the Governments to act on the social and environmental factors operating at higher levels of organization—population and societies—and in playing its condition-creating role. Government involvement in addressing the social and environmental factors operating at the community and population levels, and fulfilling their role of fostering environments that promote health, is a basic precondition for putting in place an obesity prevention strategy for the Americas and achieving health goals.

This role consists of creating and promoting a suitable environment, together with all stakeholders concerned, which encourages behaviors of individuals, families, and communities in a positive way to opt continuously for balanced nutrition and an active lifestyle:

– Implementation of a National Plan or Program which requires a clear division of tasks and sufficient structural financing.

– Allocation of specific funds for prevention of obesity in the government budgets.

– Preparation of a prevention policy document and a prevention policy enforced by the Governments, so that all actors are familiar with the prevention policy.

– An integrated approach requires that the various policy sectors, such as education, public health, sports, culture, agriculture, trade, infrastructure, youth, traffic, are all involved proactively and take responsibility, in order to influence the entire community.

– Implementation of healthy school policies, in order to support a healthy foundation for children and for teachers at school.

– Integration of messages regarding sufficient physical activity and balanced nutrition into various initiatives, and better coordination among programs.

– Advertising and marketing to children should be reviewed and World Health Assembly resolution (WHA) 63.14, restricting marketing of 'junk foods' in settings where children gather, should be implemented.

– Cooperation between actors in the social sector should be strengthened and primary and secondary prevention should be in line with each other.

– The themes 'healthy physical activity and balanced nutrition' should be integrated into the school curricula and the school environment modified to positively support these themes.

- There should be a sufficient investment in projects to support the achievement of these health objectives, which meet the criteria of sustainability, intersectoral coordination, and a structural basis.

- Countries should consider raising additional funds by increasing the excise duty on non-nutritive food and beverage products such as candy and sugar-sweetened drinks.

Strategies

The Life Course perspective: healthy children, healthy adults

There is ample evidence that many adult diseases (including obesity) originate early in life, even during fetal life. This 'developmental origins of disease' theory is supported by a number of studies in developed and developing countries. Thus, it is imperative that prevention efforts also start as early in life as possible, and takes particular consideration of the developing child and his/her environment.

This important aspect links obesity prevention with ongoing efforts to reduce child mortality and promote child health. Initiatives to promote healthy pregnancy and birth weight, exclusive breastfeeding and appropriate complementary feeding, and prevention of underweight are also critical to reduce the risk of obesity later in life.

Another key integrating element for a life course approach, because it impacts both children and adults, is the **built environment**, i.e., the conditions of everyday life, work, recreation and living spaces created by decisions and preferences of a community. It is recognized that a critical step to reduce obesity is to modify this built environment, in order to facilitate all elements of a healthy lifestyle, as discussed below.

Multi-level, multi-sectoral approaches to obesity prevention

Healthy communities

To create Healthy Communities and Cities, commitment by all stakeholders is necessary in order to change the social norms and environment. The strategies should create awareness and increase physical activity in everyday life, targeting neighborhoods, families and children. The strategies should have different activities, including diet together with physical activity and a strong educational component, focused on facilitating healthy behavior. Healthy Communities/Cities strategies should include:

- Healthy options available in restaurants.

- Transportation policies that will increase physical activity.

- Tax incentives for workplaces with wellness programs, using a whole-family approach that views parents as change agents for children.

- Access to parks, church yards, and community centers with a focus on overall physical activity & fitness rather than competitive sports.

- Core health messages in all education campaigns.

- Controls on advertising and marketing food and drinks to children.

- Front-of-Pack national food labeling systems, providing consumers with simple ways to make healthier choices.

- Mass public movement events, like the well-known Ciclovias Saludables.

Healthy schools

Schools are a key component of the built environment affecting children. Children spend a substantial portion of the day at school, providing opportunities for education, direct intervention and peer learning. It is also common for children to consume food during school time, either brought from home or purchased on the premises. In some countries, federal programs provide food assistance at schools, giving another opportunity to influence diet quantity and quality. We must recognize, however, that these opportunities have been used so far to a limited extent. The main initiatives in this environment have been well defined, and include:

- Provide only food options that meet the healthy dietary guidelines of the country in school cafeterias.

- Introduce policy for exclusive healthy offerings in vending machines.

- Restructure feeding programs to recognize the threat of excess weight, and not just underweight.

- Support for physical activity throughout the day, and not only as a specific subject in the curriculum (i.e., physical education). At the same time, formal physical education time must be initiated, supported and protected.

- Assist teachers to include healthy lifestyle and healthy eating content in their curriculum.

- Encourage organized parental involvement in physical activity at school.

- Settings where children gather should be free from all forms of marketing of foods high in fats, sugars and salt or otherwise low in nutritional value.

The workplace

National and local governments should frame policies and provide incentives to encourage physical activity and healthy behavior at work. The workplace is an ideal venue to offer employees structured and planned activities to improve their health. Programs that are accessible, sustainable, and economical and that include the whole family can provide maximum health benefits for employees, and reduce the burden of poor health on employers.

- Promoting balanced nutrition and sufficient physical activity.

- Education for the employees on raising healthy and fit children (self-care skills).

- Creating areas for breast feeding and storing breast milk.

- Encouraging mothers to eat well during pregnancy, and throughout the duration of breastfeeding.

- Including healthy canteens and healthy options in vending machines.

- Promoting the possible cooperation between companies, so that smaller companies can participate in larger projects.

- Promoting company sports and tournaments.

- Family days, during which the entire family exercises and learns how to eat healthy - also stimulating healthy food/nutrition classes in the workplace.

The living environment of infants and young children

The first year of life is of crucial importance to a healthy life. Babies who are breastfed have health benefits in the short term, such as a reduced risk of acute otitis media, atopic dermatitis, gastrointestinal infections, lower respiratory tract infections, asthma, and necrotizing enterocolitis (this last only in premature children). In the long term, breastfeeding protects against chronic disorders, such as obesity, diabetes mellitus, celiac disease, and leukemia. Multifaceted interventions are notably effective, when they are focused on the beginning, the duration, and the exclusiveness of breastfeeding.

- Promoting healthy birth weight by providing pregnant women with appropriate prenatal advice and monitoring.

- Promoting exclusive breastfeeding for at least six months.

- Providing support in the transition from breastfeeding to healthy eating habits.

  • The first years of life are important to acquire a healthy lifestyle with balanced and varied eating habits and sufficient physical activity. Childcare is the main factor of influence, combined with the parents and extended families, in the child's immediate social environment. Therefore, additional attention should be paid to the role these influences can play in promoting a healthy environment for young children. Young children should have sufficient possibilities and opportunities to exercise and develop physically.

– Legislation that guarantees healthy child daycare centers with supervision over the quality and contents of childcare programs.

– Programs to educate the daycare providers on healthy food and physical activities and minimizing sedentary behaviors.

The health care sector

The health care delivery models in the Americas are diverse, still evolving, and present critical challenges; these need to be considered beyond the scope of this paper. But one cannot ignore the central role that the health care system plays in the fight against obesity. For many citizens, the only contact with health education may be a visit to the clinic or a house visit by a health care worker. It is therefore critical that health care providers are well versed and motivated to target obesity prevention as a major public health priority.

Unfortunately, in most countries the medical education curriculum is still heavily focused on treatment rather than prevention, and this training is potentiated by a health care system largely centered around disease management as well. Thus, a sustainable obesity prevention program will have to enhance the public health skills of the healthcare providers through continuing professional development, develop alternative providers for the prevention component of health services, or implement both strategies.

Evidence suggests that the healthcare providers do not provide patients with clear, unambiguous information about overweight and obesity. To properly inform and refer people, care providers should dispense the appropriate knowledge and be able to make use of practical tools when giving advice. Therefore, it is necessary to draw up unambiguous information and to adopt guidelines for this group. As most of the prevention will depend on the first line, support to primary care practitioners is necessary.

Integration of health care services is another challenge closely linked to obesity prevention. As noted above, effective obesity prevention programs must address a healthy pregnancy and birth weight, breastfeeding, introduction of appropriate solid foods, monitoring of diet and weight during school years, and continuing tracking of indices of energy balance in adulthood.

The role of the private sector

– The private sector, in relation to overweight/obesity, should play an important role and have vital responsibility in building a healthy environment, as well as for promoting healthy choices through mass media campaigns that are accompanied by appropriate "upstream" policy support and "downstream" community based activities, usually involving a community participation approach. The companies should focus on the main domain of their activities, while promoting product information; and consumer education within the framework set by public health policy.

- Incentives vs. disincentives for healthy foods vs. alternatives.
- Nutrition labeling and consumer education.
- Consistent, coherent, simple and clear messages concerning advertisements and other public education should be communicated through many channels to the population.
- Implications for Free Trade Agreements.
- Making healthy foods available and affordable.
- Implement marketing restrictions throughout the Americas to ensure that marketing of foods high in sugar, fats, and/or salt are eliminated.

Integration of all the stakeholders

International organizations could play an important role in advocacy across international, national, regional and municipal levels; promoting and supporting healthy public policies; setting standards that encourage better living conditions; and promoting the primordial and primary prevention of obesity. Also it could promote commercial practices that consistently facilitate healthy choices which in turn may require legislative and international regulatory support to ensure that strategies are fully resourced and implemented; and that appropriate control measures are enforced.

Monitoring and evaluation of strategies

A process needs to be put in place to develop internationally comparable core-indicators for inclusion in national health surveillance systems. Monitoring and evaluation is essential to measure the effectiveness and efficiency of the program in achieving its desired outcomes. The countries should create an Alliance of Collaboration to facilitate the exchange and accumulating of knowledge on which strategies, experiences, and projects have proved effective and in which settings.

Summary

Obesity prevalence in the Americas has increased to an alarming level. This situation is threatening the economic development of the Americas, because it raises health care costs dramatically and at the same time it reduces productivity in the adult population.

Preconditions are needed as the foundation for an obesity prevention strategy in the Americas. The strategies must be based on three principles: a) that primordial and primary prevention with a life course approach should be the central component of national programs to stem the obesity epidemic, b) that the multi-level focus should be working across all sectors to modify the 'obesogenic' environment that facilitates a positive energy balance and excess weight gain, and c) that developing self care skills, meaning actions taken by the individual to protect and promote their health and the health of their children, is imperative.

The strategies must be applied in our communities, schools, workplaces and the living environments of infants and young children; considering the life course perspective (healthy children, healthy adults) and the role of thehealth care sector, private sector and the integration of all the stakeholders. Finally we have to monitor and evaluate the strategies, which will be essential for measuring the effectiveness and efficiency of our efforts.

Final note

Preventing obesity poses a pivotal challenge and opportunity for change. It's also one of humanity's most pressing obligations. Many shortcomings and contradictions come with this task, yet never before have so many political leaders, scientists, and health experts conjointly recognized their concern and need to act on this issue.

We must address it now and with the full strength of our professional knowledge, research capacity, diplomatic cooperation, and public outreach because the health and development of entire nations depend upon it.

We can prevent obesity. With the contributions of everyone concerned, let's do it right.

Appendix 2

THE PANAMERICAN CONFERENCES ON OBESITY— IDENTIFYING STRATEGIES TO PREVENT OBESITY IN THE AMERICAS— PACO 2

Theme: Let's get together to stop childhood obesity.

CONCLUSIONS AND RECOMMENDATIONS

Background:

The first Pan American Conference on Obesity, with special attention to Childhood Obesity (PACO I) was held in Aruba from June 8-11, 2011 (www.paco.aw). Experiences and lessons learned were analyzed by attendees and experts from various sectors such as health, education, sport, media, local and national government, and international institutions to send "The Aruban Call for Action on Obesity: Throughout Life . . . at All Ages" (http://www.paco.aw/pdf/20110608_20110610_the_aruba_call_for_action_on_obesity.pdf) to the United Nations Summit on Non-Communicable Chronic Diseases.

PACO I concluded that the solution to the problem of obesity requires tackling obesogenic environments through systematic, extensive multi-level and multisectorial initiatives. The Aruban Call for Action supported and complemented numerous authoritative recommendations that have been made to urge such initiatives to be undertaken in relation to obesity or obesity-related NCDs. What is pressing at this juncture is to extend the call to action to focus on specific ideas effective in the prevention of obesity and then to evaluate whether these actions are having the intended effects.

The Second Pan American Conference on Obesity, with special attention to Childhood Obesity (PACO II) was held in Aruba from June 15–16, 2012 (http://www. paco.aw/paco2conference.php#workshops), with the following objectives:

1. Develop a specific platform for the prevention of obesity, specifically childhood obesity; locally, nationally, and internationally to facilitate the implementation of actions and operational research that addresses the epidemic of obesity.

2. Strengthen the focus on non-communicable diseases (NCD's) including obesity; locally, nationally, and across the institutions of the United Nations and the Inter American System.

The conference was preceded by two international courses and seven thematic workshops (June 11–14th):

International Courses:

– Exercise is Medicine

– CDC: International Course on Physical Activity and Health

Workshops:

- Promoting Physical Activity to Prevent Childhood Obesity;

- School Environment and the Prevention of Childhood Obesity;

- Economic Cost of Obesity;

- Food- Based Dietary Guidelines in the Prevention of Childhood Obesity;

- PAHO/PAHEF Workshop on Education for Childhood Obesity Prevention: A Life Course Approach

- The Role of E-Health in the Prevention of Childhood Obesity;

- Creating Healthy Environments and Healthy People.

Other PACO II topics were genetic and alternative causes of obesity, the roles of women, agriculture, food safety, the marketing of food and beverages for children, the role of the food and beverage industry in the prevention of childhood obesity and alternative treatments for obesity.

PACO II was convened by the Minister of Health and Sports of Aruba. Participants included ministers, legislators, representatives of ministers, representatives of international agencies and organizations, policy makers, representatives of the food industry, and representatives of governments and civil society organizations from 25 countries in the Americas region, practicing health professionals, and scientists engaged in the study of various aspects of obesity.

The conference recognized that obesity and childhood obesity are a global problem, which is increasing at alarming rates in all countries with considerable health and socio economic impact. Most importantly, countries have not been able to succeed in reversing this epidemic.

Conferees agreed to focus on child growth and development emphasizing policies and interventions to promote the child's "healthy weight" goal including enabling healthy environments and education on healthy living.

To contribute to the prevention of obesity in the Americas, all the proceedings of PACO II including documents, reports, and videos of the conference will be on line at www.paco.aw.

The conclusions and recommendations will be sent to the ministers of all the countries of the Americas as well as to the Inter-American Meeting at Ministerial Level on Health and Agriculture (Chile, July 26–27, 2012) and Pan American Sanitary Conference (USA, 2012).

Conclusions and Recommendations from PACO I:

The results of the call to action from PACO I emphasized the need to support effective public policies and multi-level, comprehensive strategies to address obesity, based on three principles: 1) That primordial and primary prevention with a life course approach should be the central component of national programs to stop the obesity epidemic; 2) That the multi-level focus should be working across all sectors and societal levels to modify the 'obesogenic' environment that facilitates a positive energy balance and excess weight gain; 3) That developing self-care skills, meaning actions taken by the individual to protect and promote their health and the health of their children, is imperative. PACO I also stressed the need to create, promote, and sustain supportive environments that facilitate access to education and information, physical activity, healthy foods, and empower the individual to make decisions towards improving their quality of life. PACO II reaffirmed and built upon these recommendations.

Conclusions and Recommendations from PACO II:

1. Fund, design, and implement a study in Latin American and Caribbean countries to estimate the economic costs of obesity in children and adults in different age and sex groups. This will be essential for engaging non-health sectors in the discussions and reaching decision makers who can allocate the resources needed to address the problem.

   Hunger and undernutrition are ongoing food and nutrition problems in areas of Latin America and the Caribbean for which the high economic costs have been clearly documented. In recent years, however, the problem of overweight has increased, co-existing with under nutrition. Researchers in high income countries have estimated that obesity is responsible for a substantial economic burden in health care and other costs. Such estimates are urgently needed for Latin America and the Caribbean to generate synergies between the objectives of a) addressing the urgency of action and b) deepening understanding of the social and economic consequences for populations that come with overweight and obesity.

2. Public policies to tackle social determinants of obesity through the life course (health promotion, multi settings, multi-sectorial and multi-level interventions) Participants at the PACO II conference acknowledged that obesity and NCD's are not randomly distributed across all population groups. In fact, vulnerable groups in poor communities and developing countries carry an increasing burden of the cost and health consequences of the problem. A 'whole of society' approach, as defined by WHO, is needed to

influence the various social, economic and environmental determinants of child obesity and other NCDs.

Public policies should be based on health promotion principles to promote healthy child growth and development. The emphasis should be changing obesogenic environments through multi-level (global, regional, national, state, municipal and community) initiatives. Vertical and horizontal multi-sectorial, multi-level coordination is needed for countries to implement effective approaches for the prevention of childhood obesity based on the life course approach framework. There is a special need for closer coordination and integrated actions between the Ministries of Health, Education, Environment, Agriculture, Economy, Trade or Commerce, Transportation,Urban and Rural Infrastructure, Security, Sports, and Culture; with clear goals and accountability mechanisms.

Public policies to be considered include: exclusion of sugary drinks and unhealthy snacks from school canteens, upgrading existing school feeding programs to include more fresh foods and water, regulations on publicity/ advertising of products high in salt, sugar and saturated fat. Other policies that may not be considered obesity specific as development and promotion of urban agriculture, mass transit, and street safety, are critical complements to the above stated childhood obesity policies and should be actively pursued by the public health sector in alliance with the corresponding leading sectors as agriculture, transportation city planning and others.

As for policy development it is fundamental that the first take at the policies must come from the public sector and be based on solid scientific evidence to later move into receiving input from other stakeholders and also private sectors entities with a stake in the modifications implied in the proposed policies. Public policies should include inputs from multiple sectors, and promote interventions in multiple settings by enabling healthy environments and providing incentives for better access to healthy choices regarding healthy eating and active living.

Obesity prevention programs and interventions should address physical and virtual settings where children live, learn, eat, play, and socialize, such as homes, childcare and early education centers, schools (pre and after school programs), faith-based organizations, recreational and social media networks, and other community based facilities for children and families.

3. Strengthen education interventions into the life course approach to prevent childhood obesity

Public policy and education are key in enabling individuals to make healthy choices. Obesity prevention in education settings must be based on multidisciplinary interventions and collaboration between schools, families and the entire society. Capacity building in obesity prevention is required and should include the entire learning community, teachers, leaders, health care providers, related services personnel, university professors, and other interested community members.

a. Undertake educational interventions to reduce obesity in the preconception period, fostering appropriate weight gain during pregnancy, supporting women in avoiding the retention of excessive weight gain during the postpartum period, and promoting optimalinfant feeding practices, including breast feeding, nutritious and safe complementary feeding, and the avoidance of sugar sweetened beverages and "junk foods;"

b. Strengthen school feeding and physical activity programs at preschool, school, and after school and summer care programs with the aim to reduce screen time and increase consumption of nutritious foods and physical activity during out of school time. Educational based feeding programs must promote consumption of local available fruits and vegetables, safe water and physical activity, while restricting access to calorie-dense, fat-dense, nutrient-vacant foods and beverages. In addition, obesity prevention must be practiced in a way that is culturally sensitive and takes into account beliefs associated with body image, particularly in young women;

c. Incorporate nutrition and physical activity for healthy living content into core curricula (math, language arts, social studies, etc.) in all educational settings (schools, early childhood centers/child care centers, summer programs, etc.);

d. Establish inter-sectorial agreements to enable health promoting environments (recreational parks, gyms, game courts,), infrastructure (bike and walking paths) and transportation to promote and increase physical activity and active living during and after school and work hours;

e. Engage key community institutions outside the formal education system, including local governments, civil society organizations, local farmers, early childhood centers, churches, pediatric/family medicine clinics, and others, to support family nutrition education, access to healthy food, and daily physical activity – all of which are key to promote child "healthy weight."

Additional strategies to enable the education interventions through the life course approach should include:

• Institutionalization of an early career leadership scholars program/ network in Latin America and the Caribbean, that focuses on evidence-based approaches to childhood obesity prevention based on the life course approach;

- Promote investment in longitudinal research to explore effectiveness, replicability, sustainability, scalability and cost of interventions to prevent childhood obesity through the life course prioritizing the preconception, pregnancy and early childhood periods;
- Childhood obesity prevention should be included as a priority into the maternal-child health and education policies and programs of international agencies including the Inter-American system;
- Innovative and attractive social marketing educational efforts should be developed to disseminate food based dietary guidelines (FBDG) and other evidence-based messages to improve nutrition and physical activity;
- Monitoring and evaluation systems to properly assess process and impact of life course national strategies, and targets for childhood obesity prevention should be included in national and regional plans.

4. Routinely incorporate obesity and related health issues into foreign policy and trade negotiations.

NCDs and obesity are significant global health concerns, which have a direct impact on economic growth and development, and therefore should be taken into account in foreign policy and trade discussions.

National governments and regional or international agencies, in negotiations of bilateral and international trading arrangements, should therefore include public health considerations including the prevention of obesity and associated conditions or diseases.

Complementary to this recommendation, governments and agencies should also identify and take full advantage of opportunities to focus on obesity and NCD health issues as part of the foreign policy agenda. This will support core foreign policy goals of co-operation and progress among states.

Existing international trade policies in the areas of market access, sanitary and phyto-sanitary measures, technical barriers to trade, and innovation and intellectual property are examples of instruments that may be used in achieving these objectives.

To be most effective, these trade policy measures should be used in concert with educational, fiscal, and agricultural initiatives.

The focus of these interventions in trade and other policy spheres should be to promote availability of nutrient-rich, lower-salt, lower-sugar, and less-fatty foods that should replace many of the calorie-dense, fat-dense, nutrient-vacant foods that are traded and consumed across the region.

5. Limit marketing of foods and non-alcoholic beverages containing high amounts of fat, sugar, salt, and low in essential nutrients.

A strong and convincing body of evidence points to the critical importance of public policies limiting the marketing of unhealthy foods and beverages to children and youth, as they are not yet rational economic decision makers. Both WHO and PAHO have published clear recommendations to this effect. All governments should commit to implementing these recommendations, enforced by law.

Reducing advertising of unhealthy foods to children will be most effective when accompanied by industry actions to reformulate foods to reduce fat, salt and sugar, and to make available healthier choices. Transparent front of pack information should also be provided to aid consumer's choices. Civil society and academia can have a clear role in advocating for and monitoring some of these actions.

6. Reframe the leadership role of women regarding family health to include fathers as an active participant in the implementation of healthy home environments.

PACO II sees the role of women as of overarching importance when seeking solutions and proposing recommendations to curb the impending rise of childhood obesity in the Americas. As with all other aspects of the "whole of society" approach, the role of women in society needs to be analyzed and its substance highlighted when formulating policy aimed at arresting childhood obesity.

Major societal changes resulting from socio-economic inequalities, advances in education, and increased equality for women have propelled the incorporation of women into full labor force participation. Parallel to these changes or possibly resulting from them, the number of female–headed households has exponentially increased, while concomitantly the presence of husbands and fathers within the households has decreased. This is important since female headed households are usually below poverty income guidelines and it is well known that income level and obesity are very much related; income has an impact on the availability of quality foods in the household, health care and quality time spent with children. Labor policies are needed that address the participation of women in the labor force and that provide suitable options to satisfactorily respond to their dual roles of mothers and workers.

Moreover, there exists a lack of correspondence between the noted structural changes and the evolution of appropriate values and norms. This is especially the situation for the various social roles that women play in society; and particularly as mothers, no longer centered only within the household. The multifaceted roles that women now play in and outside the household must be revisited since understanding the latter can make an important contribution toward the improvement of childhood obesity. This leads to the following recommendations:

1. Policy makers in multiple sectors need to initiate a public dialogue to redefine the new emerging roles of men and women within the family and society;

2. Policies are needed to actively support family practices of healthy eating, increased physical activity and the promotion of good health;

3. Policies are very much needed to promote equal pay for men and women, paid maternity leave and flexible work schedules, in order to facilitate parents' engagement in their children eating habits and physical activity;

4. Increased public and private sector support for the construction of parks and other recreational spaces that facilitate physical activity and promote a holistic approach to family recreation and healthy eating;

5. Increased public and private sector support for low cost fresh fruits and vegetables;

6. Increased public and private sector to promote the full participation of women in policy-making;

7. Providing seminars and other support to promote leadership skills in women.

7. Tailor the content, regulatory, and operational frameworks of food based dietary guidelines.

Food based dietary guidelines (FBDG) should be: a) institutionalized as part of public policies related to food and nutrition security; b) supported by national food and nutrition education plans; c) included at the regular programs of Ministries of Health, Education, Agriculture and Social Development, as well as in the First Ladies' Agenda, as a tool to promote healthy diet.

Besides developing general FBDG, there should be guidelines for the following age groups: infants and preschool children, school age children, and adolescents.

It is also is essential to develop regulatory frameworks to support the implementation of the FBDG's recommendations. These should include: a) appropriate legislation to support and promote exclusive breastfeeding; b) legislation to regulate foods in the schools environment (food advertising, food available in the school); c) use of FBDG to define school feeding programs; d) appropriate legislation for mandatory nutritional labels that are simple and easily to be understood by lay people.

Countries need support to develop and implement effective communication strategies for different context and audiences. It is crucial that both, professionals from different sectors as well lay people are trained in the content, application and use of the FBDG.

8. Develop and pilot test initiatives to identify and utilize local food sources and promote adult and youth consumers' appreciation for the natural origins of available foods.

Over consumption of heavily processed foods and a lack of information and availability of more nutritious alternatives is directly resulting in a new "malnutrition" among the people of the Americas. Detachment from food production further limits what people have available to eat. Through community agricultural programs people can be persuaded to better their environment, develop community and produce healthy food locally for their own use and as a source of (supplemental) income. Ultimately when people eat food that is produced locally there are many benefits including; access to fresher food, money that stays at home (instead of going to an overseas merchant) and spin off economies. The promotion of novel xerophytic (desert) crops adapted to dry tropical environments may be an essential element to success in some countries in the region.

9. Food safety and nutrition

The safety, quality and nutritional value of the food we eat is of fundamental importance to our health and wellbeing. Food safety and nutrition are therefore strongly associated. Risk factors associated with an unsafe diet and the need to improve dietary quality and at same time the importance of improving food safety should be recognized. It was discussed that the food safety concept should be expanded from the typical microbiological or chemical contaminants to focus on poor nutritional quality. Recommendations for how to address these issues are as follows.

a. Establish a link between the food safety concepts and nutrition;

b. Articulate policies at country and regional levels considering healthy and safe food;

c. Promote the local food culture in each region or place;

d. Promote multi-sectorial policies to improve food safety, education, water and sanitation, and access to health services;

e. Promote good manufacturing practices of food;

f. Educate children with the five keys for safer food along with the five keys for healthy diet of WHO.

10. Develop complementary and integrative actions to increase physical activity across whole communities.

Physical activity is an independent risk factor for non-communicable diseases. Therefore it demands a population-based, multi-sectorial, multi-disciplinary, and culturally relevant approach. The evidence base on physical activity interventions is large and has grown exponentially in the last decade with a considerable number of published studies from middle income countries in Latin America. The evidence shows that there are different types of interventions that can be implemented which encompass the primary care settings; public spaces; mass media campaigns; school and workplace settings and active transport among others.

a. Primary care settings should routinely assess physical activity, provide patients with advice and counseling on physical activity (exercise prescription) and refer to or provide additional resources (e.g., health education, group activities, fitness professionals) with the aim to increase physical activity;

b. Increase training of primary health care professionals on how to promote physical activity; increase staff to integrate physical activity counseling into the routine practice in busy primary care settings; increase provision of and access to community based facilities or programs on physical activity linked with primary care; ensure resources and capacity to deliver ongoing patient support in person, by phone, email or other communication methods;

c. There is strong evidence that mass media campaigns that aim to raise community awareness, inform and change attitudes towards being active are effective. Mass media campaigns were identified as "Best-buys" by WHO and use a combination of mass media components and multiple channels including television and radio adverts, as well as print media, often linked with community events and programs. One major barrier to these interventions is the cost component of developing and executing campaigns in the most popular media at the most popular coverage time;

d. Schools are common settings for effective interventions aimed at increasing physical activity in children and young adults. Interventions include changes to the school curriculum to increase time and activity levels in PE classes, classroom physical activity sessions, recess in primary schools, after school activities based within the school context, and active travel to school. There is a moderate to strong evidence base on the effectiveness of school based interventions aimed at increasing physical activity;

e. Safe Routes to School interventions need to have the involvement of teachers, parents, transportation officials, and the community, combining promotional activities with safety, environmental, and structural improvements, such as sidewalk and signage enhancements;

f. Transport policies can promote active and safe methods of travelling such as walking or cycling. Results show positive effects can be achieved from multicomponent cycling interventions. It is important to ensure that walking, cycling and other forms of physical activity are accessible to and safe for all. Therefore work with urban planners is important and needs to be proactively led by the health sector. Mass public events that incentivize physical activity such as Ciclovías, have been implemented in recent years in many countries in the Americas and have shown to increase physical activity in the population. These interventions need the necessary supportive infrastructure (e.g. bike lanes, cycle tracks, bike boxes, traffic signals, sidewalks, cycle parking and storage);

g. Proximity to parks, public open space, and private recreation facilities are related to use of those facilities and total physical activity. Thus, policies to ensure access to recreation facilities in all neighborhoods are important throughout the life course. Group activity programs in public spaces have been shown to be popular and effective in Latin America and can be implemented at modest cost;

h. To build capacity for physical activity promotion, public health departments at the national, regional, and local levels are encouraged to hire appropriately trained staff to coordinate this work.

11. Enhance the use of eHealth to support obesity prevention. All governments in the Americas should adapt the framework of the PAHO Strategy and Plan of Action on eHealth, which was approved by all the Member States in the Region on September 2011, to any development related to eHealth and programs against obesity. Specifically, Member States are urged to undertake the prevention of obesity through the following initiatives:

a. Produce and disseminate through the Internet information to target different audiences, such as health workers, parents, teachers, and others;

b. Develop in collaboration with the Pan American Health Organization and the Pan American Health and Education Foundation, a Virtual Health Library on the topic of obesity;

c. Map initiatives, projects and campaigns that work against obesity and create an electronic repository with this information;

d. Promote the use of information and communication technologies as effective tools against obesity and physical inactivity;

e. Use mHealth, such as the ¨Get the message¨ initiative, to reach citizens through mobile devices http://www.healthycaribbean.org/get-the-message.php;

f. Use social networks to engage target audiences and to build networks;

g. Develop virtual courses for diverse audiences about the prevention of obesity;

h. Launch pilot projects on teleconsultations to monitor/follow up with obese patients.

Following the commitments established by the United Nations (UN) member states, at the UN High-Level meeting on Non-Communicable Diseases, in New York, in September 2011, the PACO II international meeting, held in Aruba, in June 2012 was instrumental in raising awareness and bringing stakeholders together around the child obesity and NCDs challenge in the Region.

The PACO initiative convened by the Ministry of Health and Sports of Aruba, with the support of the Government of Aruba, the Pan American Health Organization (PAHO)/World Health Organization (WHO), Food and Agriculture Organization (FAO), the Latin American Economic Commission (in Spanish CEPAL), the International Olympic Committee (IOC), International Association for the Study of Obesity (IASO), the World Council of University Academics (COMAU), the Pan American Health and Education Foundation (PAHEF), International Organization of School Sports (IOSS), the Caribbean Public Health Agency (CARPHA), the Centers for Disease Control and Prevention (CDC), worked in collaboration with 209 participants in the PACO II meeting .

The participants left the meeting with a commitment to evaluate and build upon the successes of this initiative and strengthen political leadership and actions against child obesity across the Region of the Americas.

Appendix 3

THE PANAMERICAN CONFERENCES ON OBESITY— IDENTIFYING STRATEGIES TO PREVENT OBESITY IN THE AMERICAS— PACO 3

CONCLUSIONS

The PACO III conference was extraordinary because Ministers of Health were involved from Aruba, Bermuda, British Virgin Islands, Dominica, Grenada, Montserrat, Saint Lucia, Surinam, and Turks and Caicos Island, and the Secretary of Health of Colima State (Mexico): the Representative of the First Lady of Chile; Representatives of the Ministers of Health of the Bahamas, Barbados, Bolivia, Costa Rica, Dominican Republic, Ecuador, El Salvador, Mexico, Puerto Rico, St. Kitts & Nevis, St. Maarten; the General

Director of PARLATINO; the Director of Food Agency of Santa Fe, Argentina; the Representatives of Guayas, Santa Elena, Los Rios, Bolivar and Galapagos Provinces, Ecuador; experts from Belgium, Brazil, Canada, Colombia, Cuba, France, Guatemala, The Netherlands, UK, USA; the President of IASO; Representatives of WHO, PAHO, FAO, PAHEF, CARICOM, CARPHA, ALAPE, Inter American Cardiologist Association, FLASO and the World Bank as well as Coca Cola and PepsiCo in detailed discussions and debate. They developed a series of conclusions relating to what they themselves as Ministers of Health could do directly and what they would plan to do as part of their leadership role for public health within government.

Conclusions:

1. Ministers of Health through their leadership role will seek to prioritize at an international, national and local level the inclusion of obesity as an important topic in the political agenda within WHO, PAHO, World Bank, FAO and other international organizations.

2. Ministers of Health need to change doctors' and health professionals' understanding of the dietary and physical activity basis of NCDs and their management by changing the curriculum of both undergraduate and postgraduate programs.

   Physicians and other health workers need to understand and publicize the rapid and substantial benefits of:

   a. Physical activity for both children and adults with pre-existing health problems. Physical activity induces rapid benefits particularly in those with serious health problems such as diabetes, high blood pressure, heart disease, depression and several other mental health disorders; dietary change with modest weight loss is also a very cost-effective change with clear benefits in terms of both morbidity and mortality.

   b. Doctors and other health workers in the Health Services need to change the way they practice and should operate as community leaders to promote effective dietary change and increased physical activity within the community. They should also introduce a cooperative service with other providers e.g. weight loss and exercise/sports groups in the community;

   c. "Walk the talk:" health care professionals in health services need to reduce their own obesity rates, by eating healthily and by their commitment to daily exercise thereby serving as role models for their peers and followers;

   d. Promote the need for families as a whole to change their dietary and physical activity patterns. This is particularly important for avoiding obesity in families gaining weight

e. Enforcing hospital breast feeding promotion practices;

f. Removing soft drink and fast food provision from hospital and all Ministry of Health premises and ensuring that physical activity facilities exist within the medical facilities such as hospitals.

3. Ministers of Health must become ambassadors or diplomats engaging other Ministers to change government policies. Thus, in accordance with the UN General Assembly Recommendations of September 2011 Ministers of Health should take the lead by interacting with the following major Departments of government:

A. Education:

 I. Re-orient the curriculum of both medical students and postgraduate doctors and also paramedical professions;

 II. Preschool nursery food and activity regulations need to be addressed to remove all fast foods and confectionary and soft drinks from the premises and to promote active play and learning and communal eating rather than snacking;

 III. Introduce national regulations to halt all forms of food marketing in schools, aligned with WHO designated Policy Frameworks;

 IV. Change the curriculum on food with practical experience of food growing and preparation whilst ensuring the recognition of the value of farming and food provision in society. This is important for ensuring the future importance of a high quality food chain and the economic value of agriculture.

B. Transport: Policy Changes need to promote permanent change in the national infrastructure to:

 I. Reduce car use for any access to schools

 II. Increase walking and cycling to and from school with appropriate facilities

 III. Close roads on weekends and public holidays to promote communal physical activity

 IV. Re-orient public infrastructure to promote active travel by providing facilities for safe physical activity such as the provision of cycle lanes and public spaces for physical activity at the population level

 V. Subsidize public transport and reduce car use whenever possible. This, with marked improvements in the public domain, reduces crime as well as promoting physical activity as shown by the remarkable changes in Bogota, Colombia.

C. Finance:

    I. Taxation—Increase the opportunity to change the relative prices of fats and sugars (currently cheap) and expensive fruits and vegetables the price of which have been known for years to induce behavioral change and alter purchasing and consumption patterns;

    II. Provide financial incentives for behavioral change allowing for the regressive effect of some changes on the poorest in society.;

    III. Promote new local/farm/food/physical activity industries by setting out plans and incentives for the next 5–10 years;

D. Business:

    I. Use Public Private Partnerships to improve the well-being of the society and request accountability of the private sectors by government led leadership;

    II. Create new opportunities for recreation and changes in the canteen food systems within and associated with companies.

    III. Import businesses in food should be asked to describe and then improve the nutritional criteria of foods purchased for import within a defined time scale for change.

    IV. Retail food businesses should consider new proposals for labeling retail areas based on healthy foods only and the opportunities for a business led progressive nutritional changes in the usual provision of take-away foods and drink. Company led financial incentives for improved purchasing habits can also be profitable.

E. Agriculture and Food:

    I. Increase opportunities to promote local industry with use of suitable barriers to imported poor quality food. . Increase the opportunity for import policy changes using the CARICOM expertise which includes an understanding of the unused opportunity for making coherent health promoting changes in food import policies within the important WTO framework.

    II. Link local farmers to the provision of food for schools and government facilities. This brings great benefits to local agriculture as well as children and a community's valuing local produce. This has been done very successfully in Chile.

III. Consider regulating all publicly supported facilities including local government, military, police as well as educational facilities to change food provision with healthy preferably local food options as the priority initially before these become the exclusive options thereby altering the economics of the food chain as well as changing public perceptions of appropriate food and drink. These programs and their justification relate to the High Level Meeting of Ministers of Health in Aruba on 6 June 2013.

RECOMMENDATIONS OF THE HIGH LEVEL MEETING IN ARUBA ON CHILDHOOD OBESITY

We, the Ministers of Health of Aruba, Bermuda, British Virgin Islands, Dominica, Grenada, Montserrat, Saint Lucia, Surinam, Turks and Caicos Island, the Secretary of Health of Colima State (Mexico), Representative of the First Lady of Chile, Representatives of the Ministers of Health of the Bahamas, Barbados, Bolivia, Costa Rica, Dominican Republic, Ecuador, El Salvador, Mexico, Puerto Rico, St. Kitts & Nevis, St. Maarten, the Director of Food Agency of Santa Fe, (Argentina); Representative of Guayas, Santa Elena, Los Rios, Bolivar and Galapagos Provinces, (Ecuador); President of IASO and Representatives of WHO, PAHO, CARICOM, CARPHA and the World Bank and Coca Cola, who participated in the High Level Meeting on Childhood Obesity on Thursday 6 June 2013 within the framework of the Third Pan American Conference on Obesity with special attention to Childhood Obesity held in Aruba between the 6thand 8thof June 2013,

Acknowledge:

- That particular attention must be given to childhood obesity.

- That overweight and obesity affect about two thirds of children and adolescents in the Region of the Americas, which results in important health risks such as chronic non-communicable diseases and psychological problems that all have serious economic and social consequences for individuals, their families, communities and for society at large, even limiting growth and development in our countries.

- That, in general, obesity is a multi-causal problem requiring integrated and concerted multi-sectorial interventions at all levels (global, regional, sub regional, national and local) including agriculture, education, media and communication, infrastructure, transport, urbanization, industry, trade, finance, tourism, security, health, development and social protection, which is why we believe it is necessary to include "Health and Wellbeing in all Policies."

– The 2007 Port of Spain Declaration on Non Communicable Diseases, The Aruba Call for Action on Obesity as well as the global and regional mandates relating to the prevention and control of chronic non-communicable diseases.

– That, apart from a multi-sectorial approach, obesity prevention must target the entire lifespan, including health and nutrition before, during and after pregnancy, adequate eating practices for babies and small children and adequate eating habits and healthy lifestyles in all stages of life. That during the time before and after pregnancy, childhood and adolescence interventions must be implemented to prevent and control overweight and obesity.

– That due to globalization, modernization, urban living and economic growth a significant change has occurred in our population's eating patterns and its lifestyles, as they consume more processed and over-processed foods containing high levels of saturated fats, trans fatty acids, sugars and salt, and are less active physically. As a result, regional and subregional approaches are needed to undo the negative effect of the obesogenic environment in which we live.

– That even though our countries have developed policies, legislative and regulatory frameworks, programs and interventions to contain the childhood obesity epidemic, analysis of the available data indicates that the epidemic continues to advance in our Region and that the actions that have already been undertaken turn out to be insufficient.

Considering, the participants of the High Level Meeting on Childhood Obesity recommend the following:

1. Re-emphasize leadership and stewardship of the Ministries and Secretariats of Health and increase efforts to combat childhood overweight and obesity by providing policies and national programs with legislative and regulatory frameworks, infrastructure, human and financial resources, planning and programming instruments, and systems that allow for monitoring, evaluation, accountability and financing for maximal impact.

2. Incorporate actions for the prevention and control of malnutrition in all its forms and in "all policies," including agriculture, education, media and communication, infrastructure, transport, urbanization, industry, commerce, finance, tourism, security, health, development and social protection.

3. Establish formal leadership of the Pan-American Conference on Obesity among regional and sub regional countries and establish a regional platform that allows for dialogue and multisectoral consultation, mobilization of resources, awakening of political and social recognition of the importance and consequences of overweight and obesity, research on and identification of needs, project management and execution, exchange of best practices and lessons learned and training of human resources and community leaders.

4. To incorporate or adjust existing trade regulations and establish or adjust national and regional regulatory frameworks in different sectors (e.g. impose taxes on unhealthy food products, subsidize local farmers, regulate advertising, labeling and the commercialization of processed foods with high caloric density such as sugary foods and drinks targeting children and adolescents).

5. Provide comprehensive programs on a national scale for overweight and obesity prevention in educational institutions (child care facilities, kindergartens, elementary and secondary schools), for which we reiterate the need for stronger inter-ministerial coordination and further development of supporting policies for education, sports, agriculture, trade and health, providing for legislative and regulatory frameworks, infrastructure, human and financial resources, planning and programming instruments, content and curricular and extracurricular activities, and systems for monitoring, evaluation and accountability.

6. Provide programs on a national scale for the promotion of physical activity, for which we reiterate the need for stronger inter-ministerial coordination and further development of supporting policies for urban planning and development, transport, security, education, sports, recreation and health, providing for legislative and regulatory frameworks, infrastructure, human and financial resources, planning and programming instruments, sports and recreational activities, and systems for monitoring, evaluation and accountability.

7. Integrate the inspection of food, nutrition and the determinants within the national systems for food inspection, monitor and evaluate programs and interventions, establish accountability systems and utilize the information gathered to develop and guide national and regional public policies.

8. Promote safe and healthy tourism, by creating healthy environments and boosting healthy eating, physical activity and recreation.

9. Encourage solidarity, collaboration, exchange and adoption of policies and programs that are harmonized among countries and regions.

10. We request from:

   a. PAHO/WHO to develop models for public policy, legislative and regulatory frameworks and to provide to its Member States effective interventions to be adopted and adapted to the epidemiological and social context of our countries, as well as provide clear rules to establish a dialogue with the private sector and with industry, while protecting the interest of the population.

b. All interested parties to provide our countries with resources allowing for the implementation at the national scale of programs and interventions that have proven to be effective.

c. Industry to reformulate its food products and its commercial policies taking into account nutritional properties that promote and safeguard the health and development of children, adolescents and the population at large.

Foreword by: Dr. Richard Visser

The High-Level Meeting of PACO reunites 13 Ministers and delegates from 23 countries, different organizations: WHO, PAHO, PAHEF, CARPHA, CARICOM, IASO, the World Bank, among others, and we are also accompanied by several companies from the private sector, to deconstruct and reconstruct the way in which we have been working. PACO wants to bring together the lessons learned and shared experiences for our continent and region.

Normally, the pharmaceutical industry and governments only want to focus on achievements and do not desire to look back at the failures. The airline industry, for instance, has perfected this idea and has in place a failure analysis that is phenomenal and which requires of a cross-sectional group of specialists to work properly. When a plane falls down, through this analysis, they deconstruct every little detail until they find what went wrong, instead of throwing the whole airplane out. As leaders in this continent and as people who can get things moving, we need to cross-train ourselves on failure analysis, because through it we can learn critical issues about failure. Otherwise, many ideas will continue to be thrown out, with the ensuing waste of time, money, knowledge, energy and human resources. We have to pull failures back and analyze them, relook at what failed in our countries with a new breed of crossed-trained people that through this analysis can tell us what detail we missed and where we went wrong, before we throw whole ideas outs, helping us see how to renew these different ideas, and grow and move forward exponentially on them, instead of constantly trying to reinvent the wheel.

It is therefore necessary to look at cross-training in all different areas, to create a new breed of scientists, a new breed of investigators, a new breed of people that lead, and this in turn requires for us to study what other disciplines are doing. Biology, for example, is doing this through systems biology, bringing people in with different disciplines to solve the big questions, thus becoming more effective.

There is a strong need for us to perform different analysis, look at how the micro affect the macro and learn from this research happening in different fields and bring back this acquired intelligence to our work. Ask ourselves how we can replicate what we do on a micro level on a population level, how we can create a "swarming" effect on a population level, where there is no leader, just movement and group intelligence, that is bigger than that of mere individuals, and where there is trust. We see it in our populations, if there is a certain amount of mass in an idea, then, all of a sudden it goes and becomes its own movement. Now, how do we create that? How do we, instead of forcing things on our people, can simulate the swarm movement?

I think in Aruba we've seen this in the way people move. In a little more than 4 years, we've been able to go from 9 to 39% in mass movement, and we've done this, sometimes by accident, but it's been an impulse from all sides. So we have impulses that we have stimulated from the private sector, impulses stimulated from inside, from the schooling sector, from the sport sector, etcetera, and we have had to create the infrastructure to motivate the swarming. In Aruba we also have a universal care system that is pretty unique. We do an 11% GDP, and market GDP is around 9%. It is a complete health care system where everyone gets care and medicines free. We have had a growth in the last three years that we've been able to keep at 4% growth, average, compared to the international average of 5 or 6%. So we're not bad for an island, we're doing pretty well, but it still needs work. On an island you're always working and analyzing what you keep here and what you send out. We do 1.8 guilders a month sending patients out to Colombia, to specialized centers. It's been working real well for us. We use private hospitals there, together with also, of course, the help from PAHO, Holland, and the region, the US, and we are really able to move this, with technology.

Through that we have noticed, as have all the countries, that our biggest challenge is Chronic Non-Transmittable Diseases, due to its complexities and extent of consequences. This is something where we stand shoulder to shoulder with the World Health Organization, with PAHO, and it is something that we will champion. If you look outside, you'll see a "Bus di Salud", a health bus; it's a clinic on wheels with air conditioning, a doctor, nurses, and a nutritionist. This Bus performs NCDs' screening through our neighborhoods. We do this, for we know that the driver and the solution need a platform, NCDs, obesity and childhood obesity need their own platform, and that is also one of the important things we are pursuing here, pushing for a platform for NCDs, and specially for obesity and childhood obesity. It is something for which the First Lady of the United States is creating a wave, and we need to ride this wave. I think NCDs, childhood obesity and obesity in general can largely benefit from this.

As leaders we need to create these environments where we do system analysis, where we do failure analysis, create these environments where we simulate systems biology on a population level, an environment for our populations so that they start moving in swarms, and we have to calculate what is that required mass and what stimuli do they need for this to happen. This is achieved by looking at how people move and react in a group - and as a group - under different situations, and analyze how that group develops intelligence, with the aim at understanding better how to motivate our population, how to get them to eat healthier, get them to move, to catch on to healthy lifestyles.

It's all about the masses that you get going and for such an end we have to do an analysis of what is already working and how we can grow on that. That's where new ideas come in, and so, in this PACO, one of the things that we want to do is share information, share experiences, and also failures. We're here to bring in people that usually don't sit with us, people that will change the direction of how we think. We have a medical futurist that will be talking, we have a 20 year old inventor who is already getting deals from NIKE and others, got a prize from the Michelle Obamafoundation, and invented a way—on a platform that's gaming—for kids to eat vegetables and buy fruit.

We're looking at how to teach from different platforms, looking far beyond those environments in which we were trained in, and thus consider the use of items such as smart phones, wearable apps and the gaming platform. We need to use technology. Wearable apps, for instance, are going to revolutionize what we do and how we do things in the care sector, in the physical fitness sector, in the movement sector, in everything. These are the platforms that we need to be looking at, the ones we need to be using. These platforms are inexpensive, and although many countries argue with reason that in their countries people do not have computers because of the countries' economic situation, when we analyze those same countries in Latin America and the Caribbean, we can see that every single person has a cell phone, working or not, and even if it is not connected and the bills are unpaid, the apps will still work, and Wi-Fi will be available somewhere, and kids use these phones, and hand them down, and we are really looking at more phones than people. So, when we talk about wearable apps, we are talking about a technology that can spread the information, if used on the correct platform, so rapidly and effectively that it will really force us to change the way we do what we do.

It's time to update if we want to compete. It is not how much money we have, it is about how smart we can move and how fast we can move, and using cross-training to get our teams ready. This is another thing that we are here for: to really look at what we need to force the changing. PACO is not just a conference, we also have workshops going on, and we are, among other things, also introducing "Exercise is medicine" into our electronic patient files, which all our physicians are on.

Success lays in what we can do together. Let's make this a success for all of us, let's promote sharing and exchange during and after the conference and let's grow from this.

Thank you!

www.ingramcontent.com/pod-product-compliance
Lightning Source LLC
Chambersburg PA
CBHW061134030426
42334CB00003B/33